Lecture Notes of the Institute for Computer Sciences, Social Informatics and Telecommunications Engineering 440

More information about this series at https://link.springer.com/bookseries/8197

Xinbo Gao · Abbas Jamalipour · Lei Guo (Eds.)

Wireless Mobile Communication and Healthcare

10th EAI International Conference, MobiHealth 2021
Virtual Event, November 13–14, 2021
Proceedings

Springer

Editors
Xinbo Gao
Chongqing University of Posts
and Telecommunications
Chongqing, China

Abbas Jamalipour
The University of Sydney
Sydney, NSW, Australia

Lei Guo
Chongqing University of Posts
and Telecommunications
Chongqing, China

ISSN 1867-8211 ISSN 1867-822X (electronic)
Lecture Notes of the Institute for Computer Sciences, Social Informatics
and Telecommunications Engineering
ISBN 978-3-031-06367-1 ISBN 978-3-031-06368-8 (eBook)
https://doi.org/10.1007/978-3-031-06368-8

This Springer imprint is published by the registered company Springer Nature Switzerland AG
The registered company address is: Gewerbestrasse 11, 6330 Cham, Switzerland

Preface

We are delighted to introduce the proceedings of the 10th European Alliance for Innovation (EAI) International Conference on Wireless Mobile Communication and Healthcare (MobiHealth 2021). This conference brought together researchers, developers, and practitioners around the world who are leveraging and developing wireless communications, mobile computing, and healthcare applications. The technical program of MobiHealth 2021 consisted of 23 full papers, including two invited papers, at the main conference tracks: Medical, Communications, and Networking; Biomedical and Health Informatics; and Signal/Data Processing and Computing For Health Systems. Aside from the high quality technical paper presentations, the technical program also featured two keynote speeches given by Yan Zhang, University of Oslo, Norway, and Bin Hu, Lanzhou University, China.

Coordination with the steering chairs, Imrich Chlamtac, James C. Lin, and Michael O'Grady, was essential for the success of the conference. We sincerely appreciate their constant support and guidance. It was also a great pleasure to work with such an excellent organizing committee team for their hard work in organizing and supporting the conference. In particular, we are grateful to the Technical Program Committee, who completed the peer-review process of technical papers and helped to put together a high-quality technical program. We are also grateful to Conference Manager Rupali Tiwari for her support and all the authors who submitted their papers to the MobiHealth 2021 conference.

We strongly believe that the MobiHealth conference provides a good forum for all researchers, developers, and practitioners to discuss all science and technology aspects that are relevant to wireless mobile communication and healthcare. We also expect that the future MobiHealth conferences will be as successful and stimulating as this year's, as indicated by the contributions presented in this volume.

May 2022

Xinbo Gao
Abbas Jamalipour
Lei Guo

Preface

Organization

Steering Committee

Imrich Chlamtac (Chair)	University of Trento, Italy
James C. Lin	University of Illinois at Chicago, USA
Michael O'Grady	University College Dublin, Ireland

Organizing Committee

General Chairs

Xinbo Gao	Chongqing University of Posts and Telecommunications, China
Abbas Jamalipour	University of Sydney, Australia

Technical Program Committee Chair

Lei Guo	Chongqing University of Posts and Telecommunications, China

Web Chair

Jianbo Zheng	University of Hong Kong, China

Publicity and Social Media Chair

Nannan Wang	Xidian University, China

Workshops Chair

Miaowen Wen	South China University of Technology, China

Sponsorship and Exhibit Chair

Xiaojie Wang	Chongqing University of Posts and Telecommunications, China

Publications Chair

Xin Liu	Dalian University of Technology, China

Tutorials Chair

Qingyang Song	Chongqing University of Posts and Telecommunications, China

Local Chair

Zhaolong Ning	Chongqing University of Posts and Telecommunications, China

Technical Program Committee

Abbas Aljuboori	University of Information Technology and Communications, Iraq
Amr Tolba	King Saud University, Saudi Arabia
Azizur Rahim	National University of Sciences and Technology, Pakistan
Cheng Guo	Dalian University of Technology, China
Chengming Li	Shenzhen Institute of Advanced Technology, CAS, China
Guangjun Wu	Institute of Information Engineering, CAS, China
Ke Zhang	University of Electronic Science and Technology of China, China
Laisen Nie	Macau University of Science and Technology, China
Lu Sun	Dalian Maritime University, China
Minqiang Yang	Lanzhou University, China
Peiran Dong	Hong Kong Polytechnic University, China
Wei Wang	Sun Yat-sen University, China
Weijing Qi	Chongqing University of Posts and Telecommunications, China
Xiangjie Kong	Zhejiang University of Technology, China
Yao Yu	Northeastern University, China
Yueyue Dai	Nanyang Technological University, Singapore
Chen Chen	Fudan University, China
Eleni Boumpa	University of Thessaly, Greece
Zhicheng Yang	PAII Inc., USA

Contents

Biomedical and Health Informatics

Signal/Data Processing and Computing For Health Systems

Invited Session

A Health Status Evaluation Method for Chronic Disease Patients Based on Multivariate State Estimation Technique Using Wearable Physiological Signals: A Preliminary Study

Haoran Xu[1,2], Zhicheng Yang[3], Ke Lan[4], Wei Yan[5], Zhao Wang[1], Jiachen Wang[1], Yaning Zang[6], Jianli Pan[7], Muyang Yan[5(✉)], and Zhengbo Zhang[8(✉)]

[1] Medical School of Chinese PLA, Beijing, China
[2] Affiliated Hospital of Medical Sergeant School, Army Medical University, Shijiazhuang, Hebei, China
[3] PAII Inc., Palo Alto, CA, USA
[4] Beijing SensEcho Science & Technology Co., Ltd., Beijing, China
[5] Department of Hyperbaric Oxygen Therapy, The First Medical Center, Chinese PLA General Hospital, Beijing, China
yanmy301@sina.com
[6] Shanghai University of Sport, Shanghai, China
[7] University of Missouri - St. Louis, St. Louis, MO, USA
[8] Center for Artificial Intelligence in Medicine, Chinese PLA General Hospital, Beijing, China
zhengbozhang@126.com

Abstract. Since chronic disease has become one of the most profound threats to human health, effective evaluation of human health and disease status is particularly important. In this study, we proposed a method based on Multivariate State Estimation Technique (MSET) by using physiological signals collected by a wearable device. Residual was defined as the difference between the actual value of each observed parameter and the estimated value obtained by MSET. The high-dimensional residual series were fused into a Multivariate Health Index (MHI) using a Gaussian mixture model. To preliminarily validate this method, we designed a retrospective observational study of 17 chronic patients with coronary artery disease combined high risk of heart failure whose Brain Natriuretic Peptide (BNP) had changed significantly during hospitalization. The results show that the distribution of residuals estimated by MSET had some regularity, in which the Pearson correlation coefficients between

Haoran Xu and Zhicheng Yang—Equally contributed to this work.
This work was done during Zhicheng Yang's internship at Beijing SensEcho Science & Technology Co., Ltd., Beijing, China, when he was a Ph.D. candidate at University of California, Davis, CA, USA.

X. Gao et al. (Eds.): MobiHealth 2021, LNICST 440, pp. 3–18, 2022.
https://doi.org/10.1007/978-3-031-06368-8_1

Cohen Standardized Mean Difference (SMD) and Overlapping Coefficient (OVL) of MHI and the change of BNP examination results reached 0.786 and 0.835, with their p-values less than 0.001, respectively. We preliminarily demonstrated that the model can reflect the level of change in human health status to some extent. This MSET-based approach shows great potential for applications of treatment effect evaluation, and provides abundant information from physiological signals in chronic disease management.

Keywords: Health status evaluation · Chronic disease management · Multivariate state estimation technique · Physiological signals

1 Introduction

Chronic disease has become one of the most profound threats to human health [18,27]. For example, a well-known chronic disease, Chronic Obstructive Pulmonary Disease (COPD), has become the third leading cause of death worldwide in the last decade [4]. Furthermore, according to a report in 2018, two-fifths of deaths in China are attributed to cardiovascular diseases (CVD), which affects about 290 million patients [18]. While chronic diseases have brought great medical burden, family burden and social burden across the world, this situation has gotten even worse since the COVID-19 pandemic. How to treat and manage chronic diseases has become an urgent problem that remains unsolved. For chronic disease management (CDM), effective evaluation of human health and disease status is particularly important.

Currently, the widely used clinical method to evaluate a patient's health and disease status still largely relies on lab test results [3]. It compares a patient's several key lab examination values with those values of the pre-defined reference ranges, which are obtained from a healthy population [7,10]. However, this evaluation method has three main shortcomings. First, the lab examination normal intervals formed by large-sample healthy people are not always appropriate for everyone when individualized medicine is considered [26,29]. Second, the lab examination-based evaluation method lacks timeliness to some extent, because many results need half or even more days to be available. Third, in general wards, the frequency of lab result collection is significantly lower than that of physiological signal collection. For example, a hospitalized patient in China hardly takes daily lab examination due to unnecessary over-collection and expensive out-of-pocket cost. Furthermore, the timing that a patient takes lab examination is mostly determined by a physician's experience, which aggravates the uncertainty of estimating the patient's condition.

In the era of the Internet of Things and Digital Medicine, wearable technology enables people to collect physiological signals continuously, enjoying the merits of easy accessibility, real-time acquisition, and high sampling rate. Physiological signals such as electrocardiogram (ECG), heart rate (HR), breathing rate (BR) contain rich medical information that has a great potential for disease early warning, rehabilitation assessment and CDM [1,9,20]. Several research groups have proposed various methods to solve the problem of health status recognition based on physiological signals: Li-wei H. Lehman et al. conducted a series of studies that analyzed the dynamical behaviors in cardiovascular variables which can be used to recognize the state of a patient [12,13,15]. In [5], Principal Component Analysis and a Hidden Markov Model were adopted to recognize the abnormalities in physiological signals to realize health status recognition.

Due to the high complexity of human body, each individual has her/his specific physiological wave patterns. Most of the previous studies are based on large sample specific population, reflecting population characteristics while individual differences are largely eliminated in population analysis. Moreover, chronic disease patients are often elderly and suffered from multiple chronic diseases at the same time, entangling the analysis of their health status conditions. Furthermore, their individual differences pose a challenge for in-depth mining of physiological signals and research on state identification. Thus, how to establish a physiological-signal-based method to individually evaluate the health status of chronic disease patients is still a problem that needs investigation.

To resolve the above problems, the Multivariate State Estimation Technique (MSET) can be used, which is first proposed by Singer R M et al. at 1997 [23]. MSET measures the difference between the observed status of the system and historical status when the system running normally. This algorithm is often used to realize fault early warning of electron devices or equipment and has been successfully deployed in several industrial scenarios [16,28,33]. The advantages of MSET has been proved in fast training and accurate prediction. In medicine domain, R. Matthew Pipke et al. [21] used MSET to conduct individualized non-parametric modeling for patients with heart failure. They collected HR, BR, Pulse Transit Time (PTT), Pulse Pressure Index (PPI), blood oxygen saturation, etc. by a wearable device, and finally realized the effective identification of dynamic changes in these physiological signals of patients. Richard L. Summers et al. [25] verified that the dynamic threshold of cardiovascular hemodynamic parameters predicted by MSET can achieve early warning compared with the traditional fixed threshold method by using simulated data. Recently, Josef Stehlik et al. [24] used an individualized physiological signal analysis platform based on MSET to predict readmission time in patients with heart failure. The platform was able to detect the worsen heart failure caused readmission with 76% to 88% sensitivity and 85% specificity in 100 patients. The median time between initial alarm sent from the platform and readmission was 6.5 (4.2–13.7) days.

Previous studies provide great inspiration and have shown the potential to apply MSET to the CDM. In this study, we aim to establish a process for analyzing the physiological signals collected by a medical-grade wearable device, to build an MSET-based model, and preliminarily verify the effectiveness of MSET to indicate the health condition change of a cohort who has specific chronic diseases. Our key contributions are summarized as follows:

- We preliminarily demonstrate that MSET is able to unveil the latent relationship between the lab examination results and time-series physiological

signals, indicating that physiological signals and MSET promisingly supply added values to the lab examination.
- We leverage the kernel density estimation to characterize the distribution of the residuals obtained from the MSET-based model. Changes in patient health status were quantified by measuring the difference between the two kernel density curves.
- We adopt Cohen Standardized Mean Difference (SMD) [2] and Overlapping Coefficient (OVL) [8] to effectively highlight the difference among the distributions.

2 Materials and Methods

2.1 Multivariate State Estimation Technique (MSET)

MSET is a non-parametric modeling method that estimates the current state of the system based on its historical data, which was originally used for temperature sensor monitoring [23] and further various medical applications [21,24,25]. The core idea of MSET is similarity measurement. It first learns the relationships among parameters of the historical data when the system is running properly. Once a new observation value comes, MSET then leverages the most similar state learned from the historical data to estimate the current state. The key steps of MSET can be formulated as follows:

Step 1: Build the history matrix H based on the historical data.

$$\mathrm{H} = [\mathbf{x}(1), \mathbf{x}(2), \mathbf{x}(3), \ldots, \mathbf{x}(k)] = \begin{bmatrix} x_1(1) & \cdots & x_1(k) \\ \vdots & \ddots & \vdots \\ x_n(1) & \cdots & x_n(k) \end{bmatrix}, \tag{1}$$

where k is the number of observation; $\mathbf{x}(i)$, representing the observation vector at the time i, is defined as:

$$\mathbf{x}(i) = [x_1(i), x_2(i), x_3(i), \ldots, x_n(i)]^{\mathrm{T}}, \tag{2}$$

and $x_n(i)$ denotes the n-th observation value at the time i.

Step 2: Build the memory matrix D. When a new observation vector $\mathbf{x}^{\mathrm{obs}}$ arrives, m observation vectors are selected from H to construct D (set as 10 in our method).

$$\mathrm{D} = [\mathbf{d}_1, \mathbf{d}_2, \ldots \mathbf{d}_m] = \begin{bmatrix} d_{11} & \cdots & d_{1m} \\ \vdots & \ddots & \vdots \\ d_{n1} & \cdots & d_{nm} \end{bmatrix}. \tag{3}$$

Step 3: Calculate the estimation vector $\mathbf{x}^{\mathrm{est}}$.

$$\begin{aligned} \mathbf{x}^{\mathrm{est}} &= \mathrm{D} \cdot \mathbf{w} \\ &= [\mathbf{d}_1, \mathbf{d}_2, \ldots \mathbf{d}_m] \cdot [w_1, w_2 \ldots w_m]^{\mathrm{T}} \\ &= w_1\mathbf{d}_1 + w_2\mathbf{d}_2 \ldots + w_m\mathbf{d}_m \end{aligned} \tag{4}$$

It means that $\mathbf{x}^{\text{est}}$ can be represented as the linear combination of the m historical vectors in D. $\mathbf{w}$ can be obtained by minimizing the residual vector $\boldsymbol{\varepsilon}$, which is defined as:

$$\boldsymbol{\varepsilon} = \mathbf{x}^{\text{obs}} - \mathbf{x}^{\text{est}}. \tag{5}$$

We then detail the derivation process of $\mathbf{w}$ using the least squares method.

$$\begin{aligned}\sum_{i=1}^{n} \varepsilon_i^2 &= \boldsymbol{\varepsilon}^T \cdot \boldsymbol{\varepsilon} = \left(\mathbf{x}^{\text{obs}} - \mathbf{x}^{\text{est}}\right)^{\text{T}} \cdot \left(\mathbf{x}^{\text{obs}} - \mathbf{x}^{\text{est}}\right) \\ &= \left(\mathbf{x}^{\text{obs}} - \text{D} \cdot \mathbf{w}\right)^{\text{T}} \cdot \left(\mathbf{x}^{\text{obs}} - \text{D} \cdot \mathbf{w}\right) \\ &= \sum_{i=1}^{n} \left(x^{\text{obs}}(i) - \sum_{\text{j}=1}^{m} w_j d_{ij}\right)^2 .\end{aligned} \tag{6}$$

The partial derivatives of $\sum_{i=1}^{n} \varepsilon_i^2$ in Eq. 6 with respect to $w_1, w_2, \ldots, w_m$ respectively are set equal to 0.

$$\frac{\partial \sum_{i=1}^{n} \varepsilon_i^2}{\partial w_q} = -2 \sum_{i=1}^{n} \left(x^{\text{obs}}(i) - \sum_{\text{j}=1}^{m} w_j d_{ij}\right) d_{iq} = 0, \tag{7}$$

therefore,

$$\sum_{i=1}^{n} x^{\text{obs}}(i) d_{iq} = \sum_{i=1}^{n} \sum_{j=1}^{m} w_j d_{ij} d_{iq} = \sum_{j=1}^{m} \left(\sum_{i=1}^{n} d_{ij} d_{iq}\right) w_j. \tag{8}$$

Equation 8 can be rewritten as the following format:

$$\text{D}^{\text{T}} \cdot \text{D} \cdot \mathbf{w} = \text{D}^{\text{T}} \cdot \mathbf{x}^{\text{obs}}, \tag{9}$$

$$\mathbf{w} = \left(\text{D}^{\text{T}} \cdot \text{D}\right)^{-1} \cdot \left(\text{D}^{\text{T}} \cdot \mathbf{x}^{\text{obs}}\right). \tag{10}$$

Nevertheless, if there exists linear correlation among the vectors in D, $\text{D}^{\text{T}} \cdot \text{D}$ is always not invertible, failing to solve Eq. 10. To resolve this issue, $\mathbf{d}_j$ of D can be projected to a higher dimensional space by the function $\Phi : \mathbb{R}^n \to \mathbb{R}^z$.

$$\Phi(\text{D})^{\text{T}} \cdot \Phi(\text{D}) \cdot \mathbf{w} = \Phi(\text{D})^{\text{T}} \cdot \Phi\left(\mathbf{x}^{\text{obs}}\right), \tag{11}$$

where $\Phi(\text{D})$ is a $z \times m$ matrix ($z > m$). Therefore, Eq. 9 can be rewritten as:

$$\mathbf{w} = \left(\Phi(\text{D})^{\text{T}} \cdot \Phi(\text{D})\right)^{-1} \cdot \left(\Phi(\text{D})^{\text{T}} \cdot \Phi\left(\mathbf{x}^{\text{obs}}\right)\right). \tag{12}$$

Since $\text{D}^{\text{T}} \cdot \text{D}$ and $\text{D}^{\text{T}} \cdot \mathbf{x}^{\text{obs}}$ can be implemented by a kernel function. We here use kernel function computation ($\otimes$) to update the matrix multiplication in Eq. 12:

$$\mathbf{w} = \left(\text{D}^{\text{T}} \otimes \text{D}\right)^{-1} \cdot \left(\text{D}^{\text{T}} \otimes \mathbf{x}^{\text{obs}}\right). \tag{13}$$

Therefore, the estimation of the current observation value is:

$$\mathbf{x}^{\text{est}} = \mathrm{D} \cdot \left(\mathrm{D}^{\mathrm{T}} \otimes \mathrm{D}\right)^{-1} \cdot \left(\mathrm{D}^{\mathrm{T}} \otimes \mathbf{x}^{\text{obs}}\right), \tag{14}$$

Regarding the kernel function, we select the Gaussian kernel function

$$K(\mathbf{x}, \mathbf{y}; h) = \sum_{i=1}^{n} \frac{1}{\sqrt{2\pi}h} \exp^{-\frac{(x_i - y_i)^2}{2h^2}} \tag{15}$$

Furthermore, we use the regularization to improve the performance of MSET [6]. Equation 13 and Eq. 14 can be revised as follows:

$$\mathbf{w} = \left(\mathrm{D}^{\mathrm{T}} \otimes \mathrm{D} + \lambda \mathrm{I}\right)^{-1} \cdot \left(\mathrm{D}^{\mathrm{T}} \otimes \mathbf{x}^{\text{obs}}\right), \tag{16}$$

$$\mathbf{x}^{\text{est}} = \mathrm{D} \cdot \left(\mathrm{D}^{\mathrm{T}} \otimes \mathrm{D} + \lambda \mathrm{I}\right)^{-1} \cdot \left(\mathrm{D}^{\mathrm{T}} \otimes \mathbf{x}^{\text{obs}}\right). \tag{17}$$

where λ denotes the parameter of regularization; I represents the L2 regularization term.

Step 4: Calculate the residual of the i-th observation value and estimation value.

$$\varepsilon_i = x_i^{\text{obs}} - x_i^{\text{est}}. \tag{18}$$

We then focus on the residual distribution, which is an important measure of the state change.

Step 5: Compute the log-likelihood value using Gaussian mixture model. The authors in [21] designed an indicator based on high-dimensional residual sequence, named Multivariate Health Index (MHI). MHI represents the probability of a new residual vector belonging to the residual distribution of D. That is, we consider the MHI as a *lumped* parameter that is able to represent the overall health status change of the patient.

$$\text{MHI}(\boldsymbol{\varepsilon}) = \log_{10} \frac{1}{\hat{f}(\boldsymbol{\varepsilon})} \tag{19}$$

where

$$\hat{f}(\boldsymbol{\varepsilon}) = \frac{1}{m(2\pi)^{d/2}h^d} \sum_{i=1}^{m} \exp\left(-\frac{\|\boldsymbol{\varepsilon} - \mathbf{r}_i\|}{2h^2}\right), \tag{20}$$

m is the number of columns of D; $\boldsymbol{\varepsilon}$ refers to the residual of the current observation vector; $\mathbf{r}_i$ represents the residual of the i-th column of D; h indicates the width of window; d is the dimension of the observation vector.

2.2 Data Source

We continuously collect the physiological signals of 657 voluntary patients from the general wards of the hyperbaric oxygen department in our hospital using the medical-grade wearable multi-sensor system *SensEcho*, which has been widely used and validated in our previous work [14,17,22,30–32,34,35]. The ECG, chest

& abdominal respiratory waves and triaxial acceleration information of patients were synchronously collected. We collect every patient's physiological data at least at the beginning day and the end day during she/he is hospital. Every collection lasts at least 24 h. The total number of valid physiological series is 1,297, in which 404 patients are collected twice or more. Every participant complied with the protocol approved by the IRB review board (IRB number: S2018-095-01) and signed the printed informed consent. This study was also conducted according to the Declaration of Helsinki. Demographic information was collected by a questionnaire, including age, gender, height and weight.

Since our focus is chronic disease, in this study, the patients who have coronary heart disease with potentially chronic heart failure will construct our in-house dataset of chronic disease patients. According to clinicians' recommendation, we select Brain Natriuretic Peptide (BNP) as the reference lab examination measure because it is an important indicator of heart disease [11,19]. For healthy subjects, the results of BNP examination should be less than 100 pg/ml. On the one hand, physicians suggest that if a patient's BNP decreases by more than 80 pg/ml, the patient is well treated in the hospital. On the other hand, if a patient's BNP ascends more than 200 pg/ml, we believe the treatment effectiveness is not obvious. Thereby, we design the following rules to select satisfactory patient candidates.

- A patient has two or more BNP results;
- The patient's first BNP value is larger than 100 pg/ml;
- The physiological signals of the patient are collected and valid twice or more;
- The patient has at least one BNP result within 2 days before or after the physiological signal collection. If multiple BNP results are available, we include the last one only;
- The descending or ascending level of patient's BNP results is larger than 80 or 200 pg/ml, respectively.

As a result, a total of 17 patients are selected, in which 14 patients' BNP results are improved and 3 patients get worse.

We choose the first collection of physiological signals of patients as the historical data. First, 200 30-second windows of signals are randomly selected to calculate the historical residual values, while the remaining 30s windows of signals construct H. Second, we select 6 representative observation parameters/features (shown in Table 1) to model MSET and then compute the lumped parameter MHI using a Gaussian mixture model (by Eq. 19 and Eq. 20). Third, the last collection of physiological signals of patients is regarded as our test observation data. We extract valid windows of signals and calculate the respective historical and observation residuals. Last, the difference of residual distribution of historical and observation data is measured.

2.3 Data Preprocess and Filtration

The human body is often in a complex dynamic balanced steady-state situation. To ensure the matrix H contains as much health state information as possible,

Table 1. List of six observation physiological parameters

Parameter/Feature	Description
HR mean	Mean heart rate
HR range	Heart rate range
HR std	Heart rate standard deviation
BR mean	Mean breath rate
RESP iqr	Respiratory wave interquartile range
ACT mean	Mean activity level

Table 2. BNP change and SMD/OVL correlation of residual distribution of various physiological parameters

	SMD		OVL	
Parameter	coefficient ρ	p	coefficient ρ	p
HR mean	0.402	0.109	0.495	**0.043**
HR range	0.571	**0.017**	0.590	**0.013**
HR std	−0.088	0.738	0.587	**0.013**
BR mean	−0.670	**0.003**	0.604	**0.010**
RESP iqr	−0.280	0.277	0.395	0.117
ACT mean	0.082	0.754	0.753	**<0.001**
MHI	0.786	**<0.001**	0.835	**<0.001**

it is necessary to preprocess and filter the data first to weaken the influence of noise and remove the moving segment. In this study, we design the following procedures:

- Perform median filtering on HR and BR;
- Detrend the respiratory wave signals, and then filter them by using the fifth-order low-pass IIR Butterworth filter, whose cut-off frequency was set 2 Hz;
- Split the current signal by non-overlapping sliding window according to preset 30 s observation window;
- The activity level of the subject per second is calculated according to the triaxial acceleration signals, and the activity state of the subject is divided into resting and active according to the numerical value. The observation window will be dropped if the patient status is considered as a movement in this 30s observation window;
- Extract the observation parameters/features of the signals in the remaining observation windows in chronological order and incorporate them in the matrix H;
- Normalize the matrix H by using Min-Max scaling.

2.4 Statistical Method

We leverage kernel density estimation to describe the residual distribution. SMD [2] and OVL [8] are adopted to measure the difference of residual distribution of historical and observation data. In particular, a higher SMD value indicates the difference of two distributions is larger. OVL measures the overlap of two distributions, ranging between 0 (not overlapped) and 1 (fully overlapped). Moreover, for all involved patients, we calculate the BNP change[1] and the SMD & OVL joint distribution of residual distribution of physiological observation values, and compute the Pearson correlation coefficient ρ and its corresponding statistical p-value.

3 Experiment Results

3.1 Group Analysis

Table 2 shows the Pearson correlation coefficient ρ and statistical p-values of SMD and OVL of residual distribution of observation parameters and BNP change. We illustrate the 9 statistically significant parameters ($p < 0.05$) in Fig. 1. As we can see, there exist relationships between BNP change and the residual distribution of these parameters, indicating the possibility of using physiological parameters to infer a patient's state. Specifically, the parameter MHI has the most significant correlation with BNP change. We also find that both SMD and OVL of the BR mean parameter has a high correlation with BNP change. This exposes that a patient's BR has been improved during the second physiological data collection. In addition, the high correlation of ACT mean and BNP change implies the different activity levels between the first and second physiological data collection. When BNP is improved, a patient's activity level rises. This observation is also consistent with the professional consensus about BNP.

3.2 Case Analysis

In this section, we analyze two representative cases in detail.

Case 1. Case 1 is Patient 01 (male, 89 years old, 168 cm, 45 kg). He was in hospital from Oct. 13, 2018 to Oct. 29, 2018. He was diagnosed with heart failure, coronary heart disease, diastolic heart dysfunction, hypertension III, and chronic kidney dysfunction. Figure 2 depicts the timeline of his BNP and physiological signal collection. This patient had the first BNP examination on Oct. 13, 2018 (Day 1), reporting 1685 pg/ml. On Oct. 15, 2018 (Day 3) and Oct. 24, 2018 (Day 12), the first and second collections of this patient's physiological signals were conducted, respectively. On Oct. 26, 2018 (Day 14), the second BNP result

[1] BNP change is computed by subtracting the second BNP examination result from the first one.

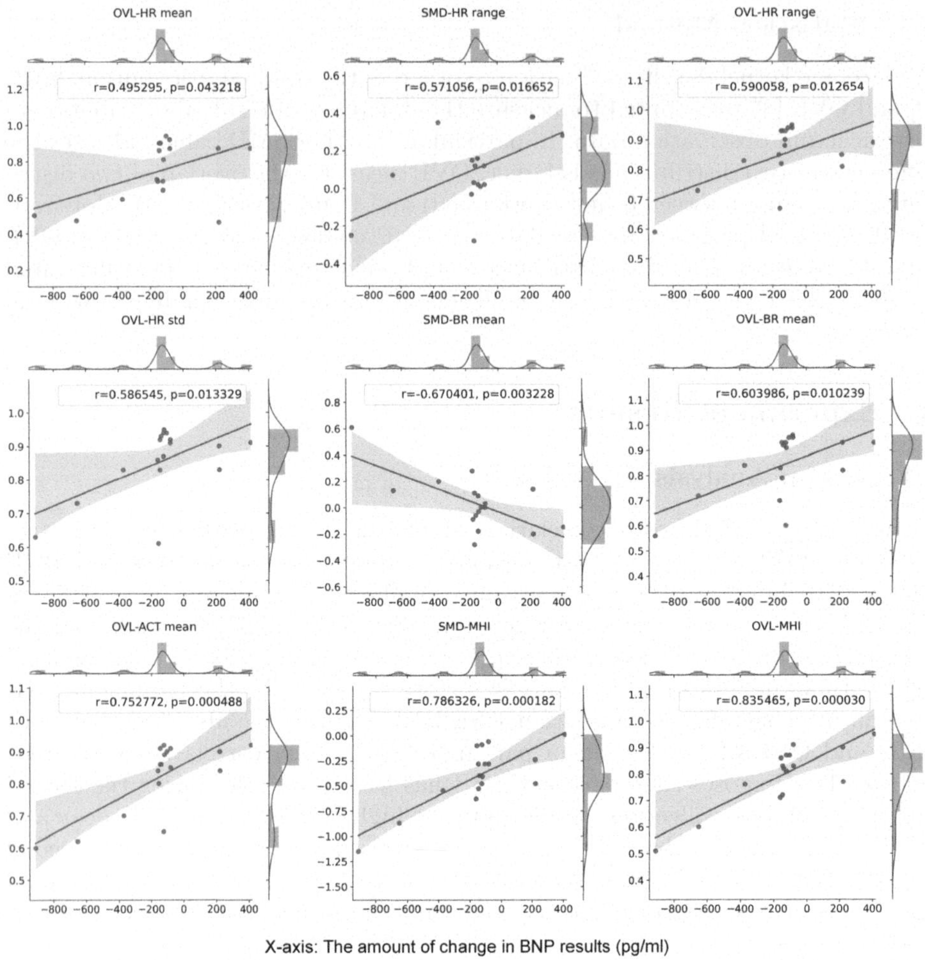

Fig. 1. Joint distribution of SMD and OVL of the residual parameter of observation values and BNP changes

was 772.2 pg/ml, reporting a decrease of 912.8 pg/ml compared with the very first one. During the last 3 hospitalized days, unclear reasons were making the patient's situation worse, but this observation is out of the scope of our protocol described in Sec. 2.2. Figure 3 illustrates the probability density of the residual distribution of various observation parameters, reflecting the difference of the patient's health state during the two physiological signal collections.

Case 2. Case 2 is Patient 15 (male, 84 years old, 167 cm, 62 kg). He was in hospital from Mar. 12, 2019 to Apr. 21, 2019. He was diagnosed with coronary heart disease, ischemic cerebrovascular disease, hypertension II, bronchiectasis coinfection, heart dysfunction, kidney dysfunction, liver dysfunction, moderate ane-

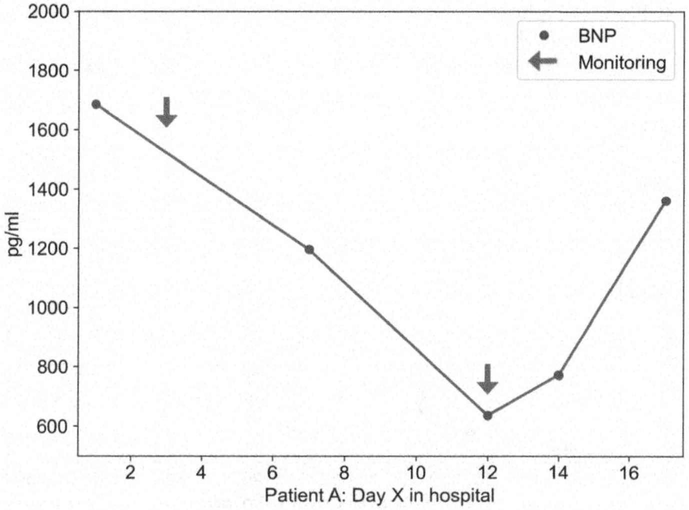

Fig. 2. BNP and physiological signal collection of Patient 01 during his inpatient residence

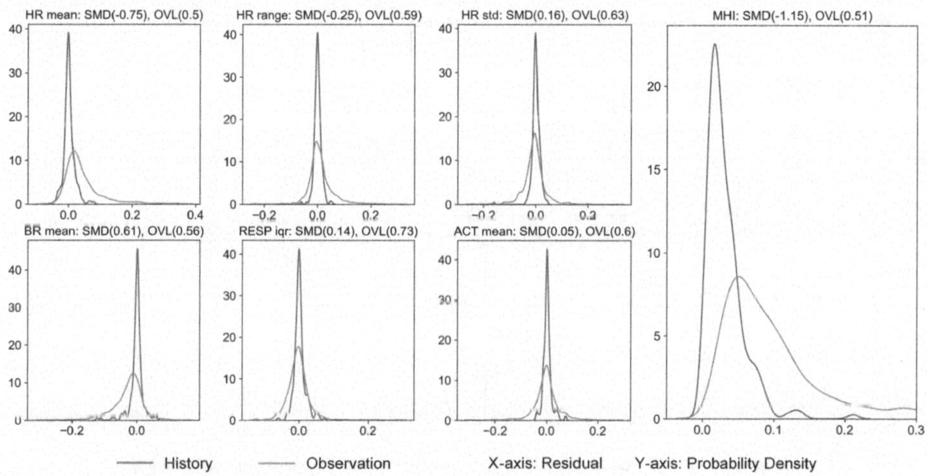

Fig. 3. Residual distribution of historical data and observed data of Patient 01

mia, hypoalbuminemia, and multiple abdominal cavity space-occupying lesions. Figure 4 shows the timeline of his BNP and physiological signal collection. On Mar. 13, 2019 (Day 2), this patient had the first BNP examination, reporting 102.2 pg/ml, and the first physiological signal collection. On Mar. 25, 2019 (Day 14) the second collection of this patient's physiological signals and BNP examination was conducted, reporting 411.3 pg/ml. Unfortunately, we were not able to collect the patient's physiological data since Mar. 25, 2019 (Day 14), even

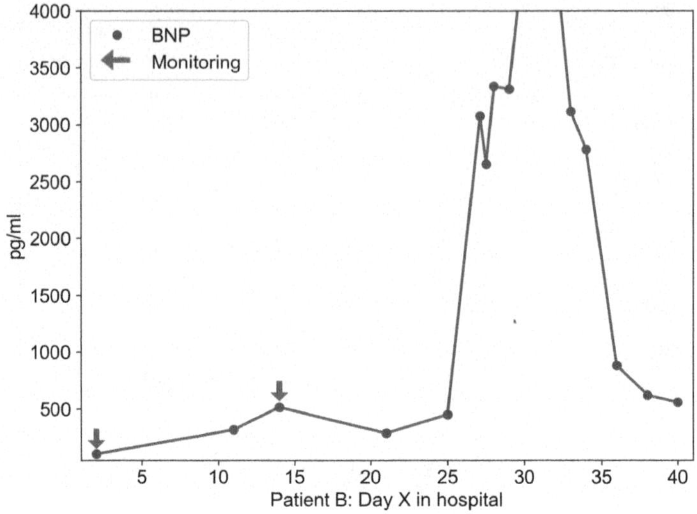

Fig. 4. BNP and physiological signal collection of Patient 15 during his inpatient residence

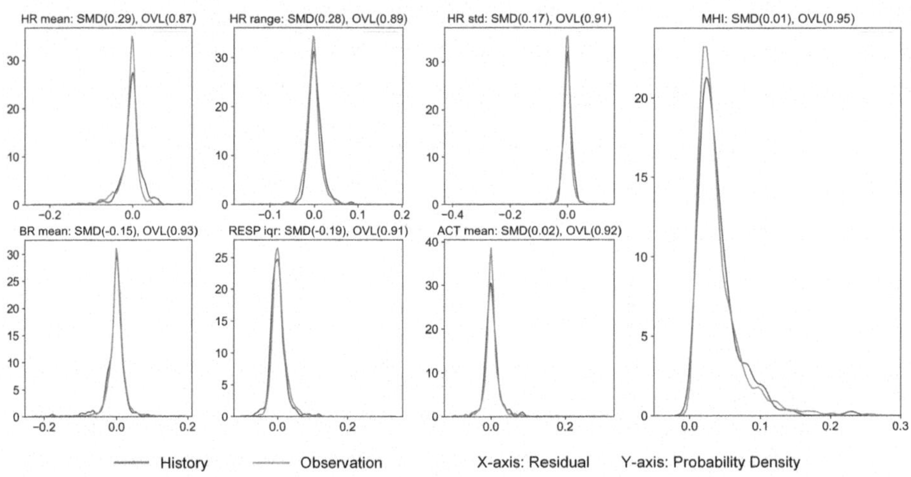

Fig. 5. Residual distribution of historical data and observed data of Patient 15

though his BNP had a dramatic change afterward. This was because he was transferred to the intensive care unit (ICU), where our wearable device was not available. However, we believe that during the two physiological data collections (Day 2–Day 14), the patient's state was not turning better. Figure 5 presents the probability density of residual distribution of various observation parameters, where no significant difference of historical and observation distributions is found.

4 Discussion

This study attempts to evaluate the change of human health and disease status based on physiological signals, which contain a large number of individualized disease and health information. The results preliminarily validate the relationships between physiological signals and lab test results using group and case analysis.

However, different from the industrial mechanical/electronic systems, there is no doubt that human body is a much-complicated system, because a human body is in a dynamic balance of improvement/deterioration all the time. Nowadays, the overall assessment of human health in medicine is based on the combined assessment of multiple laboratory tests (or some specific clinical scale). Nevertheless, the examination timing of these lab tests largely depends on the physician's experience and is difficult to be mathematically quantified. In this pilot study, the lab examination results of BNP were used to approximately indicate the health status of the patients who have the high risk of heart failure, and the change of BNP approximately reveals the change of the health status.

In this paper, we preliminarily explore the efficacy of MSET on a cohort with chronic disease. The experiment results show that a promising relationship between patients' BNP examination values and SMD & OVL of MSET residual distribution. Specifically, MHI has the most significant linear correlation in our results, reporting a coefficient of 0.835 and a p value less than 0.001. The case study indicates that the great potential of using MSET residual distribution as an indicator to distinguish a patient's condition gets better or worse. Our findings suggest that when a patient is admitted to our hospital, her/his physiological signals can be collected on the first day as the baseline, then her/his change of health and disease status is dynamically evaluated afterward. It is expected that this MSET-based approach is highly promising for treatment effect evaluation, as well as providing more abundant information from physiological signals for physicians in CDM.

There also exist some limitations in this study. First, the modeling parameters we used were selected based on experience. More modeling parameters to express the health and disease status of chronic disease patients can be further systematically studied, such as automatic determination of screen parameters of time-series physiological signals. Second, since our data were collected from patients in general wards of the hyperbaric oxygen department, the patients' recovery phase data has a lack of the information from the high dependency unit (HDU) and the intensive care unit (ICU) if the patient's status gets worse, or a lack of the wearable data when the patient is discharged from our hospital. The current data thus does not support us to investigate the model performance when the patient's condition gets worse. Third, chronic disease in the real world is very complicated and patients in the hyperbaric oxygen department always have complex comorbidities, making the cohort volume in the study is relatively small with inevitably confounding factors.

5 Conclusions

In this paper, we conduct a preliminary study to explore the efficacy of MSET on a cohort with chronic disease. The experiment results show that a promising relationship between patients' BNP examination values and SMD & OVL of MSET residual distribution. Specifically, MHI has a more significant linear correlation, reporting a coefficient of 0.835 and a p-value less than 0.001. The case study indicates that the great potential of using MSET residual distribution as an indicator to distinguish a patient's condition gets better or worse. Currently, we are continuously collecting data to expand our in-house dataset, and a more comprehensive analysis will be further performed.

Acknowledgment. This work is supported by The National Natural Science Foundation of China (62171471); Beijing Municipal Science and Technology (Z181100001918023); Big Data Research & Development Project of Chinese PLA General Hospital (2018MBD-09).

References

1. Baig, M.M., GholamHosseini, H., Moqeem, A.A., Mirza, F., Lindén, M.: A systematic review of wearable patient monitoring systems – current challenges and opportunities for clinical adoption. J. Med. Syst. **41**(7), 1–9 (2017). https://doi.org/10.1007/s10916-017-0760-1
2. Cohen, J.: Statistical Power Analysis for the Behavioral Sciences. Academic Press, UK (2013)
3. Cohen, N.M., et al.: Personalized lab test models to quantify disease potentials in healthy individuals. Nat. Med. **27**(9), 1582–1591 (2021)
4. Fernandez-Granero, M.A., Sanchez-Morillo, D., Leon-Jimenez, A.: An artificial intelligence approach to early predict symptom-based exacerbations of COPD. Biotech. Biotechnol. Equipment **32**(3), 778–784 (2018)
5. Forkan, A.R.M., Khalil, I.: Peace-home: probabilistic estimation of abnormal clinical events using vital sign correlations for reliable home-based monitoring. Pervasive Mob. Comput. **38**, 296–311 (2017)
6. Hines, J.W., Usynin, A.: MSET performance optimization through regularization. Nucl. Eng. Technol. **37**(2), 177–184 (2005)
7. Hoffmann, R.G.: Statistics in the practice of medicine. Jama **185**(11), 864–873 (1963)
8. Inman, H.F., Bradley, E.L., Jr.: The overlapping coefficient as a measure of agreement between probability distributions and point estimation of the overlap of two normal densities. Commun. Stat.-Theor. Methods **18**(10), 3851–3874 (1989)
9. Kamei, T., Kanamori, T., Yamamoto, Y., Edirippulige, S.: The use of wearable devices in chronic disease management to enhance adherence and improve telehealth outcomes: a systematic review and meta-analysis. J. Telemedicine Telecare **28**(5), 342–359 (2020). https://doi.org/10.1177/1357633X20937573
10. Katayev, A., Balciza, C., Seccombe, D.W.: Establishing reference intervals for clinical laboratory test results: is there a better way? Am. J. Clin. Pathol. **133**(2), 180–186 (2010)

11. Krüger, S., Graf, J., Kunz, D., Stickel, T., Hanrath, P., Janssens, U.: Brain natriuretic peptide levels predict functional capacity in patients with chronic heart failure. J. Am. Coll. Cardiol. **40**(4), 718–722 (2002)
12. Lehman, L.W.H., et al.: A physiological time series dynamics-based approach to patient monitoring and outcome prediction. IEEE J. Biomed. Health Inform. **19**(3), 1068–1076 (2015). https://doi.org/10.1109/JBHI.2014.2330827
13. Lehman, L.W.H., Mark, R.G., Nemati, S.: A model-based machine learning approach to probing autonomic regulation from nonstationary vital-sign time series. IEEE J. Biom. Health Inform. **22**(1), 56–66 (2018). https://doi.org/10.1109/JBHI.2016.2636808
14. Li, P., et al.: Mobicardio: a clinical-grade mobile health system for cardiovascular disease management. In: 2019 IEEE International Conference on Healthcare Informatics (ICHI), pp. 1–6. IEEE (2019)
15. Li-wei, H.L., Nemati, S., Mark, R.G.: Hemodynamic monitoring using switching autoregressive dynamics of multivariate vital sign time series. In: 2015 Computing in Cardiology Conference (CinC), pp. 1065–1068. IEEE (2015)
16. Liang, Y., Aihua, L., Zhenren, Z.: On cylinder pressure recognition of internal combustion engines by hilbert-huang transform and multivariate state estimation technique. Mech. Sci. Technol. **27**(4), 494 (2008)
17. Liu, X., et al.: Top-net prediction model using bidirectional long short-term memory and medical-grade wearable multisensor system for tachycardia onset: algorithm development study. JMIR Med. Inform. **9**(4), e18803 (2021)
18. Ma, L.Y., Chen, W.W., Gao, R.L., Liu, L.S., Zhu, M.L., Wang, Y.J., Wu, Z.S., Li, H.J., Gu, D.F., Yang, Y.J., et al.: China cardiovascular diseases report 2018: an updated summary. J. Geriatr. Cardiol.: JGC **17**(1), 1 (2020)
19. Morita, E., et al.: Increased plasma levels of brain natriuretic peptide in patients with acute myocardial infarction. Circulation **88**(1), 82–91 (1993)
20. Patel, S., Park, H., Bonato, P., Chan, L., Rodgers, M.: A review of wearable sensors and systems with application in rehabilitation. J. Neuroeng. Rehabil. **9**(1), 1–17 (2012)
21. Pipke, R.M., Wegerich, S.W., Saidi, A., Stehlik, J.: Feasibility of personalized non-parametric analytics for predictive monitoring of heart failure patients using continuous mobile telemetry. In: Proceedings of the 4th Conference on Wireless Health, pp. 1–8 (2013)
22. Shi, Y., et al.: Robust assessment of ecg signal quality for wearable devices. In: 2019 IEEE International Conference on Healthcare Informatics (ICHI), pp. 1–3. IEEE (2019)
23. Singer, R.M., Gross, K.C., Herzog, J.P., King, R.W., Wegerich, S.: Model-based nuclear power plant monitoring and fault detection: Theoretical foundations. Technical Report, Argonne National Laboratory, IL (United States) (1997)
24. Stehlik, J., et al.: Continuous wearable monitoring analytics predict heart failure hospitalization: the LINK-HF multicenter study. Cir.: Heart Fail. **13**(3), e006513 (2020)
25. Summers, R.L., Pipke, M., Wegerich, S., Conkright, G., Isom, K.C.: Functionality of empirical model-based predictive analytics for the early detection of hemodynamic instabilty. Biomed. Sci. Instrum. **50**, 219–224 (2014)
26. Tyler, P.D., et al.: Assessment of intensive care unit laboratory values that differ from reference ranges and association with patient mortality and length of stay. JAMA Netw. Open **1**(7), e184521 (2018)

27. Bai, C., et al.: Prevalence and risk factors of chronic obstructive pulmonary disease in china (the china pulmonary health [CPH] study): a national cross-sectional study. Lancet **391**(10131), 1706–1717 (2018)
28. Wang, Z., Liu, C.: Wind turbine condition monitoring based on a novel multivariate state estimation technique. Measurement **168**, 108388 (2021)
29. Xu, H.: Varying association of laboratory values with reference ranges and outcomes in critically ill patients: an analysis of data from five databases in four countries across Asia, Europe and North America. BMJ Health Care Inform. **28**(1), e100419 (2021)
30. Xu, H., et al.: Study on the accuracy of cardiopulmonary physiological measurements by a wearable physiological monitoring system under different activity conditions. Sheng wu yi xue gong cheng xue za zhi= J. Biomed. Eng.= Shengwu yixue gongchengxue zazhi **37**(1), 119–128 (2020)
31. Xu, H., et al.: Construction and application of a medical-grade wireless monitoring system for physiological signals at general wards. J. Med. Syst. **44**(10), 1–15 (2020). https://doi.org/10.1007/s10916-020-01653-z
32. Xu, H.: Assessing electrocardiogram and respiratory signal quality of a wearable device (sensecho): semisupervised machine learning-based validation study. JMIR mHealth uHealth **9**(8), e25415 (2021)
33. Zhang, W., Liu, J., Gao, M., Pan, C., Huusom, J.K.: A fault early warning method for auxiliary equipment based on multivariate state estimation technique and sliding window similarity. Comput. Ind. **107**, 67–80 (2019)
34. Zhang, Y., et al.: Breathing disorder detection using wearable electrocardiogram and oxygen saturation. In: Proceedings of the 16th ACM Conference on Embedded Networked Sensor Systems, pp. 313–314 (2018)
35. Zhang, Y., et al.: Automated sleep period estimation in wearable multi-sensor systems. In: Proceedings of the 16th ACM Conference on Embedded Networked Sensor Systems, pp. 305–306 (2018)

Security and Privacy Concerns for Healthcare Wearable Devices and Emerging Alternative Approaches

Eleni Boumpa[1(✉)], Vasileios Tsoukas[1], Anargyros Gkogkidis[1], Georgios Spathoulas[2], and Athanasios Kakarountas[1]

[1] Intelligent Systems Laboratory, Department of Computer Science and Biomedical Informatics, University of Thessaly, Lamia, Greece
{eboumpa,vtsoukas,agkogkidis,kakarountas}@uth.gr

[2] Department of Information Security and Communication Technology, Norwegian University of Science and Technology (NTNU), Gjovik, Norway
georgios.spathoulas@ntnu.no

Abstract. The wide use of wearable devices rises a lot of concerns about the privacy and security of personal data that are collected and stored by such services. This concern is even higher when such data is produced by healthcare monitoring wearable devices and thus the impact of any data leakage is more significant. In this work a classification of the wearable devices used for healthcare monitoring is conducted, and the most prominent relevant privacy and security issues and concerns are presented. Furthermore, a brief review of alternative approaches that can eliminate most of such issues, including federated learning, homomorphic encryption, and tinyML, is presented. The aim of this work is to present the privacy and security concerns in healthcare monitoring wearable devices, as well as some solutions in hot topics about these issues.

Keywords: Privacy · Security · Wearable devices · Healthcare

1 Introduction

Wearable Devices (WDs) have already become an integral part of our lives. Research and development in relevant fields, such as the Internet of Things (IoT), Artificial Intelligence (AI), and Machine Learning (ML) continuously evolve, affecting WDs that in turn penetrate more and more in people's daily lives. The main fields of use of WDs can be generally classified as i) wellness and/or healthcare monitoring [1], ii) entertainment [2], and iii) gaming [3].

The field of WDs for healthcare monitoring is very interesting and promising from both research and industry points of view. Furthermore, the use of WDs for healthcare monitoring becomes more and more popular among users, as they can use them for various purposes, such as improving their wellness, reducing

X. Gao et al. (Eds.): MobiHealth 2021, LNICST 440, pp. 19–38, 2022.
https://doi.org/10.1007/978-3-031-06368-8_2

their stress, and monitoring their vital signals. A classification of the WDs for healthcare monitoring is proposed in [4]. As depicted in Fig. 1 the three main categories are i) e-textiles, ii) e-patches, and iii) accessories. While the last category could also be sub-classified as i) wrist-worn, ii) head-mounted, and iii) other WDs. It is observed that in the category of e-textiles, WDs mainly use smart fabric to monitor users' health. Many applications have been proposed, such as paper [5], which explores the pedestrians' safety via shoe-mounted inertial sensor. Also, the authors in [6] present a wearable accelerometer network for recognition of muscle activation in high-motion exercising.

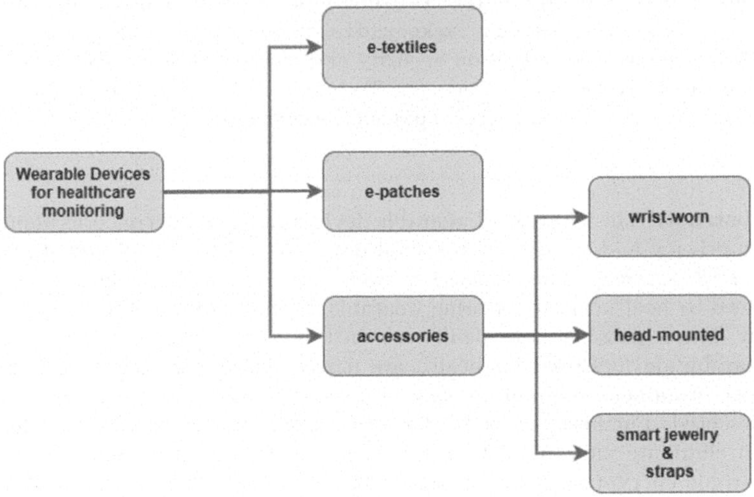

Fig. 1. The classification of WDs for healthcare monitoring as proposed by S. Seneviratne et al. [4].

The category of e-patches is the latest entry in WDs for healthcare monitoring. This category includes the sensor patches and the e-tattoo/e-skin. A research team [7] developed a patch for 24/7 health monitoring. The patch monitors electrocardiogram (ECG) and electroencephalogram (EEG) signals and transmits them in real-time, without intervening in people's daily life. An e-tattoo was proposed by Kim et al. [8]. The proposed wearable is an alcohol bio-sensing system for non-invasive alcohol monitoring via sweat.

The last category is further classified into three subcategories. The wrist-worn devices include smartwatches and wrist bands. A plethora of such WDs, that monitor users' activities and their vital signals, has been designed and produced both from research teams and the industry. A characteristic example of these WDs is presented in work [9], a smartwatch that monitors Cardiopulmonary Resuscitation (CPR). In the sub-category of head-mounted WDs, most common systems are smart eye-wear devices, such as Google Glass [10]. Many research teams have developed extensions and applications for Google Glass for healthcare reasons, such as the authors in [11]. In this work, a real-time augmented-reality system for people suffering from color blindness has been proposed. Another type of devices that belongs in this sub-category is headsets/earbuds devices. Such a device was developed in [12], which regulates inflammation and treats rheumatoid arthritis by delivering electrical fields in the outer ear. Lastly, examples of devices that belong to the sub-category of other WDs are smart jewelry and straps. A ring [13] has been developed to monitor users' health conditions, while a custom-built microphone capturing different body vibrations from body surface has also been proposed in [14]. This WD captures and recognizes non-speech body sounds, helping in various health conditions, like respiratory physiology.

It is obvious that all WDs collect data to facilitate the services they offer, however healthcare WDs tend to monitor and collect data that are more frequently characterized as sensitive and confidential. Some characteristic examples of collected data from those WDs are location, quality of surrounding air, activity, movement, sleep, body temperature, heart rate, blood pressure, blood oxygen, and measuring cognitive functions [15]. Depending on the type and the context of each application, the confidentiality and/or the integrity of such data can be critical and thus leaking and/or tampering with those can induce high risks. This is both a big issue and a challenge for security and privacy researchers. The main focus of the present paper is to identify the highest security and privacy concerns with respect to healthcare WDs, enumerate corresponding threats, and propose alternative approaches that can significantly reduce the attack surface area of such systems.

The contribution of this work is to review the emerging approaches for securing WDs regarding healthcare applications. A classification of WDs used in healthcare monitoring is conducted, and a taxonomy of threats and attacks for those devices is presented. The main focus is to highlight the privacy concerns in sensitive healthcare information and suggest several emerging technologies as alternative possible solutions. The remainder of this paper is organized as follows: In Sect. 2 a brief review of privacy and security concerns in WDs is presented; Sect. 3 provides a classification of threats and attacks in the WDs; Sect. 4 reviews some related works about security and privacy in WDs; in Sect. 5 several solutions are presented about security and privacy in WDs; while Sect. 6 concludes the review's findings.

2 Privacy and Security Concerns in Wearable Devices

Statista's global consumer survey in 2021 estimated the number of WDs users per country. The survey reported that the users of WDs for the United Kingdom, United States, Sweden, China, and India were above 30% [16]. Only in Russia, consumers purchased four million WDs in the first nine months of 2021, while annual WDs sales increased by 400 thousand devices between the years 2019 and 2020 [17]. Moreover, in 2020 the market value of wearable medical devices in Latin America was around 665 million U.S dollars. In 2021, it is projected to amount to 777 million U.S dollars, and it is forecasted to skyrocket to a value of 1.4 billion U.S dollars by the end of the year 2025 [18]. It is noticed that this data is being increasingly collected and processed to provide health monitoring and tracking [19]. Health-related data is identified as personal data and, more precisely, as sensitive data and the most confidential information among all types of personal data [20]. This data must be protected, transmitted only to trusted third parties, and securely stored [21]. The procedure of collecting, transmitting, and storing health-related data can raise many privacy and security concerns due to user behavior, attacks, and data breaches [22]. Furthermore, users are able to use several of those WDs to make payments, something that adds more security concerns to the aforementioned. In conclusion, the three main issues regarding security and privacy in health WDs are user behavior and perception, health-related data transfer, and data storage. A brief description follows of the aforementioned issues as they are presented in the literature [15,23,24].

2.1 User's Behavior

In 2020 a survey [25] showed that people in the fourth decade, or more, of their life, have less understanding of what sensitive data is and the importance of securing it. Another interesting finding was that many users chose not to use any authentication method to secure their devices, and the majority of them thought that they had no sensitive information stored in the devices. The users are prominent actors in the procedure of protecting their information regarding the way they use the device and protect it. Several studies revealed that users are not in a position to protect their devices due to a lack of knowledge or understanding [25–28] on how to achieve it. This raises the need for awareness campaigns and training especially to users aged 50+, on the importance of securing devices and protecting sensitive data. In 2018, a survey about the willingness to share wearable health device information among U.S. citizens 18+ years old was conducted by Statista. The results revealed that 90% of the respondents would share the information with their doctor. A 76-percentage answered that they would share data with a friend or family member, whereas almost 47% would share sensitive data with other communities or app users [29]. Another survey [23] revealed that users have a poor perception of danger and threats and cannot comprehend meanings such as security and privacy. Users tend to trust every application and wearable manufacturer with their sensitive data. The survey concludes with the conjecture that the user could possibly be the weakest link regarding security. Finally, a study [15] of 106 users, owning a health-related WD, showed that half of them were unaware of the need to protect their health information. Additionally, interviewees have a gap in knowledge about the privacy concerns associated with the data acquired by WDs.

2.2 Data Transfer

Most health-related WDs gather data and send it to the cloud for processing. The reason behind the need for transferring data to the cloud is due to the nature of the process data must go through. The high complexity of Deep Learning (DL) algorithms and ML models requires more power and computational resources than those a small WD can provide. Moreover, most WDs collect health-related data such as heart rate, body temperature, oxygen saturation, blood pressure, and more, every few minutes or even while the user is asleep. This results in a vast amount of data that is impossible to store inside the device. WDs are configured to connect to other smart devices via Bluetooth or Wi-Fi. The data under transmission most of the time is not encrypted, and the devices under consideration have insufficient or even no wireless security mechanisms. Furthermore, when a user connects his/her private devices to work networks, may prove dangerous. WDs may act as a starting node that can open a network backdoor, due to device vulnerabilities in stealing corporate data. WDs are always connected to a network, intranet, internet, or a mesh network with other smart devices. Due to limited resources, computational power, and cost minimization requirement, WDs are not developed with security in mind. Hackers attempt to find their weakest and most vulnerable point in order to gain access or even alter data and manage the communication [30]. Moreover, despite the main advantages of bluetooth, this technology suffers from many threats and vulnerabilities with attacks such as Denial of Service (DoS), Man-in-the-middle (MITM), and eavesdropping attacks, or bluetooth-specific attacks such as bluesnarfing [31].

2.3 Data Storage

The third step of the data procedure, after capturing and transferring, is storing data in the cloud. Once data is stored in the cloud, the user does not have a clear image of how this data is manipulated and used. Additionally, this data may now be owned by the company that maintains the server and not the actual owner (the user), giving them the opportunity to use the data in ways they disclose in the user terms and agreement [32]. Two of the most common issues regarding data storage on the cloud are the DoS attacks, which could hinder data availability, and data breaches leading to sensitive information exposure. According to a study by WebsitePlanet and independent cybersecurity expert Jeremiah Fowler, over 61 million fitness tracker records from Apple and Fitbit were leaked in a data breach. The researchers determined that the data leak originated with GetHealth, a health and wellness startup that enables customers to consolidate their data from WDs, medical devices, and apps. The disclosed data belonged to users of WDs distributed around the world and included data such as their names, birth dates, weight, height, gender, and geographical location. There was no password or any cryptographic means to protect the database, and the content in plain text was easily recognizable. Fitbit was cited in more than 2,700 recordings, while Apple's Healthkit was mentioned more than 17,000 times. Additionally, researchers determined that the files included information of the location of the data on the storage medium, as well as a blueprint of the network's backend operations, making it an exceedingly simple target for attackers [33].

3 Threats and Attacks

In this section, a classification of the most common security threats and attacks is provided. Each threat is categorized in three different layers as mentioned above, about the user, data transfer, and data storage. Additionally, the impact, the likelihood for the attack, and its consequences to the triad of confidentiality-integrity-availability properties (CIA) are reported. Confidentiality is related to prohibiting access to information for unauthorized users, integrity ensures that the information is correct and unaltered, and availability guarantees that the information and/or service are always available.

Wearable Device: The first threat has to do with the device itself, and it belongs to the first layer, the user. The user may lose the device, or a malicious user could steal it. This threat has low to high impact, depending on the user; it is easy and highly possible to happen and can impact confidentiality and integrity.

Social Engineering: It also belongs in the first layer of the data procedure and involves attackers that attempt to gain the confidence of users to get the necessary information. In summary, social engineering is the skill of persuading others into disclosing sensitive information. Hackers may get information by impersonating other individuals through email, chat, or even in-person. The impact is moderate and could hinder confidentiality and integrity [34].

Brute Force Attack: This type of attack often happens as a subsequent step of previous attacks. The hacker must have physical access to the device and possibly some information about the user. What follows is many attempts based on trial and error to get access. The hacker can use an automated process with malicious software or enter random sequences of characters by hand. This type of attack could happen for access in the WD or access to the data storage infrastructure. The possibility for a successful attack can be identified as moderate, and the impact of the damage is high. This type of attack can hinder all three aspects of information security. A similar type of attack is dictionary attacks, where the attacker uses a list of the most common passwords [35–37].

Malware/Ransomware: Malicious software can be installed in the WD and access or alter sensitive information. This type of threat has a moderate impact; it is not that common and could hinder confidentiality and integrity [38]. Another similar attack is ransomware, in which the attacker uses software to encrypt the user's sensitive information and asks for a ransom to release the decryption key. A common type of attack with high impact that affects all three pillars of information security [39].

Denial of service (DoS): With this type of attack, the hacker attempts to bring a computer or network to a halt, rendering it unreachable to its authorized users. DoS attacks make this possible by flooding the target with traffic or by providing information that causes the target to crash. In all cases, the DoS attack denies genuine users access to the service or system. DoS attacks may be classified into two broad categories: flooding services and crashing services. Flood attacks occur when the system gets an excessive amount of traffic that the server cannot buffer, leading it to slow down and finally cease operation. The most popular flood assaults are:

- *Buffer overflow* is the most used DoS attack. The goal is to send more traffic to a network address than the system's developers intended. Buffer overflow includes two other types of attacks, i) Internet Control Message Protocol (ICMP) and ii) Synchronization (SYN) flood. i) ICMP flood - takes advantage of any misconfiguration that may appear in network devices by delivering packets to every device on the targeted network, rather than just one. ii) SYN flood - initiates a request for connection with a server but never completes it. This process is repeated until all open ports are inundated with requests, and none are accessible to genuine users.
- *DoS attacks* are forming the second category, the crashing type, the attacks simply exploit flaws in the target system or service, causing it to crash. These attacks send input that exploits flaws in the target system, crashing or severely destabilizing it to the point where it cannot be accessed or utilized.
- *Distributed Denial of Service (DDoS)* assault is another category of DoS attacks. A DDoS happens when numerous systems coordinate a DoS attack on a single target. The critical distinction is that the victim is attacked simultaneously from several sites rather than being targeted from a single place.

In general, DoS attacks are common; it is an easy way to disrupt services due to automated software and may have a high impact on data storage by hindering their availability [40–43].

Rogue access point: A rogue access point is a threat deployed on a network without the consent of the network's owner. The attacker who controls the rogue access point may intercept personal and sensitive information transferred through the network. There are two categories of interception, active and passive. In the active interception, the attacker can receive the user's data, alter it, and then deliver the updated user data to the target endpoint. In the passive interception, the hacker may read the user's private information, but there is no possible way to alter the information for other malicious usages. This threat occurs in the second step of the data procedure, data transfer, it is not a common threat, and the impact is high, affecting the integrity and confidentiality [44–46].

Man in the middle attack: The man in the middle (MITM) is a kind of attack in which the attacker discreetly transmits and maybe modifies messages between two users who are under the impression that they are communicating directly with one another. A type of MITM attack is eavesdropping which is a real-time illegal interception of private communication between two parties. Another type of MITM attack is the replay attack, where the attacker intercepts the communication between users and then delays or resends messages. These attacks occur in data transfer. They are easy to perform, with a high impact on confidentiality and integrity [4, 47–49].

SQL injection: Attackers insert SQL statements in input fields to gain access to private information, alter it or even delete it. An SQL injection attack could destroy a database or even a system. It is a common attack, easily achievable since the hacker only needs to type SQL statements, with high impact and affecting all three security information pillars [50,51].

In Table 1 a taxonomy of threats/attacks in the three layers of the user, the data transfer, and the data storage in WDs is depicted. The layer of the user is divided into two categories, that of the user and the device, as there are some differences in the attacks between them. Also, the CIA properties affected are pointed out for every threat/attack. Furthermore, the impact of each threat/attack, on a 3-grade scale (low, moderate, high), as well as the difficulty of every threat/attack, on a 3-grade scale (easy, medium, hard), are highlighted.

Table 1. Taxonomy of the threats and attacks in wearable devices.

Threat/Attack	User	Device	Data transfer	Data storage	Impact	Difficulty	Confidentiality	Integrity	Availability
Theft/Lost	•	○	○	○	Moderate	Easy	•	•	○
Social	•	○	○	○	Moderate	Medium	•	•	○
Brute	○	•	○	•	High	Medium	•	•	•
Guessing	○	•	○	•	High	Hard	•	•	•
Dictionary	○	•	○	•	High	Easy	•	•	•
Malware	○	•	○	•	Moderate	Medium	•	•	•
Ransomware	○	•	○	•	High	Medium	•	•	•
DoS	○	○	•	○	High	Easy	○	○	•
Rogue	○	○	•	○	High	Hard	•	•	○
MITM	○	○	•	○	High	Easy	•	•	○
Replay	○	○	•	○	High	Easy	•	•	○
Eavesdropping	○	○	•	○	High	Easy	•	•	○
SQL injection	○	○	○	•	High	Easy	•	•	•

4 Related Works

This section provides a brief review of previously accomplished works regarding the security and privacy issues in WDs. The works are reported in chronological order.

A brief review of security and privacy issues both in electronic healthcare records and wearable healthcare monitoring devices is explored in [52]. While these technologies provide many benefits for healthcare delivery to all the involved, such as patients, doctors, and familiars, some privacy and security issues, like data storage, data transfer, and data analysis rights, raise privacy and security concerns and are examined in this work.

Safavi and Shukur [53] proposed a privacy and security framework for WDs in healthcare. The developed framework can be embedded in every operating system for WDs, while it comprises ten principles for the WDs users' privacy protection.

From another point of view, Wang et al. [54] examined security concerns in WDs and suggested a multi-layered security architecture for WDs. The proposed architecture aims to prevent the system's security enemies from "breaking through" the security in all system layers. A security analysis of WDs is presented in [42]. After a brief review of the security and privacy attacks in WDs, the authors also evaluated three WDs to understand their security and privacy vulnerabilities. While the authors of work [55] conducted a survey about the lack of users' understanding regarding the security and privacy of wearable healthcare monitoring devices that they use. The respondents showed a poor understanding of threats about their recorded health data. Furthermore, the authors present a method to mitigate the results of users' security and privacy threats, through their education about this issue.

Seneviratne et al. [4] analyzed the communication security threats of WDs. They classified these threats, regarding network security, into three categories according to confidentiality, integrity, and availability. Furthermore, they presented some approaches that address these threats.

The authors of the paper [22] highlight the importance of the deployment of a framework for effective privacy, equity, and protection of users of wearable wellness and/or healthcare devices. This is a result of the fact that more and more people that live in the United States use wearable health monitoring devices. This issue raises one of the most challenging public health problems, which is a serious individual privacy concern. Also, the authors of the paper [56] conducted an ethical survey about the use of WDs in healthcare. The survey's results show that the users are concerned about their data and their usage of them from third parties. The aim of this work is to be proposed an ethical framework that considers users' privacy.

Finally, a discussion about the various privacy and security problems from the use of WDs is presented in [57]. Additionally, this work proposed both the adoption of different policies from the companies for their consumers' privacy issues and the awaken of users about the misuse of WDs and their data leakage.

5 Emerging Approaches

The model under which health monitoring service providers offer their services usually requires WDs to constantly collect health/medical-related data on the side of the user and transmit such data to their side to process for monitoring, prognosis, and/or prevention. When it comes to prognosis it is common for service providers to use ML models, which can either be user-specific or generic, to which such data is fed. While health related data is considered as very sensitive, the aforementioned model of processing set as prerequisites the transmission of such data to the service provider and the processing of that (potentially after integration with data of others), in order to produce models that will enable decision taking on the side of the user.

It is obvious that this increased flow of information from WDs to the service provider and vice versa, increases the risk of sensitive data leakage either through cases of direct data breaches or even through cases of personal data inference from trained models [94,95]. In the present section an analysis of alternative approaches that enable the training of models in more privacy conscious workflows is presented. The emerging approaches of Federated Learning (FL), Homomorphic Encryption (HE), and Tiny Machine Learning (TinyML) have been employed to minimise data privacy issues in the last two steps of the data procedure in WDs, the data transfer and the data storage. A brief description of the aforementioned approaches and several applications of those in the field of healthcare monitoring are described in the rest of the Section.

5.1 Federated Learning

Federated Learning is an emerging technology with great scientific interest, especially in the field of healthcare [58–67]. With FL, participants are able to train ML models collaboratively by only exchanging parameters of trained models, instead of exchanging sensitive information for each participant. The approach enables the training of personalised models for each participant through a secure workflow. FL can also contribute to a better understanding of data and produced models. Additionally, FL reduces network bandwidth requirements as only parameters required for aggregation must be transmitted to the server. The technology can be classified into three main categories, horizontal FL, vertical FL, and federated transfer learning. In the first category, participants share different records of a data-set; in the second participants share different features of the same samples; and finally, in the third and last category, the participants attempt to transfer trained models between completely heterogeneous sets of data. Finally, FL can protect against known network and device attacks, while there are enhancements that ensure that no connected actor is malicious [68–72].

A team of researchers proposed FL4W [71], a FL system for WDs aiming at human activity recognition. The system's architecture is the classic client-server architecture, where the server orchestrates the devices in four different steps. In the first step devices are registered to the system. Then the server specifies the appropriate tasks and hyperparameters to broadcast to the WDs. The third step contains the local model training where every device uses data without uploading anything to the server. Finally, the parameter tables of the updated models are sent to the server, which aggregates the local models with federated averaging [73] algorithm.

FedHealth [74] is a framework for healthcare WDs. The framework utilizes the technology of FL and aims to achieve accurate personal healthcare without compromising privacy. Four different procedures are required to create intelligent WDs. To begin, a server-side cloud model is trained using publicly available data. This model is then distributed to all users, who may start training their own models using data from their devices. The user model may then be uploaded to the server to be used for the training of a new global model. It is worth mentioning that no user data or information are uploaded to the sever apart from the encrypted model parameters in this phase. The parameters are encrypted with HE, which is going to be discussed later on. Finally, any user may train personalized models by combining the cloud model with his or her previous model and data. The system may update both the user and the cloud models concurrently in response to the latest user data. As a result, the more time a user spends with the service, the more tailored for the user the model may be. Finally, the future plans for the system are to be extended so it can be in a position to detect Parkinson's disease and developed in a way so it can be deployed in hospitals.

Finally, in work [75], an edge-based FL framework is being proposed. According to the authors, the system could aid healthcare practitioners by offering data-driven insights for illness diagnosis and prognosis by analyzing mobility levels and behaviors obtained from WDs. The suggested framework is organized into three modules: cloud, edge, and application. The cloud module will be administered by a model owner who will be responsible for coordinating different cloud-based duties such as patient registration, database maintenance, and model uploading. It consists of two primary components: a controller, which provides alerts when possibly updated global models become available, and a master aggregator, which uses techniques such as federated averaging. The global model is being trained using publicly accessible datasets so that users' sensitive information is safe. The edge module comprises three essential components: a FL server, a local-storage controller, and an aggregator. This module improves the overall training process by personalizing the models on each corresponding device. Finally, the application module enables the addition of any device capable of generating health-related data. In conclusion, the framework could be extended to support disease prevention, addiction and mental health tracking, and real-time health monitoring.

5.2 Homomorphic Encryption

Homomorphic Encryption is a technique that enables mathematical operations on encrypted data without requiring the decryption of such data. The outcome of the aforementioned actions is an encrypted result. The result in its decrypted form corresponds to the outcome of operations done on the raw data [76]. HE systems are classified into two broad types according to the sort of operations they support: HE and partially HE [77]. A system is identified as fully homomorphic if it exhibits both additive and multiplicative properties of homomorphism [78]. Although the first system was described in 1978, the first feasible fully homomorphic system was developed in 2009 [79]. While fully homomorphic schemes are believed to be safer than partially homomorphic schemes, they need much more computer resources and have a higher overhead. The somewhat HE schemes are a subcategory of the Fully Homomorphic Encryption (FHE) schemes. They include addition and multiplication, but only specific operations are permitted, and calculations are limited as the cipher-text size expands [80]. Partially homomorphic systems may allow just one type of operation at a time, either addition or multiplication and are identified as a more practicable option than fully homomorphic systems.

In work [81] the authors suggest a four-layer mobile healthcare network, which includes a WD part, a preprocessing section, a cloud server section, and a physician diagnostic portion. Then, three secure medical calculations are defined: the average heart rate, the identification of long QT syndrome, and the chi-square testing. To perform calculations on the ciphertext, the encryption of the health data is accomplished using FHE.

Using data acquired from WDs, a team [82] presented a smart responsive software that may advise in real-time patients, physicians, emergency teams, and carers. Depending on the patient's health, the relevant user will be notified to act as required and take care of the situation. To safeguard the private and sensitive information of patients undergoing treatment and care, they discuss a secure HE technique that will maintain data encryption throughout the data gathering, collecting, and processing stages.

Researchers in [83] presented a wireless sensor network for healthcare in which data is encrypted utilizing the technique of HE. The system ensures secure communication and data storage by dividing the original data into two or three portions. Additionally, the system enables forwarding nodes to transmit encrypted sensor data without decrypting it. As a consequence, even if a forwarding node is hacked, the attacker will be unable to eavesdrop on the data, providing far more privacy than older healthcare systems.

The authors of work [84] propose an end-to-end encrypted security architecture that enables safe data collection from embedded medical devices, protected processing on this data in a low-cost commodity cloud environment, and restricted delegation of access to this data to selected recipients. This solution capitalizes on recent advances in HE and Proxy Re-Encryption (PRE) to address the practical demands of a secure medical data architecture's data collection, processing, and dissemination. According to the authors this architecture reduces the cost of healthcare data systems by securely outsourcing computation to cloud computing environments, while also reducing vulnerabilities to some of the most pernicious security threats, such as insider attacks, and enabling additional cost savings through the use of lower-cost embedded medical devices.

In study [85] a privacy-preserving solution based on HE for preventing attackers from accessing medical plaintext data is suggested. Computations are spread to numerous edge virtual nodes and all arithmetic operations are masked, preventing untrusted cloud servers from knowing about the actions done on the encrypted patient data. Virtual edge nodes use cloud computing resources to perform computationally difficult mathematical operations, and minimize data transmission latency between devices and edge nodes. A comparison to prior research revealed that homomorphically encrypted data kept at the edge protects the privacy and integrity of the data.

A team in [86] proposed a privacy-preserving protocol for healthcare systems that makes use of WDs and implemented it on the Raspberry Pi, in order to determine the real efficiency of FHE over WDs. The authors developed the protocol using two FHE libraries, HElib and SEAL, on a Raspberry Pi, and a network simulator in order to quantify the computational and communication costs associated with wireless body area networks. The results indicate that the protocol with SEAL has a lower communication overhead than the protocol with HElib. The protocol with SEAL has almost identical transmission costs to the simple protocol, which is the one that lacks encryption. SEAL was able to do more homomorphic operations per unit of plaintext than HElib. As a result, Helib, which is faster, is well suited for applications requiring low time complexity, while SEAL is well suited for applications requiring a large number of homomorphic operations.

5.3 Tiny Machine Learning

Tiny Machine Learning is one of the fastest-growing domains, attracting increased attention from the healthcare sector. TinyML is a hardware-software hybrid that allows ML models and DL algorithms to be deployed on small, reasonably inexpensive, and power-efficient devices. These devices will pave the way for new services and technologies that do not require costly and energy-intensive Graphics Processing Units (GPUs) or cloud systems that are constrained by significant restrictions with respect to security, latency, and bandwidth. A typical TinyML workflow is composed of three major phases. The first step is to train the ML model on a workstation with sufficient processing capability. Following that, the model is optimized through using model reduction methods such as pruning and quantization. Finally, the refined TinyML model is ready to be implemented in the healthcare WDs in the last stage [87–89]. ML on device is a helpful step in preventing consumers from losing or leaking data and from waiting for results due to latency and load difficulties. WDs will be used to gather, analyze, and extract data. This data is not communicated to other devices or servers, resulting in safer and more private devices. Additionally, microcontrollers are considered to be ultra-low-power devices. They typically operate in less than one mWatt and can deliver machine intelligence for the cost of a battery. TinyML may be the field that revolutionizes how we see healthcare applications today by introducing several new devices and apps that the whole healthcare research community may use. Wearable gadgets for health monitoring and prevention seem to have the highest promise for TinyML applications. They will provide real-time analysis and possible alerts without requiring data transmission or significant computational power, resulting in autonomous, intelligent, safe, and efficient devices in the form factor of a wristwatch or earwear.

The authors in [90] created a wrist device that monitors vital indicators such as body temperature, breathing pattern, and blood oxygen saturation in order to aid in the prioritization of COVID-19 patients in the emergency room. The neural network that evaluates respiration operates locally on the WD, preventing data transfer to the cloud, using TinyML technology, and protecting the privacy of patient-sensitive information.

The work [91] discusses the fields of AI, low-power wide-area network and TinyML for new safe and intelligent WDs. The research demonstrates the unique properties of these cutting-edge paradigms, concluding that the future generation of WDs will enable a broad range of fresh services and applications.

In another study [92], TinyML is recommended for customized home healthcare with the goal of assisting patients in rehabilitation, patients with chronic and acute diseases, but also caregivers' physical and emotional well-being during times of extreme stress, such as the COVID-19 pandemic.

To conclude, in [93] proposed a novel TinyML framework for healthcare is capable of the following: 1) selection or customization of ML models, 2) enhancing optimization for improved decision making, and (3) learning and adapting for improved performance. Additionally, the system will be sufficient to support a variety of e-health applications, including symptom tracking, hygiene monitoring, body scanning, and mental health.

Finally, in Table 2 a taxonomy of the aforementioned applications of emerging approaches is presented. Also, the system's type (framework, network, model, scheme, protocol, and device), as well as the Technology Readiness Lever (TRL) of each work is depicted.

Table 2. Taxonomy of the emerging approaches for security and privacy issues.

Work	Type	Federated learning	Homomorphic encryption	TinyML	TRL
[71]	Framework	●	○	○	5
[74]	Framework	●	●	○	5
[75]	Framework	●	○	○	1
[81]	Network	○	●	○	3
[82]	Model	○	●	○	3
[83]	Network	○	●	○	2
[84]	Framework	○	●	○	2
[85]	Scheme	○	●	○	2
[86]	Protocol	○	●	○	4
[90]	Device	○	○	●	6
[91]	Device	○	○	●	5
[92]	Device	○	○	●	1
[93]	Framework	○	○	●	1

6 Conclusion

This work aims to provide a brief literature review on wearable healthcare devices. However, the wide use of these devices, especially for healthcare purposes, arises several concerns about data privacy and security. The security threats and attacks that wearable devices are exposed to were identified and categorized, while the corresponding impact and difficulty were assessed. Also, the confidentiality, integrity, and availability effect of each threat has been highlighted. Furthermore, the existing emerging approaches for processing data collected in multiple WDs that strengthen security and privacy, like Federated

Learning, Homomorphic Encryption and TinyML are reviewed. A taxonomy of the proposed emerging approaches for security and privacy issues is presented. Overall, the review provides to the researchers an evaluation on security and privacy issues concerning the healthcare wearable devices that are quite common to our daily life.

References

1. Lu, L., et al.: Wearable health devices in health care: narrative systematic review. JMIR Mhealth Uhealth **8**(11), e18907 (2020)
2. Olson, J.S., Redkar, S.: A survey of wearable sensor networks in health and entertainment. MOJ Appl. Bionics Biomech. **2**(5), 280–287 (2018)
3. Future Marketing Insights. https://www.futuremarketinsights.com/reports/wearable-gaming-technology-market. Accessed 21 Oct 2021
4. Seneviratne, S., et al.: A survey of wearable devices and challenges. IEEE Commun. Surv. Tutorials **19**(4), 2573–2620 (2017)
5. Jain, S., Borgiattino, C., Ren, Y., Gruteser, M., Chen, Y., Chiasserini, C.F.: Lookup: enabling pedestrian safety services via shoe sensing. In: Proceedings of the 13th Annual International Conference on Mobile Systems, Applications, and Services, pp. 257–271 (2015)
6. Mokaya, F., Lucas, R., Noh, H.Y., Zhang, P.: Myovibe: vibration based wearable muscle activation detection in high mobility exercises. In: Proceedings of the 2015 ACM International Joint Conference on Pervasive and Ubiquitous Computing, pp. 27–38 (2015)
7. ILLINOIS.EDU. https://news.illinois.edu/view/6367/233722. Accessed 21 Oct 2021
8. Kim, J., et al.: Noninvasive alcohol monitoring using a wearable tattoo-based iontophoretic-biosensing system. Acs Sens. **1**(8), 1011–1019 (2016)
9. Gruenerbl, A., Pirkl, G., Monger, E., Gobbi, M., Lukowicz, P.: Smart-watch life saver: smart-watch interactive-feedback system for improving bystander CPR. In: Proceedings of the 2015 ACM International Symposium on Wearable Computers, pp. 19–26 (2015)
10. Google Glass. https://www.google.com/glass/start/. Accessed 21 Oct 2021
11. Tanuwidjaja, E., et al.: Chroma: a wearable augmented-reality solution for color blindness. In: Proceedings of the 2014 ACM international joint conference on pervasive and ubiquitous computing, pp. 799–810 (2014)
12. Nēsos - Treat diseases by harnessing the power of the brain to regulate immune function.https://nesos.com. Accessed 21 Oct 2021
13. Ōura ring: accurate health information accessible to everyone.https://ouraring.com. Accessed 21 Oct 2021
14. Rahman, T., et al.: BodyBeat: a mobile system for sensing non-speech body sounds. In: MobiSys, vol. 14, no. 10.1145, pp. 2–594 (2014)
15. Cilliers, L.: Wearable devices in healthcare: privacy and information security issues. Health Inf. Manag. J. **49**(2–3), 150–156 (2020)
16. Wearable device usage 2021. (n.d.). Statista. https://www.statista.com/forecasts/1101110/wearables-devices-usage-in-selected-countries. Accessed 22 Oct 2021
17. Wearables sales volume in Russia 2021. (n.d.). Statista. https://www.statista.com/statistics/1243485/number-of-wearables-sold-in-russia/. Accessed 22 Oct 2021

18. Wearable medical devices market Latin America 2025. (n.d.). Statista. https://www.statista.com/statistics/800329/wearable-medical-devices-market-value-latin-america/. Accessed 22 Oct 2021
19. Khan, S., Parkinson, S., Grant, L., Liu, N., McGuire, S.: Biometric systems utilising health data from wearable devices: applications and future challenges in computer security. ACM Comput. Surv. (CSUR) **53**(4), 1–29 (2020)
20. Mehraeen, E., Ghazisaeedi, M., Farzi, J., Mirshekari, S.: Security challenges in healthcare cloud computing: a systematic. Glob. J. Health Sci. **9**(3) (2017)
21. Celdrán, A.H., et al.: PROTECTOR: towards the protection of sensitive data in Europe and the US. Comput. Netw. **181**, 107448 (2020)
22. Montgomery, K., Chester, J., Kopp, K.: Health wearables: ensuring fairness, preventing discrimination, and promoting equity in an emerging Internet-of-Things environment. J. Inf. Policy **8**, 34–77 (2018)
23. Bellekens, X.J., Nieradzinska, K., Bellekens, A., Seeam, P., Hamilton, A.W., Seeam, A.: A study on situational awareness security and privacy of wearable health monitoring devices. Int. J. Cyber Situational Aware. **1**(1), 74–96 (2016)
24. Els, F., Cilliers, L.: Improving the information security of personal electronic health records to protect a patient's health information. In: 2017 Conference on Information Communication Technology and Society (ICTAS), pp. 1–6. IEEE (2017)
25. Tsoukas, V., Gkogkidis, A., Kakarountas, A.: A survey on mobile user perceptions of sensitive data and authentication methods. In: 24th Pan-Hellenic Conference on Informatics, pp. 346–349 (2020)
26. Cilliers, L., Viljoen, K.L.A., Chinyamurindi, W.T.: A study on students' acceptance of mobile phone use to seek health information in South Africa. Health Inf. Manag. J. **47**(2), 59–69 (2018)
27. Wiercioch, A., Teufel, S., Teufel, B.: The authentication dilemma. J. Commun. **13**(8), 443–449 (2018)
28. Cherapau, I., Muslukhov, I., Asanka, N., Beznosov, K.: On the impact of touch id on iphone passcodes. In: Eleventh Symposium on Usable Privacy and Security (SOUPS 2015), pp. 257–276 (2015)
29. Sharing of wearable health device data U.S. 2018. (n.d.). Statista. https://www.statista.com/statistics/829472/wearable-health-data-sharing-willingness-us-adults/. Accessed 22 Oct 2021
30. Siboni, S., Shabtai, A., Tippenhauer, N.O., Lee, J., Elovici, Y.: Advanced security testbed framework for wearable IoT devices. ACM Trans. Internet Technol. (TOIT) **16**(4), 1–25 (2016)
31. Shah, K.T.: Privacy and Security Issues of Wearables in Healthcare (Doctoral dissertation, Flinders University, College of Science and Engineering.) (2019)
32. Piwek, L., Ellis, D.A., Andrews, S., Joinson, A.: The rise of consumer health wearables: promises and barriers. PLoS Med. **13**(2), e1001953 (2016)
33. 61 M Fitbit, Apple Users Had Data Exposed in Wearable Device Data Breach. Healthitsecurity. https://healthitsecurity.com/news/61m-fitbit-apple-users-had-data-exposed-in-wearable-device-data-breach. Accessed 22 Oct 2021
34. Schlöglhofer, R., Sametinger, J.: Secure and usable authentication on mobile devices. In: Proceedings of the 10th International Conference on Advances in Mobile Computing & Multimedia, pp. 257–262 (2014)
35. Clarke, N.: Transparent User Authentication: Biometrics. Springer Science & Business Media, RFID and behavioural profiling (2011)

36. Bellovin, S.M., Merritt, M.: Augmented encrypted key exchange: a password-based protocol secure against dictionary attacks and password file compromise. In: Proceedings of the 1st ACM Conference on Computer and Communications Security, pp. 244–250 (1993)
37. Conrad, E., Misenar, S., Feldman, J.: Eleventh Hour CISSP®: Study Guide. Syngress (2016)
38. Bada, M., von Solms, B.: A Cybersecurity Guide for Using Fitness Devices (2021). arXiv preprint http://arxiv.org/abs/2105.02933
39. Garmin: the latest wearable attacked by ransomware and a controversial ransom. Panda Security Mediacenter (2020). https://www.pandasecurity.com/en/mediacenter/adaptive-defense/garmin-ransomware-attack/. Accessed 22 Oct 2021
40. What is a denial of service attack (Dos)? (n.d.). Palo Alto Networks. https://www.paloaltonetworks.com/cyberpedia/what-is-a-denial-of-service-attack-dos. Accessed 23 Oct 2021
41. Arış, A., Oktuğ, S.F., Yalçın, S.B.Ö.: Internet-of-things security: denial of service attacks. In: 2015 23nd Signal Processing and Communications Applications Conference (SIU), pp. 903–906. IEEE (2015)
42. Ching, K.W., Singh, M.M.: Wearable technology devices security and privacy vulnerability analysis. Int. J. Netw. Secur. Appl. **8**(3), 19–30 (2016)
43. Hale, M.L., Lotfy, K., Gamble, R.F., Walter, C., Lin, J.: Developing a platform to evaluate and assess the security of wearable devices. Digit. Commun. Netw. **5**(3), 147–159 (2019)
44. Forensic analysis and security. Security Today. https://securitytoday.com/articles/2018/05/01/forensic-analysis-and-security.aspx. Accessed 23 Oct 2021
45. Secure Wi-Fi For Healthcare Applications. Aruba Network (n.d.). https://www.arubanetworks.com/assets/wp/WP_Healthcare_WLAN.pdf. Accessed 23 Oct 2021
46. Rai, S., Chukwuma, P., Cozart, R.: Security and Auditing of Smart Devices: Managing Proliferation of Confidential Data on Corporate and BYOD Devices. Auerbach Publications, Boca Raton (2016)
47. Melamed, T.: An active man-in-the-middle attack on bluetooth smart devices. Safety and Security Studies, vol 15 (2018)
48. Bluetooth bug opens devices to man-in-the-middle attacks. https://threatpost.com/bluetooth-bug-mitm-attacks/159124/. Accessed 23 Oct 2021
49. Hajian, R., ZakeriKia, S., Erfani, S.H., Mirabi, M.: SHAPARAK: scalable healthcare authentication protocol with attack-resilience and anonymous key-agreement. Comput. Netw. **183**, 107567 (2020)
50. Zhang, C., Shahriar, H., Riad, A.K.: Security and privacy analysis of wearable health device. In: 2020 IEEE 44th Annual Computers, Software, and Applications Conference (COMPSAC), pp. 1767–1772. IEEE (2020)
51. Chen, K., et al.: Internet-of-things security and vulnerabilities: taxonomy, challenges, and practice. J. Hardware Syst. Secur. **2**(2), 97–110 (2018). https://doi.org/10.1007/s41635-017-0029-7
52. Meingast, M., Roosta, T., Sastry, S.: Security and privacy issues with health care information technology. In: 2006 International Conference of the IEEE Engineering in Medicine and Biology Society, pp. 5453–5458. IEEE (2006)
53. Safavi, S., Shukur, Z.: Conceptual privacy framework for health information on wearable device. PLoS One **9**(12), e114306 (2014)
54. Wang, S., Bie, R., Zhao, F., Zhang, N., Cheng, X., Choi, H.A.: Security in wearable communications. IEEE Netw. **30**(5), 61–67 (2016)

55. Bellekens, X., Hamilton, A., Seeam, P., Nieradzinska, K., Franssen, Q., Seeam, A.: Pervasive eHealth services a security and privacy risk awareness survey. In: 2016 International Conference On Cyber Situational Awareness, Data Analytics And Assessment (CyberSA), pp. 1–4. IEEE (2016)
56. Anaya, L.S., Alsadoon, A., Costadopoulos, N., Prasad, P.W.C.: Ethical implications of user perceptions of wearable devices. Sci. Eng. Ethics **24**(1), 1–28 (2018). https://doi.org/10.1007/s11948-017-9872-8
57. Alrababah, Z.: Privacy and Security of Wearable Devices (2020)
58. Liu, J.C., Goetz, J., Sen, S., Tewari, A.: Learning from others without sacrificing privacy: simulation comparing centralized and federated machine learning on mobile health data. JMIR Mhealth Uhealth **9**(3), e23728 (2021)
59. Rieke, N., et al.: The future of digital health with federated learning. NPJ Digit. Med. **3**(1), 1–7 (2020)
60. Huang, L., Shea, A.L., Qian, H., Masurkar, A., Deng, H., Liu, D.: Patient clustering improves efficiency of federated machine learning to predict mortality and hospital stay time using distributed electronic medical records. J. Biomed. Inf. **99**, 103291 (2019)
61. Lee, J., Sun, J., Wang, F., Wang, S., Jun, C.H., Jiang, X.: Privacy-preserving patient similarity learning in a federated environment: development and analysis. JMIR Med. Inf. **6**(2), e7744 (2018)
62. Brisimi, T.S., Chen, R., Mela, T., Olshevsky, A., Paschalidis, I.C., Shi, W.: Federated learning of predictive models from federated electronic health records. Int. J. Med. Inf. **112**, 59–67 (2018)
63. Sheller, M.J., Reina, G.A., Edwards, B., Martin, J., Bakas, S.: Multi-institutional deep learning modeling without sharing patient data: a feasibility study on brain tumor segmentation. In: Crimi, A., Bakas, S., Kuijf, H., Keyvan, F., Reyes, M., van Walsum, T. (eds.) BrainLes 2018. LNCS, vol. 11383, pp. 92–104. Springer, Cham (2019). https://doi.org/10.1007/978-3-030-11723-8_9
64. Farhad, A., Woolley, S., Andras, P.: Federated learning for AI to improve patient care using wearable and IoMT sensors. In: 2021 IEEE 9th International Conference on Healthcare Informatics (ICHI), pp. 434–434. IEEE (2021)
65. Li, W., et al.: Privacy-preserving federated brain tumour segmentation. In: Suk, H.-I., Liu, M., Yan, P., Lian, C. (eds.) MLMI 2019. LNCS, vol. 11861, pp. 133–141. Springer, Cham (2019). https://doi.org/10.1007/978-3-030-32692-0_16
66. Fang, L., et al.: Bayesian inference federated learning for heart rate prediction. In: Ye, J., O'Grady, M.J., Civitarese, G., Yordanova, K. (eds.) MobiHealth 2020. LNICST, vol. 362, pp. 116–130. Springer, Cham (2021). https://doi.org/10.1007/978-3-030-70569-5_8
67. Xiao, Z., Xu, X., Xing, H., Song, F., Wang, X., Zhao, B.: A federated learning system with enhanced feature extraction for human activity recognition. Knowl. Based Syst. **229**, 107338 (2021)
68. Xu, J., Glicksberg, B.S., Su, C., Walker, P., Bian, J., Wang, F.: Federated learning for healthcare informatics. J. Healthc. Inf. Res. **5**(1), 1–19 (2021). https://doi.org/10.1007/s41666-020-00082-4
69. Li, T., Sahu, A.K., Talwalkar, A., Smith, V.: Federated learning: challenges, methods, and future directions. IEEE Signal Process. Mag. **37**(3), 50–60 (2020)
70. Hao, M., et al.: Efficient and privacy-enhanced federated learning for industrial artificial intelligence. IEEE Trans. Industr. Inf. **16**(10), 6532–6542 (2019)
71. He, X., Su, X., Chen, Y., Hui, P.: Federated learning on wearable devices: demo abstract. In: Proceedings of the 18th Conference on Embedded Networked Sensor Systems, pp. 613–614 (2020)

72. Yang, Q., Liu, Y., Chen, T., Tong, Y.: Federated machine learning: concept and applications. ACM Trans. Intell. Syst. Technol. (TIST) **10**(2), 1–19 (2019)
73. McMahan, B., Moore, E., Ramage, D., Hampson, S., yArcas, B.A.: Communication-efficient learning of deep networks from decentralized data. In: Artificial intelligence and statistics, pp. 1273–1282. PMLR (2017)
74. Chen, Y., Qin, X., Wang, J., Yu, C., Gao, W.: Fedhealth: a federated transfer learning framework for wearable healthcare. IEEE Intell. Syst. **35**(4), 83–93 (2020)
75. Hakak, S., Ray, S., Khan, W.Z., Scheme, E.: A framework for edge-assisted healthcare data analytics using federated learning. In: 2020 IEEE International Conference on Big Data (Big Data), pp. 3423–3427. IEEE (2020)
76. Yi, X., Paulet, R., Bertino, E.: Homomorphic encryption. In: Homomorphic Encryption and Applications. SCS, pp. 27–46. Springer, Cham (2014). https://doi.org/10.1007/978-3-319-12229-8_2
77. El Makkaoui, K., Beni-Hssane, A., Ezzati, A.: Cloud-ElGamal and fast cloud-RSA homomorphic schemes for protecting data confidentiality in cloud computing. Int. J. Digit. Crime Forensics (IJDCF) **11**(3), 90–102 (2019)
78. Biksham, V., Vasumathi, D.: Homomorphic encryption techniques for securing data in cloud computing: a survey. Int. J. Comput. Appl. **975**, 8887 (2017)
79. Gentry, C.: A Fully Homomorphic Encryption Scheme. Stanford university, California (2009)
80. Sathya, S.S., Vepakomma, P., Raskar, R., Ramachandra, R., Bhattacharya, S.: A review of homomorphic encryption libraries for secure computation (2018). arXiv preprint http://arxiv.org/abs/1812.02428
81. Sun, X., Zhang, P., Sookhak, M., Yu, J., Xie, W.: Utilizing fully homomorphic encryption to implement secure medical computation in smart cities. Pers. Ubiquit. Comput. **21**(5), 831–839 (2017). https://doi.org/10.1007/s00779-017-1056-7
82. Farooqui, M., et al.: Improving mental healthcare using a human centered internet of things model and embedding homomorphic encryption scheme for cloud security. J. Comput. Theor. Nanosci. **16**(5–6), 1806–1812 (2019)
83. Wang, X., Zhang, Z.: Data division scheme based on homomorphic encryption in WSNs for health care. J. Med. Syst. **39**(12), 1–7 (2015). https://doi.org/10.1007/s10916-015-0340-1
84. Rohloff, K., Polyakov, Y.: An end-to-end security architecture to collect, process and share wearable medical device data. In: 2015 17th International Conference on E-health Networking, Application & Services (HealthCom), pp. 615–620. IEEE (2015)
85. Salim, M.M., Kim, I., Doniyor, U., Lee, C., Park, J.H.: Homomorphic encryption based privacy-preservation for IoMT. Appl. Sci. **11**(18), 8757 (2021)
86. Prasitsupparote, A., Watanabe, Y., Shikata, J.: Implementation and analysis of fully homomorphic encryption in wearable devices. In: The Fourth International Conference on Information Security and Digital Forensics. The Society of Digital Information and Wireless Communications, pp. 1–14 (2018)
87. David, R., et al.: TensorFlow lite micro: embedded machine learning for TinyML systems. Proc. Mach. Learn. Syst. **3**, 800–811 (2021)
88. Gorospe, J., Mulero, R., Arbelaitz, O., Muguerza, J., Antón, M.Á.: A generalization performance study using deep learning networks in embedded systems. Sensors **21**(4), 1031 (2021)
89. Han, S., Pool, J., Tran, J., Dally, W.J.: Learning both weights and connections for efficient neural networks (2015). arXiv preprint http://arxiv.org/abs1506.02626

90. Fyntanidou, B., et al.: IoT-based smart triage of Covid-19 suspicious cases in the Emergency Department. In: 2020 IEEE Globecom Workshops (GC Wkshps), pp. 1–6. IEEE (2020)
91. Sanchez-Iborra, R.: LPWAN and embedded machine learning as enablers for the next generation of wearable devices. Sensors **21**(15), 5218 (2021)
92. Yamanoor, S., Yamanoor, N.S.: Position paper: low-cost solutions for home-based healthcare. In: 2021 International Conference on Communication Systems & NETworkS (COMSNETS), pp. 709–714. IEEE (2021)
93. Padhi, P.K., Charrua-Santos, F.: 6G enabled tactile internet and cognitive internet of healthcare everything: towards a theoretical framework. Appl. Syst. Innov. **4**(3), 66 (2021)
94. Papernot, N., McDaniel, P., Sinha, A., Wellman, M.P.: SoK: security and privacy in machine learning. IEEE Eur. Symp. Secur. Priv. (EuroS&P) **2018**, 399–414 (2018). https://doi.org/10.1109/EuroSP.2018.00035
95. Yeom, S., Giacomelli, I., Fredrikson, M., Jha, S.: Privacy risk in machine learning: analyzing the connection to overfitting. In: 2018 IEEE 31st Computer Security Foundations Symposium (CSF), pp. 268–282 (2018). https://doi.org/10.1109/CSF.2018.00027

Medical, Communications, and Networking

A CNN-Based Computer Vision Interface for Prosthetics' Control

Emanuele Lindo Secco[1(✉)], Daniel David McHugh[1], and Neil Buckley[1,2]

[1] Robotics Laboratory, School of Mathematics, Computer Science and Engineering, Liverpool Hope University, L16 9JD Liverpool, UK
{seccoe,13005235,bucklen}@hope.ac.uk

[2] AI Laboratory, School of Mathematics, Computer Science and Engineering, Liverpool Hope University, L16 9JD Liverpool, UK

Abstract. In this paper we present a CNN-based Interface for the control of prosthetic and robotic hand: a CNN visual system is trained with a set of images of daily life object in order to classify and recognize them. Such a classification provides useful information for the configuration of prosthetic and robotic hand: following the training, in fact, a low cost embedded computer combined with a low cost camera on the device (i.e. a prosthetic or robotic hand) can drive the device in order to approach and grasp whatever object belong to the training set.

Keywords: Prosthetics · AI · CNN · Auto-grasping

1 Introduction

In today's world, there are more than 2.1 million people in the US alone that live with a prosthetic limb this number is expected to double by 2050 in recent studies the number of people each year that become an amputee in the US is 185,000. This results in around 300 to 500 amputations performed every day, with this many people becoming amputees the need for smarter and better prosthetics is a must as more people become amputees (Access Prosthetics, 2020).

One of the possible ways that prosthetics can become smarter is with the use of *Artificial Intelligence* (AI) this area in computer science is growing massively as the number of useful applications that stem of AI are endless. For example, most car industries now use robotics and AI to build cars as they are far quicker than humans and are more accurate this results in better produces for the business this is one of many uses that AI can offer. Another very important part of AI is the creation of intelligent machines that react and learn as humans do so when combined with prosthetics the idea of smart prosthetic that can move and think without the user having to interact with the device becomes a very real possibility.

This paper will highlight how AI and prosthetics could be used together to create smarter prosthetics that will help users interact with the real world better by improving these devices. Amputees could be given a better quality of life with the help of AI not only that, but with the help of AI the field of prosthetics could advance must quicker leading to better prosthetics devices for amputees.

X. Gao et al. (Eds.): MobiHealth 2021, LNICST 440, pp. 41–59, 2022.
https://doi.org/10.1007/978-3-031-06368-8_3

2 Materials and Methods

In this section of the paper, the techniques of controlling a prosthetic will be listed this will give information about what they are and how they are used in prosthetics then the two projects that the researcher has done will be explained in detail explaining what the project is and how it works.

2.1 Current Techniques for Controlling a Prosthetic

Prosthetics have been around for many years now and have changed many different times as our technology advances to become more precise and general smarter devices overall, the main aim for prosthetics is to mimic a real limb both in function and appearance so the user has the same freedom as a real limb would. One of the main advancements over the years within prosthetics is how the user can control a prosthetics. In this part of the paper, threepossible methods are discussed on how a prosthetics can be controlled.

1 – EMG- The first method that will be discussed is myoelectric prosthetics this has been used in prosthetics for many years now as it is one of the easiest and best ways to identify movement within the arm and translate it to the prosthetics limb. Myoelectric prosthetics are unique in the way they allow the user to control their limb as once the prosthetic is attached to the user it starts to detect and collect muscle and nerve activity from the body which then is translated to the limbs motors to perform the action that the user requires in a natural way that looks realistic and performs well. The way the prosthetic detects muscle and nerve activity from the body is a method know as *Electromyography* (EMG) this is when one or more small needles which are called electrodes are inserted into the arm and attached to the muscle.

When these electrodes detect electrical activity within the muscle, a wave is created on an oscilloscope (which is a monitor that displays electrical activity) from these waves the person can see if the user is moving their whole hand or just one finger by the number of waves on the screen. Also, these electrodes allow us to detect how intense this electrical activity is which tell us the amount of muscle contraction, which is happening.

One device that has been used for prosthetics that use's EMG is called MyoBand it was created by ThalmicLabs which is a band that is made from eight EMG sensors that when worn on the arm will start to read electrical activity this data then will be sent over Bluetooth to a dongle that will be inserted into another device like a computer that will read the transmitted data and perform the action that relates to what the user is doing with their arm. This device works just the same as one that would be attached to a prosthetic limb as proven by (McHugh, D. 2019). In which the MyoBand was connected to a prosthetics hand, and by detecting certain gestures using EMG, the prosthetic hand would move to different grasp types (Fig. 1).

2 – Computer Vision - The second method we want to focus on, is *Computer Vision* (CV): this is the method that most researchers are using to create smarter prosthetics this method has been used for many years now in different fields and given great results. An example would be most robotic arms in the manufacturing industry have computer vision as this allows them to see with the help from a camera and allows them to detect an object in their vision also they will be able to recognize different objects.

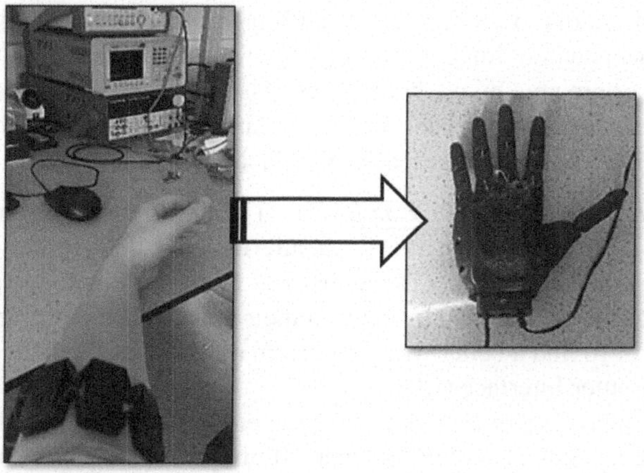

Fig. 1. The MyoBand connected to the open bionicsrobotic hand

As Computer Vision has been used for many years within robotics it's only natural that researchers would try to use it on prosthetics given the results when applied to robots, two main areas within computer vision that are being explored for prosthetics hands are object recognition/detection and gesture recognition. These are very important areas within prosthetics as by mastering these fields the ideal that smarter prosthetics could become more mainstream looks more realistic. Object recognition/detection is one of the main areas within prosthetics with the focus of giving prosthetic hands/arms the ability to see an object this should allow the hand/arm to be able to change into one of the set grasp types in order for the user to interact with the object more naturally and should result in faster response's times. When compared to a human this is the same with gesture recognition as well, but instead of using an object to get the hand/arm to perform the action the user will make a certain gesture that will tell the hand/arm to move in a certain way.

How this is done is using Artificial intelligence or AI to tell the hand that when certain object is in view it should perform this grasp type in order to interact with this object but a simple AI wouldn't be able to perform to the degree that is required for the hand to grasp an object properly, so certain methods within AI are used to make the AI perform better and allow it to handle complex tasks which increases its speed when compared to other methods. This method is called deep learning which use's artificial neural networks to be able to determent what the object is based on certain criteria for example; one network that could be used is a *Convolutional Neural Network* or CNN. This is one model that is used to automatically learn an object's features in order to identify that object this is done by feeding the model thousands of training images of different objects and getting the model to learn the different feature that makes certain objects different this is called feature extraction and is used in many different models.

For gesture recognition, the same model and the same methods can be used this is because feature extraction can work with any object like hands so it can be used for gestures as well. Some example work that other researchers have done can be seen here (Hu et al., 2018) and (Ghazaei et al., 2017). Another method that is used alongside feature extraction is edge detection this is an image processing technique for finding boundaries of objects within images this helps the feature extraction as it highlights that an object is in a certain area by the boundaries. Also, the model will be able to classify the object at the same time this is another important part of a deep learning model as it speeds up the process of correctly identifying objects.

3 – Brain Computer Interface (BCI or BMI) - The third method is one of the newest out of all three; it has been used mostly in the medical field to help with neuronal rehabilitation among other subjects in the medical field. But due to the potential of this topic, many researchers have tried to use it in their areas to solve problems that current technology can't or to find a better way to perform a solved problem, and this method is called Brain Computer Interface (BCI).

One of these fields is prosthetics as researchers believe that with BCI technology users will have better control of their prosthetic limb that is just as responsive as a human limb would be not only that but if this technology can be mastered then many people that have lost their function in one limb could be restored using a prosthetic. BCI works by acquiring electrical activities from the brain and nerves this step is very complex as the volume of signals that the brain fires off in a single second is unimaginable, so the task to read and understand what signals control muscle movement in the hand is very difficult. But with the help from AI, this task is possible to some degree this involves using deep learning with big data to gather vast amounts of data then trying to understand and classify what each signal means.

In one study the use of BCI and Myoelectric has been used together to create a system where the user could control the prosthetic by thought with the help of a MyoBand to collect the electrical signals (Hotson et al., 2016) not only this. But other researchers have tried to bring the sense of touch into prosthetics using BCI, which is on a different level compared to the other two methods (Kwok, 2013).

2.2 Convolutional Neural Networks (CNN)

It is important to understand how the CNN works to understand how the AI can detect and recognize each gesture as the CNN is the brain of the AI, to do these certain layers are used to extract the feature needed in order for the AI to make the right choice. Something to note with CNNs are they aren't all the same, some will have different steps, and some will have fewer steps it depends on how complex the CNN is, the database of images that were collected will be inputted into the CNN for training so the model can make a prediction when it sees the same gesture being performed by the user but that doesn't mean all images will be used for training some are used to test if the AI can correctly identify the gesture.

A simple overview of a CNN for classification could have this kind of architecture:

- *Input layer* - This will hold the pixel values of the images.
- *Convolution layer* - This will compute the output of neurons that are connected to the inputs, each computing the dot product of the inputs.
- *Pooling layer* - This will perform a down-sampling operation along the spatial dimensions.
- *Fully-connected layer* - This will compute the class scores, which provides the AI will the answer.

In this project each image has been pre-processed meaning the images have been turned into greyscale images so the pixel values have a range of 0 to 255 this means if you placed a pixel matrix over one of the images used you would be able to see its pixel values which help the AI understand what that pixel is. Another smaller matrix of numbers is created to perform convolution on the image, how convolution is done is by overlaying the smaller matrix over the image matrix and multiplying the numbers to create the dot of that value this will be saved into a new table called the convolved feature or feature map which is the most important information from that image that the AI will use later on.

Unlike with a normal CNN were each neuron is connected to all neurons, it would be better to use a method called Local Connectivity which connects each neuron to only a local region of input volume. The spatial extent of this connectivity is a hyper-parameter called the Receptive Field of neuron which is the size of the filter which is used by the CNN this is important to understand as the connectivity along the depth axis is always equal to the depth of the input volume it is also important to remember the asymmetry in spatial dimensions, e.g. (height and width) and the depth dimension.

An example of this could be that, suppose that the input has the sizes of [32 × 32 × 3], and the receptive field or filter size has a size of [5 × 5] then each neuron in the Conv layer should have a weight of [5 × 5 × 3] this totals into 75 weights and + 1 bias parameter also it's important the notice that the extent of the connectivity along the depth axis must be 3 since this is the depth of the input in this case.

To compute the spatial size of the output, a function can be performed which is the input size (*W*), the receptive field size/filter size (*F*), the stride which has been applied (*S*) and the amount of zero-padding that has been used (*P*). The formula below calculates how many neurons can fit

$$(W - F + 2P)/S + 1 \tag{1}$$

Parameter Sharing is a scheme to control the number of parameters in the neural network. By using this scheme the number of parameters used can be strongly reduced

$$W_2 = (W_1 - F + 2P)/S + 1 \tag{2}$$

where $H_2 = (H_1 - F + 2P)/S + 1$ and $D_2 = K$. Pooling layer this step is between the convolution layer and is used to reduce the dimensionality of the feature map as using higher dimensions can cause some issues as it confuses the CNN in later steps with the amount of noise, so to help the AI it's better to get rid of the dimensions without losing any important information in the process.

Max pooling is one of the methods used which uses a filter matrix of any size and a stride to down-sample every depth of the input through this method around 75% of the input will be down-sampled. The formula's for pooling layer holds:

$$W_2 = (W_1 - F)/S + 1 \tag{3}$$

where $H_2 = (H_1 - F)/S + 1$ and $D_2 = D_1$. The next step is the fully-connected layer this is when the neurons have full connections to all activations in the previous layer. These activations can be computed with a matrix multiplication which is followed by a bias offset.

2.3 Gesture Recognition

Gesture recognition is the ability for computers to capture and understand human gestures as commands and perform certain actions depending on the gestures an example could be a wave of the hand to start up the system, or it could be a peace sign to put the system to sleep. The amount of gestures a human can do is unlimited as a gesture is defined as any physical movement, which is non-verbal; gesture recognition has been around. For many years now and has become more popular as the potential use becomes more evident in today's world some of the most popular examples of gesture recognition would be the Wii, X-box Kinect and PlayStation Move.

In our first project gesture recognition was used in order to detect five different hand gestures from the user using a live camera feed and a keyboard input from the user, when the program starts it will only display the first screen which will be used to capture the gestures from the user, but in total three screens can be displayed at once. The first screen will be a live-feed of what the camera sees with the Region of Interest (ROI) being a blue square box this is important as the user must perform the gesture within that region in order for the AI to detect what gesture the user is performing. Otherwise, the AI won't work as it will only detect within that area this is because of the amount of resource it takes for the AI to work so the ROI will be half of the main screen size, but this can be changed to fit the whole screen if the user requires it to be.

The second screen is a real-time grey-scaled camera feed this is called the Binary thresholding screen this will activate when a certain key is pressed and can be used to save new gestures that the user can use to train the AI on. This gives the user an easy way to add new gestures as some of the pre-processing is done, but the main use of this screen is when the space bar is pressed it will give the user the prediction score and the predicted gesture the AI thinks the user has performed based on what gesture was seen on the first screen in the ROI. Finally, the third screen shows the contour matrix in real-time this shows the users how the AI sees the hand and how it can detect the different gestures (Fig. 2).

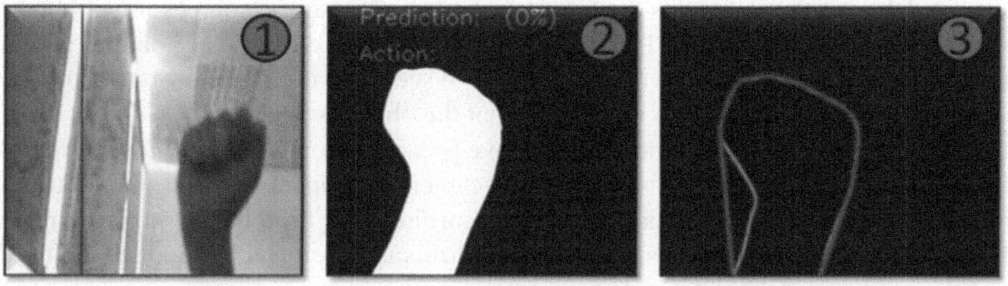

Fig. 2. Screenshots of the three stages of fist gesture recognition

Once the AI was able to predict the gesture, it would then send a character to the prosthetic hand which would then move the actuators into the correct position so that the prosthetic hand would be mimicking the user's gesture.

For this project to work three main technologies have been used these are OpenCV, Keras and TensorFlow each of these have been used to handle certain parts of the project and played an important role in the final version not only that but the model that was used is very important as it is the brain of the AI which allows it to predict the gesture the user has done.

The VGG-16 model works by sending the image through a stack of convolution layers then it uses a filter with a small receptive field normally the size is 3×3 which is the smallest size to capture all directions of the image. The convolution stride is fixed to 1 pixel the spatial padding of convolution layer input is such that the spatial resolution is preserved after convolution, i.e. the padding is 1-pixel for 3×3 convolution layer, spatial pooling is carried out by five max-pooling layers, which follow some of the convolution layers not all the convolution layers are followed by max-pooling. Max-pooling is performed over a 2×2 pixel window with stride 2.

2.4 Object Detection and Recognition

Object detection and recognition is one of the main topics when computer vision is brought up these two subjects have been used in many different applications from face recognition to live video detection normally these are used together as when used together an AI can see that an object is in view and it can understand what the object is. But they both perform very different job in object detection the AI will only be able to see if any object is present so it will highlight that an object is in view while object recognition will understand what that object is so it will tell you what the object is and normally give you a percentage score which will inform the user how accurate the AI thinks it is.

In the second project an AI was used to detect and recognise multiple objects this ranged from humans to household objects it uses a live-feed camera to detect and recognise any object in real-time that comes within view of the camera this was built using python and runs on *Jupyter notebook* which is an IDE that can be downloaded from Anaconda. When the program runs, it will start by loading up a screen, and this is what the camera can see which can be resized depending on what the user wants. In this project the screen was around half of the monitor, this was due to the amount of resources that were available on the system as the larger the screen, the more resources it would take to run the AI. When the screen is loaded, the user can then start to place objects within the view of the camera which will allow the AI to see if it can first detect that an object is present then see if the AI can recognize what the object is.

In this project, many different libraries have been used some of these are for support to help with images like Pillow or to handle the camera like OpenCV while other libraries are the main backbone of the project like TensorFlow and Protobuf. One of the main libraries that this project uses is called Protobuf this is developed by Google and used to configure the model and training parameter.

This project uses a special kind of model which is called You Only Look Once (YOLO) this is one of the newer models that has been used for object detection and has started to grow quite rapidly within the machine learning family. YOLO models are known for their speed as when compared to other models like R-CNN they often perform much faster which is one of the reasons why it was used in this project as speed is very important when you are using a real-time detection and recognition AI.

YOLO first works on splitting the input image into a grid of cells these cells are responsible for predicting the bounding box if the center of a bounding box falls within it, each cell will predict a bounding box and share its X, Y coordinate, height, width and confidence score also class prediction is based on each cell's information. While the image is being split into different bounding boxes multiply convolution layers, and max-pooling layers are processing the image to decide what the probability is that an object is inside each of the cells.

However not all bounding boxes would have an object within them if this is the case one of the jobs is to remove these bounding boxes as they can lead to producing bad results this is done based on the predicted confidence score of each cell that if the score is less than a certain threshold which is set to 0.24 then remove this cell as it should be redundant as it doesn't allow the AI to detect the object.

The first important loss function in the YOLO model is the confidence loss function this allows the model to measure the 'objectness' of each cell which will produce a value which is the confidence value for the whole boundary box. If an object is detected in the boundary box then this function will be used (Eq. 4), if no object is detected in the boundary box then this function will be used (Eq. 5).

$$\sum_{i=0}^{S2} \sum_{j=0}^{B} 1obj\ ij \left(Ci - \acute{C}i \right)^2 \tag{4}$$

where $\acute{C}i$ is the box confidence score of box j in cell i. When $obj\ ij = 1$ then the box j in cell i is responsible for detecting the object.

$$\lambda\ noobj \sum_{i=0}^{S2} \sum_{j=0}^{B} 1noobj\ ij \left(Ci - \acute{C}i \right)^2 \tag{5}$$

where $1noobj\ ij$ is the complement of $1obj\ ij$, $\acute{C}i$ is the box confidence score of box j in cell I and $\lambda\, noobj$ weights down the loss when detecting background. Another loss function in the YOLO model is the classification loss function this is used if an object has been detected; the classification loss at each cell is the squared error of the class conditional probabilities for each class (Eq. 6).

$$\sum_{i=0}^{S2} 1obj\ i \sum_{C_\varepsilon\ classes} \left(\mathrm{pi(C)} - \tilde{\mathrm{P}}\mathrm{i(C)}\right)^2 \tag{6}$$

where *1 obj i* = 1 if an object appears in cell *i*, otherwise 0 and $\widetilde{P}\, i(C)$ *denotes the conditional class probability for class C on cell i.* Finally, another loss function in the YOLO model is the localization loss which measures the errors in the boundary boxes location and sizes this function is only used when the boxes have objects within them (Eq. 7)

$$\begin{aligned} &\lambda\ coord \sum_{i=0}^{S2} \sum_{j=0}^{B} 1obj\ ij\left[(xi - Xi)^2 + (yi - Yi)^2\right] \\ &+ \lambda\ coord \sum_{i=0}^{S2} \sum_{j=0}^{B} 1obj\ ij\left[\left(\sqrt{wi} - \sqrt{Wi}\right)^2 + \left(\sqrt{hi} - \sqrt{Hi}\right)^2\right] \end{aligned} \tag{7}$$

where *1obj ij* = 1 then the box *j* in cell *i* is responsible for detecting the object and the *λ coord* increase the weight for the loss in the boundary box coordinates.

The last important function in the YOLO model is the loss function for an iteration of t which is an objective function that is a multi-part function that tells the model what to do if a bounding box doesn't have any objects within it. Its confidence of objectness needs to be reduced and shown as a first loss term this will tell the model that no object is present within this box as bounding boxes coordinate prediction need to align with prior information a loss term reducing the difference between prior and predicted is added for a few iterations. If a bounding box k is responsible for a truth box, the predictions need to be aligned with the truth values which are represented as the third loss term the **λ** values are the pre-defined weightages for each of the loss terms (Eq. 8).

$$\begin{aligned} losst = &\sum_{i=0}^{W} \sum_{j=0}^{H} \sum_{k=0}^{A} 1MaxIOU < Thresh\ \lambda noobj * (-boijk)^2 \\ &+ 1t < 12800\ \lambda prior * \sum r\varepsilon(x, y, w, h)(priorrk - brijk)^2 \\ &+ 1truthk\ (\lambda coord * \sum r\varepsilon(x, y, w, h)(truthr - brijk)^2 \\ &+ \lambda obj * (IOUktruth - boijk)^2 \\ &+ \lambda class * \left(\sum_{C=1}^{C} (truthc = bcijk)^2\right) \end{aligned} \tag{8}$$

To finalize the methodology section, both projects that have been successfully created for this paper and have been explained in great detail this includes a piece of brief information about the subject, details on how the project was created, some information about the issues faced while working on the project and finally technology used to create the project. In the next section of the paper, the results of the project will be displayed. This will include images of the projects working and a detailed explanation of each result.

3 Results

In this section of the paper, the results that have been collected from both projects will be displayed. This will demonstrate how projects have done and will show that both projects were able to work accurately.

3.1 Gesture Recognition

All of the five gestures used in this project will be displayed below this is to show how well each of the gestures is recognized by the AI after that a table will display the overall accuracy of the project for each of the gestures used in the project.

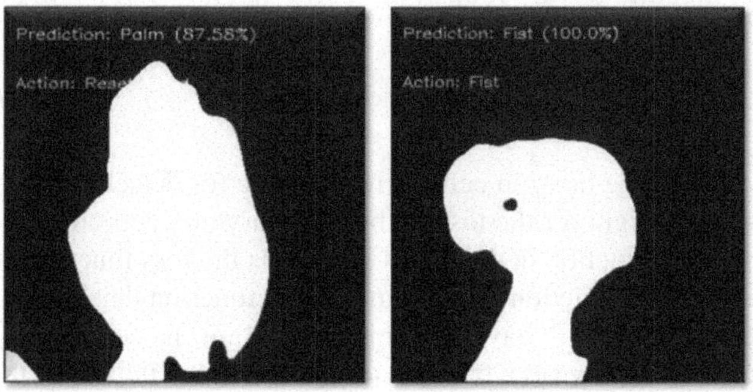

Fig. 3. On the left and right panels, the recognition of the palm and fist, respectively

As can be seen in Fig. 3 (left panel) this is the *palm gesture* that is included in the five gestures that were used in the project, as you can see when the test was performed the AI was able to correctly predict what gesture the used performed and give the researcher a very good prediction score. In this case the score was 87% which is really good this means that the AI is 87% sure that the gesture performed is the Palm gesture not only that, but the action that follows the gesture is working too as each gesture results in a different action taking place, in this case, the Palm gesture should result in the hand being reset. What this result has shown is the AI can understand what gesture the user is performing, which allows the correct action to be translated to the hand.

As can be observed in Fig. 3 (right panel) this is the *fist gesture* that is included in the five gestures that were used in the project, as you can see when the test was performed the AI was able to correctly predict what gesture the used performed and give the researcher a very good prediction score in this case the score was 100% which is great this means that the AI is 100% sure that the gesture performed is the Fist gesture. This result is unusual as getting 100% in prediction AI is not really common, if the AI is showing too many 100% it could indicate that the AI has some issues, or it could just be this one test that went really well, not only that but the action that follows the gesture is working too as each gesture results in a different action taking place, in this case, the Fist gesture should result in the hand being reset. What this result has shown is the AI can understand what gesture the user is performing, which allows the correct action to be translated to the hand.

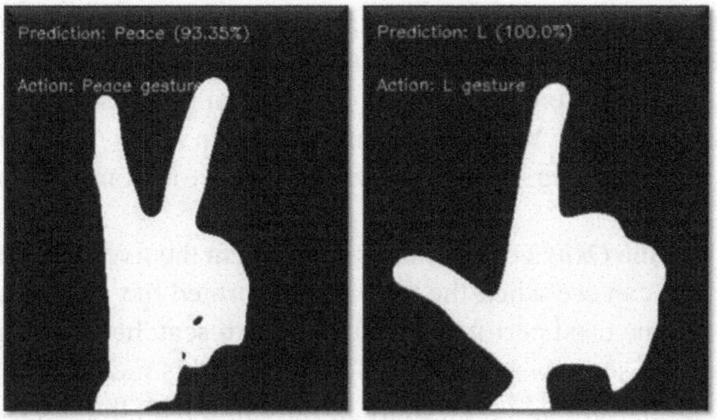

Fig. 4. On the left and right panels, the recognition of the peace gesture and L-shape gesture, respectively

In Fig. 4 (left panel) the *peace gesture* that is included in the five gestures that were used in the project, as you can see when the test was performed the AI was able to correctly predict what gesture the used performed and give the researcher a very good prediction score. In this case the score was 93% which is really good this means that the AI is 93% sure that the gesture performed is the Peace gesture not only that, but the action that follows the gesture is working too as each gesture results in a different action taking place, in this case, the Peace gesture should result in the hand being reset. What this result has shown is the AI can understand what gesture the user is performing, which allows the correct action to be translated to the hand.

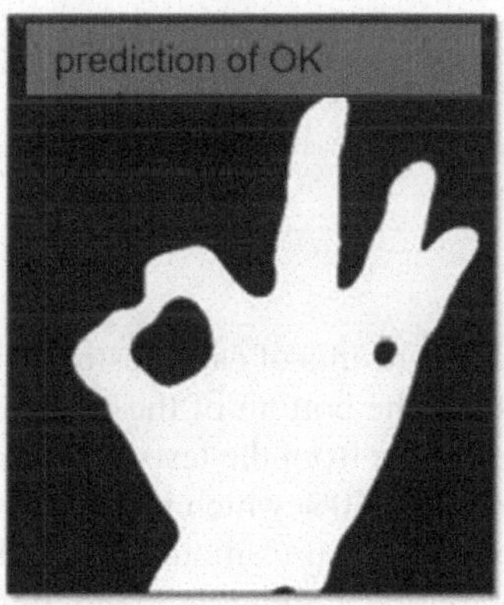

Fig. 5. Recognition of the okay gesture

Figure 4 (right panel) shows the L gesture that is included in the five gestures that were used in the project, as you can see when the test was performed the AI was able to correctly predict what gesture the used performed and give the researcher a very good prediction score. In this case, the score was 100% which is good this means that the AI is 100% sure that the gesture performed is the L gesture like with the fist gesture this could be a very good test result or something wrong with the AI more testing will confirm this to the researcher. Not only that but the action that follows the gesture is working too as each gesture results in a different action taking place in this case, the L gesture should result in the hand being reset. What this result has shown is the AI can understand what gesture the user is performing, which allows the correct action to be translated to the hand.

Figure 5 displays the *Okay gesture* that is included in the five gestures that were used in the project, as you can see when the test was performed the AI was able to correctly predict what gesture the used performed and give the researcher a very good prediction score. In this case, the score was 100% which is good this means that the AI is 100% sure that the gesture performed is the Okay gesture like with the fist gesture this could be a very good test result or something wrong with the AI more testing will confirm this to the researcher. Not only that but the action that follows the gesture is working too as each gesture results in a different action taking place in this case the Okay gesture should result in the hand being reset. What this result has shown is the AI can understand what gesture the user is performing, which allows the correct action to be translated to the hand.

Table 1. Accuracy of the five gestures' recognition [%]

Trial	Gesture 1 - Palm	Gesture 2 - Fist	Gesture 3 - Peace	Gesture 4 - L	Gesture 5- Okay
1	87	100	93	100	100
2	75	90	80	69	80
3	88	93	77	73	74
4	98	81	68	71	84
5	74	89	82	87	90
Average	84	92	80	80	86

Table 1 is a table that holds the results of each gesture that has been tested five times using our AI not only that, but at the bottom of the table, each gesture has been given an average score based on the results from the tests. All the results are quite good none of the prediction scores are less than 50% which is really good as a score which is 50% or lower tells us that the AI isn't really sure amount the prediction even if the prediction is correct, but our AI is often confident about the prediction which is why these scores are higher as the AI is confident about the result. Not only are the individually scores well the Average scores are good as well especially the Fist gesture which performed the best overall this could be because of how simple the gesture is compared to some of the others like the *Okay* and *L gesture*, or it could be that the training data was better.

Overall the gesture results have proven that the gesture recognition project was successful as the AI was able to understand what gesture the user had performed and was able to provide a good prediction score with the correct action for each of the gestures. The only part of the project that couldn't be tested was how well it would communicate with the robot hand, at the early stages of this project a robotic hand was used to see how communication could be done and the results were good the AI was able to send a letter when a certain gesture was performed and the hand would respond but this tested was done very early, and no evidence was recorded.

3.2 Objects Detection

As the number of objects that can be detected and recognized by this projects AI is many, it makes sense only to show a few objects to prove that the AI works for different objects to show that the AI works only five single objects will be shown and one multiple objects. Six results will be displayed each with an explanation about the result after that a table will show the accuracy of these five objects when tested multiple times.

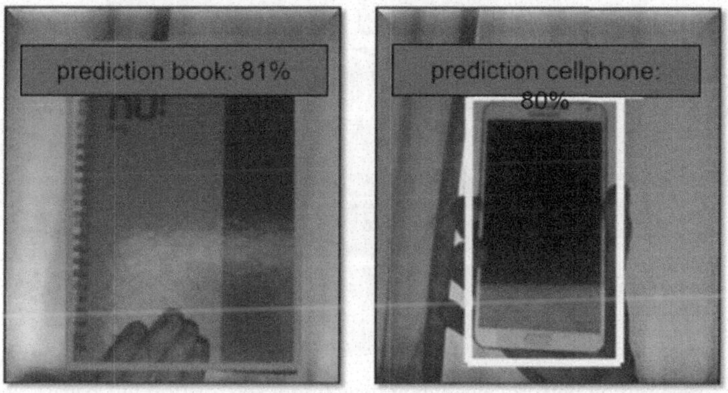

Fig. 6. Object recognition performance while detecting a book (left panel) and a mobile phone (right panel)

In Fig. 6 (left panel) which was the first object that was tested on the AI out of the five single objects as you can see from the image above the AI has been able to detect that an object is present and the AI has also been able to recognize what the object is correctly. This can be seen by the border that the AI creates around the object, in this result, the AI believes this object is a book with a confident score of 81% which is a very high score this tells the researcher that the AI is certain that this object is a book.

Figure 6 (right panel) is the second object that was tested on the AI out of the five single objects as you can see from the image above the AI has been able to detect that an object is present and the AI has also been able to recognise what the object is correctly. This can be seen by the border that the AI creates around the object, in this result, the AI believes this object is a phone with a confident score of 80% which is a very high score this result tells the researcher that the AI is certain that this object is a phone.

Figure 7 (top left panel) is the third object that was tested on the AI out of the five single objects as you can see from the image above the AI has been able to detect that an object is present and the AI has also been able to recognize what the object is correctly .

This can be seen by the border that the AI creates around the object, in this result the AI believes this object is scissors with a confident score of 69% which is still a good score not as good as the other two but still good enough for this object project this result tells the researcher that the AI is certain that this object is a pair of scissors.

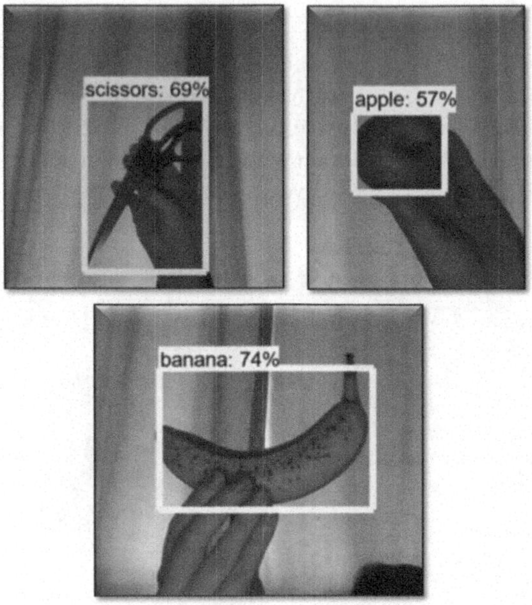

Fig. 7. Object recognition performance while detecting a scissor (top left panel), an apple (top right panel) and a banana (bottom panel)

As it can be noticed in Fig. 7 (top right panel), this was the fourth object that was tested on the AI out of the five single objects as you can see from the image above the AI has been able to detect that an object is present and the AI has also been able to recognize what the object is correctly. This can be seen by the border that the AI creates around the object, in this result the AI believes this object is an apple with a confident score of 57% which is still a good score not as good as the other two but still good enough for this object project as any score over 50% is useable this result tells the researcher that the AI is certain that this object is an apple.

As it can be observed in Fig. 7 (bottom panel), this was the 5th object that was tested on the AI out of the five single objects as you can see from the image above the AI has been able to detect that an object is present and the AI has also been able to recognise what the object is correctly. This can be seen by the border that the AI creates around the object, in this result the AI believes this object is a banana with a confident score of 74% which is a very good score not as good as the first and second objects but still good for this object project this result tells the researcher that the AI is certain that this object is a banana.

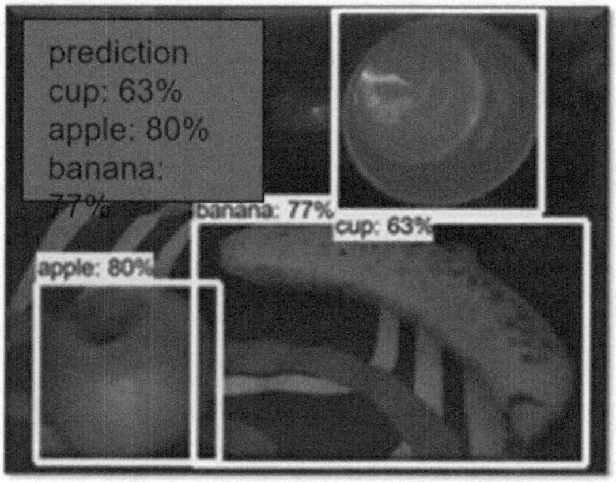

Fig. 8. Object recognition performance while detecting multiple objects

Figure 8 is the result from the multiple objects results that were taken from the AI project as you can see the AI has been able to detect that more than one object is present and has also been able to correctly recognize each of the objects that the AI can see. This can be seen by the borders that the AI creates around the objects, in this result, the AI believes that three objects are present which is an apple with an 80% confident score, banana with a 77% confident score and a cup with a 63% confident score. All these results are good scores as the AI has to work harder to understand the borders of each object and what each object is, this result tells the researcher that the AI can detect and recognize more than one object at one time.

Table 2. Accuracy of the object recognition, single object configuration [%]

Trial	Object 1 book	Object 2 phone	Object 3 scissors	Object 4 apple	Object 5 banana
1	81	80	69	57	74
2	85	95	79	66	69
3	78	82	61	73	59
4	95	72	81	86	86
5	73	77	83	69	74
Average	82	81	75	70	72

Table 2 holds the results of some of the single object which have been tested five times using our AI not only that but at the bottom of the table, each object has been given an average score based on the results from the tests. The individual scores of the objects are very good as these scores prove that the AI can accurately recognise these objects with the highest being 95% which is the phone and book object and the lowest being 57% which is the apple object. Not only are the individual scores good the average scores are very good as well this proves that the AI can understand what these objects are most of the time which is useful as it allows the researcher to know which object is easier for object recognition and which are harder.

Table 3. Accuracy of the object recognition, multiple objects configuration [%]

Test number	Book, phone & cup	Phone, apple & cup	Cup, banana & book	Apple, banana & cup	Banana, book & phone
1	72	80	84	67	70
2	68	78	76	70	88
3	69	72	60	86	81
4	91	58	79	88	63
5	70	85	68	73	87
Average	74	75	73	77	78

Table 3 holds the results of all of the multiply object that have been tested these objects have been tested five times using our AI not only that but at the bottom of the table, each object has been given an average score based on the results from the tests unlike the single objects test the individual scores here are an average of all three objects that performed in that group.

The individual scores of the multiply objects are very good as these scores prove that the AI can accurately recognize these objects with the highest being 91% which is the Book, Phone and Cup group and the lowest being 58% which is the Phone, Apple and Cup group. Not only are the individual scores good the average scores are very good as well this proves that the AI will understand what these objects are most of the time which is useful as it allows the researcher to know which object is easier for object recognition and which are harder.

By comparing Tables 2 and 3 together certain statements can be made about the AI, one of the statements that can be said is that this AI performs better at single object detection and recognition compared to multiply object detection and recognition this is shown by the average scores in both tables as in the single objects table the overall scores are higher. Which tells the researcher that single object has a higher chance of being detected and recognised by the AI not only that, but the individual scores are higher as well, which further supports this statement.

Overall the object detection and recognition project was a success it did everything that the researcher wanted it was able to detect most objects that were placed in front of the camera, and when it did detect an object, it was able to tell us what that object was with a good prediction score. The only part of the project that wasn't done was linking the AI to a robotic hand, but given that most of the work has already been done it wouldn't have been hard to write a program that could talk with the hand.

To finalize the result section, both projects have provided very good results that show how well each of the projects performed when tested this can be seen in the figures and the tables that are shown above also each of the results have been talked about in detail to explain what they mean and finally a brief overview of how the project went in terms of the results has been detailed. In the next section of the paper, the conclusion will be discussed this will summaries the projects and include the researcher's thoughts about the projects and discuss the future works of this project and the field itself.

4 Conclusion

In this section of the paper, the paper will be summarized this will include what the researcher's thoughts about the projects are also the future works of this project will be talked about plus the future works of this field will be discussed as well.

4.1 Summary

This paper set out to prove that with the help of AI, prosthetic devices could become smarter, leading to better ways that prosthetic limbs could interact with the real world. This was first shown with the gesture project by using an AI to detect and understand what each gesture did it allowed the researcher to control a robotic hand with ease this resulted in the robotic hand being able to switch to different grasp position which allowed the robotic hand to interact with different objects in the real world. The object project followed the same idea as the gesture project but used objects instead of hand gestures, using an AI to detect and recognize different objects which would then move a robotic hand so it could interact with that object in the real world.

Both projects have shown that the use of AI and prosthetics together are key in order to achieve smarter prosthetic as they far surpass any prosthetic device without AI assistants, that being said one of the main issues with AI-assisted devices at this time is how to implement the AI. Therefore it can talk with the device or how to implement the AI into the device itself as having a camera attached to the device isn't really suitable as the idea of a prosthetic is to mimic a real limb so having a visible camera closely would backfire of this idea, but other ways methods could be used in order to allow the AI to see and talk with the prosthetic limb.

The final thoughts about how the projects went now that the paper is finished are both projects did what the researcher wanted and fully prove what the paper set out to do while both projects presented certain issues while in development which is to be expected the researcher was able to overcome them and create two AI's that provide great results. Unfortunately, certain parts of the project couldn't be done due to the lack of equipment which the researcher required nevertheless both projects were still able to provide very good results this ended with the researcher feeling very satisfied with both projects.

4.2 Future Research

In terms of both projects, the next step would be to use the AI with a robotic hand to see how well both can talk to the robotic hand and to see what results can be collected from these tests this would include creating programs. So that the hand could understand the signals from the AI also another idea that could be implemented for the gesture project is having a multiple gesture recognition system like with the object project this way the user could perform two gestures at one time which could lead to more gestures being programmed into the hand. But other research that could be explored is the use of BCI with prosthetics this field is still quite new compared to the other fields as the use of thoughts to control anything is still out of our hands as researchers don't fully understand how to use thoughts to move complex objects like hands or arms, so this field is one of the most exciting for prosthetics as it opens many different doors which the other methods could not.

The possible applications from these projects are quite different as both are very different projects, from the gesture project if some UI could be created then one of the applications could be a smart home controller where one gesture could turn on the device while the other gestures control certain parameters of the device like volume, brightness, lock and unlock. Another application could be for medical use with a focus on rehabilitation as it could be used to collect data on how well the user can performing each hand gesture this would tell you if the user can perform the gesture and how well they can perform the gesture (see also Maereg et al., 2020; McHugh et al., 2020; Secco et al., 2020; Myers et al., 2021).

The performance of these systems clearly depends on the type of technology that is used vs the inter-subjects and intra-subject variability of the data: for example, in (Maereg et al., 2020) we showed that a hand gesture recognition system based on near-infrared sensing wristband allows an accuracy - over all the subjects involved in the study – of 98% with a std of 1.8%. However, such a system requires a proper training of the recognition system and a proper set-up of the sensors whose architecture involves a higher redundancy vs the proposed system in this paper.

Focusing on this CNN CNN-based Computer Vision Interface, it should be also mentioned the importance of considering the introduction of a set of features in the pre-processing of the data in order to improve the data organization and the structure of the information which are initially provided into the CNN (Buckley et al., 2021). Moreover, a proper further analysis of the Yolo drawbacks and of the advantages and disadvantages vs other techniques should be performed (Howard et al., 2022).

For the object project, many different applications could be used the first being robotics as many robots already use the same technology it could be easily integrated to work with a pick and place robot as the AI can already detect objects the only difference is some of the code would need to be changed. So, the AI knows what to do when it detects the objects. Another application could be tracking objects which could be used in surveillance so when an object comes within view of a security camera it could be able to detect what object is in front of the camera and be able to track where that object has moved this could be used on multiple cameras. So, the AI could track a person that is moving from one camera's view to another's camera view this could help identify where a person is going as the AI could highlight them making it easier to see where they are heading which could be used in police work.

Acknowledgements. This work was presented in thesis form in fulfilment of the requirements for the MSC in Robotic Engineering for the student Daniel David McHugh under the supervision of E.L. Secco from the Robotics Laboratory, School of Mathematics, Computer Science and Engineering, Liverpool Hope University.

References

McHugh, D.: Development of an interface between openbionics robotic hand and wearable Myo band. Liverpool, 1–21 (2019a)

McHugh, D.: Shows MyoBand connected to prosthetic hand (2019b). Accessed 1 July 2019

Ghazaei, G., Alameer, A., Degenaar, P., Morgan, G., Nazarpour, K.: Deep learning-based artificial vision for grasp classification in myoelectric hands. J. Neural Eng., **14**(3), 036025 (2017). Accessed 5 July 2019

Hotson, G., et al.: Individual finger control of a modular prosthetic limb using high-density electrocorticography in a human subject. J. Neural Eng. **13**(2), 026017 (2016)

Hu, Z., Hu, Y., Liu, J., Wu, B., Han, D., Kurfess, T.: 3D separable convolutional neural network for dynamic hand gesture recognition. Neurocomputing, **318**, 151–161 (2018). https://www.sciencedirect.com/science/article/pii/S0925231218309925. Accessed 5 July 2019

Maereg, A.T., Lou, Y., Secco, E.L., King, R.: Hand gesture recognition based on near-infrared sensing wristband. In: Proceedings of the 15th International Joint Conference on Computer Vision, Imaging and Computer Graphics Theory and Applications (VISIGRAPP 2020), pp. 110–117 (2020). ISBN: 978–989–758–402–2. https://doi.org/10.5220/0008909401100117

McHugh, D., Buckley, N., Secco, E.L.: A low cost visual sensor for gesture recognition via AI CNNS. In: Intelligent Systems Conference (IntelliSys), Amsterdam, The Netherlands (2020)

Secco, E.L., Scilio, J.: Development of a symbiotic GUI for robotic and prosthetic hand. In: Intelligent Systems Conference (IntelliSys), Amsterdam, The Netherlands (2020)

Myers, K., Secco, E.L.: A low-cost embedded computer vision system for the classification of recyclable objects. In: Sharma, H., Saraswat, M., Kumar, S., Bansal, J.C. (eds.) CIS 2020. LNDECT, vol. 61, pp. 11–30. Springer, Singapore (2021). https://doi.org/10.1007/978-981-33-4582-9_2

Access Prosthetics. 15 limb loss statistics that may surprise you - access prosthetics (2020). https://accessprosthetics.com/15-limb-loss-statistics-may-surprise/. Accessed 5 June 2019

Kwok, R.: Neuroprosthetics: once more, with feeling. Nature **497**(7448), 176–178 (2013)

Buckley, N., Sherrett, L., Secco, E.L.: A CNN sign language recognition system with single & double-handed gestures. In: IEEE 45th Annual Computers, Software, and Applications Conference (COMPSAC), pp. 1250–1253 (2021)

Howard, A.M., Secco, E.L.: A low-cost human-robot interface for the motion planning of robotic hands. In: Arai, K. (ed.) IntelliSys 2021. LNNS, vol. 296, pp. 450–464. Springer, Cham (2022). https://doi.org/10.1007/978-3-030-82199-9_30

A Deep Learning-Based Dessert Recognition System for Automated Dietary Assessment

Dimitrios-Marios Exarchou, Anastasios Alexiadis(✉), Andreas Triantafyllidis, Dimosthenis Ioannidis, Konstantinos Votis, and Dimitrios Tzovaras

Centre for Research and Technology Hellas, Information Technologies Institute (CERTH/ITI), 6km Charilaou -Thermi, Thessaloniki, Greece
{exarchou.dimitris,talex,atriand,djoannid,kvotis, Dimitrios.Tzovaras}@iti.gr

Abstract. Over the past few years, a significant part of scientific research has been focused on the assistance of patients who suffer from obesity or diabetes. Monitoring the food intake through self-report in diet control applications has been proven both time-consuming and non-practical and can be easily sidelined especially by children. In this paper, we propose the design and development of a novel system, which will assist obese or diabetic patients. We have implemented transfer learning as well as fine-tuning to different pre-trained CNN models to automatically distinguish dessert from non-dessert food images. For further training of these deep neural networks, a new dataset was constructed, which derived from the original Food-101 dataset. To be precise, 19 categories of desserts were used, which correspond to 19K images combined with 19K images of non-desserts. Google InceptionV3 architecture appeared to have the best performance, reaching a validation accuracy of 95.89%. To demonstrate feasibility of out platform and the independence of data biases, we constructed another data collection of food images, which was captured under challenging light and angle of capture conditions.

Keywords: CNN · Computer vision · Deep learning · Image recognition · Dessert recognition · Food Image · Image pre-processing · Diabetes · Obesity

1 Introduction

It is known that food intake is essential for the preservation of human life. The nutrients in food enable the cells in our bodies to perform their necessary functions. However, it is also proven to be an important risk factor for people who suffer from many common chronic non-communicable diseases such as obesity [1, 2], which comprises one alarming public health issue. In 2016, more than 1.9 billion adults and over 340 million adolescents were overweight according to the World Health Organization[1]. In recent years, junk food has become part of our everyday diet, especially for children [3–5].

[1] https://www.who.int/.

X. Gao et al. (Eds.): MobiHealth 2021, LNICST 440, pp. 60–70, 2022.
https://doi.org/10.1007/978-3-031-06368-8_4

Multimedia and commercial stimuli have led many young people to consume unhealthy edible products, unaware of their poor nutritional value. Serious life-threatening diseases, such as childhood obesity and diabetes emerge mainly in western countries, due to improper diet habits.

To address this situation, the nutrition industry supplied several diet plan proposals. At the same time, diet tracking applications have been developed, employing large databases of food images and their respective nutritional values. Initially, this issue was confronted by the development of applications for manual food logging and user's self-reports, which demonstrated warnings and dietary plans [6].

Nevertheless, those recording systems were often used incorrectly by the patients since they relied on manual input. They were prone to recall bias issues and could mislead, resulting in the exacerbation of patients' medical conditions. In addition, because of their complex usage, they were often easily sidelined. More specifically, children and adolescents face difficulties in self-reporting food intakes due to issues related to recall or monotonous text reporting.

This work aims to the implementation of a new technology, which will automatically identify foods containing sugar. The feasibility of these research efforts should assist in the maintenance of a healthier lifestyle by encouraging healthy food consumption at an early age. In contrast with previous research, this work probes the performance of an automated dessert recognition system under challenging image acquisition conditions.

2 Related Work

When focusing on this area, there are limitations and challenges to consider, such as the negligible intra-class differences within the food images. Data collections were soon created, playing the role of benchmarks. Food-5 K on the one hand and Food-11 on the other were used to solve the binary and the multiclass problem respectively. The preliminary approach employed hand-crafted features and the extraction of feature descriptors, such as SIFT, SURF, BRIEF, etc. [7]. However, this traditional method was outperformed by newer technological developments, such as deep learning techniques. The extraction of features is now performed by CNNs, which convolve the input image with specific kernels (also known as filters). Those visual features are reflected in the activation of internal neurons' layers. While the layers on the input side correspond to more syntactic information, the layers closer to the output convey more semantic information [8]. The two methods are illustrated in Fig. 1.

Bossard et al., [9] introduced a publicly available food image dataset, Food-101[2], with 101 food categories. They also examined a weakly supervised method to mine discriminative components with Random Forests, reaching an accuracy of 50.76%. More recently, Şengür et al. examined a feature concatenation method [10], employing the last two fully connected layers of AlexNet and VGG-16. The reported accuracy on the binary problem was 99%, while on the Food-101 challenge they achieved 79.86%. Attokaren et al. [11] leveraged the pretrained Google InceptionV3 model in combination with a multi-crop evaluation technique and obtained 86.97% accuracy. Apart from the

[2] https://data.vision.ee.ethz.ch/cvl/datasets_extra/food-101/.

general food recognition problem, the scientific community focused on the detection of unhealthy eating habits. Aiming to strengthen the motivation of children to adopt healthy diet habits, a recent work [12] proposed a social robot-based platform, based on camera images that are automatically captured by a commercially available social robot. The measured validation accuracy in a dataset of 53884 images was 99.68%.

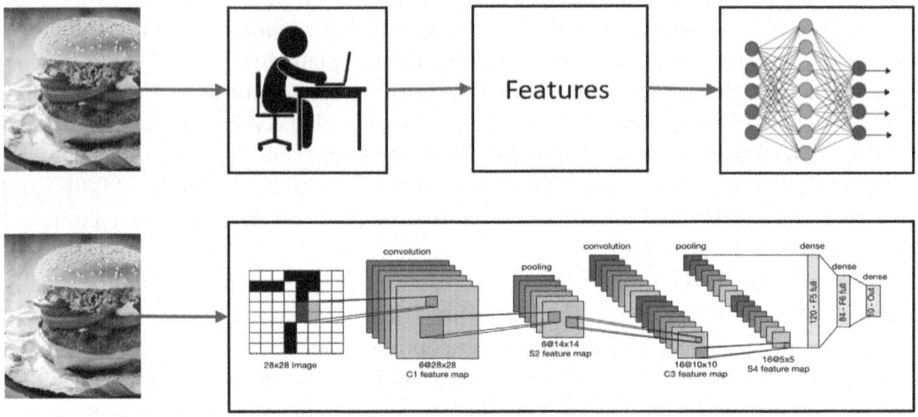

Fig. 1. (a) Traditional computer vision vs (b) Deep learning technique.

In this paper, we present the design and deployment of a dessert recognition system. The outcomes of this research are intended to contribute to the development of an end-to-end diet suggestion assistant that will address the threatening issue of childhood obesity. The structure of the paper is as follows; in the next section, we introduce the proposed methodology. Section 4 demonstrates the results and feasibility of our method. Finally, we discuss the conclusions in Sect. 5.

3 Proposed Method

In this section, we present the proposed workflow for system development. We describe our methods for dataset construction, data augmentation, transfer learning and the training process.

3.1 Dataset Construction

To the best of our knowledge, there is no previous research on the topic of automatic dessert recognition. Thus, the initial challenge was to create a dessert dataset. We gathered food images from the Food-101 dataset. Specifically, 19 categories (apple pie, baklava, beignets, carrot cake, cheesecake, chocolate cake, chocolate mousse, churros, crème brulee, cupcakes, donuts, frozen yogurt, ice cream, macarons, panna cotta, red velvet cake, strawberry shortcake, tiramisu and waffles) provided us with 19k images of desserts, while the remaining 82 categories were used to randomly sample without replacement 19k images of non-dessert images. The workflow described above resulted in a dataset of 38k images and was subsequently split into training, validation and testing partitions. 80% of the dataset was used for the training set, while validation and testing sets corresponded to the 15% and 5% of the dataset, respectively. Some samples are illustrated in Fig. 2.

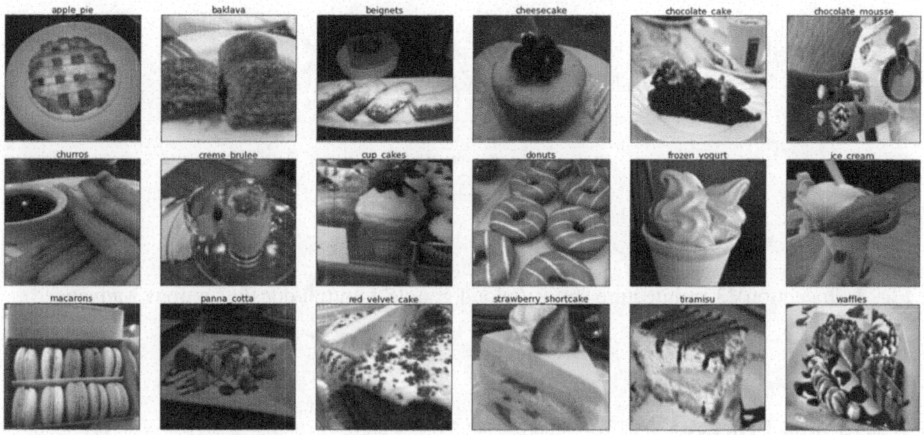

Fig. 2. Dessert images of desserts from 19 categories

3.2 Data Augmentation

To enrich the training samples and enhance the generalizability of the system, a data augmentation process was implemented. Hence, we used *torchvision*'s transforms to randomly flip the input image horizontally and vertically, to rotate it in a random angle from 0 to 45° and to adjust the color jitter. For the classification of unknown images, we used a multi-crop (10-crop) strategy, which produced 10 crops for each image (upper left, upper right, lower right, lower left, centre and their flipped versions). The images were finally normalized, according to the *ImageNet* standards.

3.3 Transfer Learning

The proposed method is based on the fine-tuning of deep pre-trained CNNs. In this paper we compare four different prestigious architectures: Google InceptionV3 [13], Resnet101 [14], VGG16 [15] and MobileNet [16] to address the problem of binary classification. The InceptionV3's architecture is shown in Fig. 3. For the implementation of the method, both *Tensorflow* and *PyTorch* frameworks were used. The output of the models was modified to the following sequential layers:

- Average Pooling 2D with output size = (1,1)
- Dropout (with different probability depending on the different architectures)

- Linear layer with 1 node, L2 regularization = 0.0005, sigmoid activation function and Xavier uniform initializer [17].

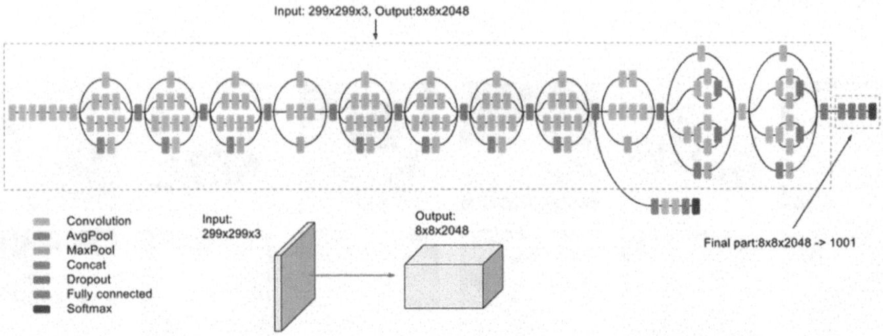

Fig. 3. InceptionV3 architecture (https://cloud.google.com/tpu/docs/inceptionv3-advanced)

3.4 Training Process

Three different strategies were considered for the fine tuning of the models described above. Firstly, the layers of the models were immediately unfrozen, while on the second case we examined a more gradual learning. Specifically, the second method included an initial training of the classifier layer, followed by the training of the entire model. Nonetheless, the impact of the interpolation of an intermediate training stage on a part of the total model's parameters was also investigated.

The optimization algorithm used was the Stochastic Gradient Descent, which is an optimizer with a good performance over large data-sets. The loss function used across all models was binary cross entropy:

$$J(w) = -\frac{1}{N}\sum\nolimits_{n=1}^{N}\left[y_n \log \hat{y}_n + (1 - y_n)\log\left(1 - \hat{y}_n\right)\right] \quad (1)$$

The hyperparameters used in each training scenario were generally different; however, the initial learning rate was 0.008 and after a certain number of epochs it was decreased by half for each training stage. The momentum was set to 0.9. The hyperparameters of the InceptionV3 model, which achieved the highest accuracy in our evaluation set, are the following:

- Initial learning rate = 0.008
- Momentum = 0.9
- Decreasing learning rate by half every 10 epochs.
- Trained to binary cross-entropy loss 0.0910 after 27 epochs.

4 Results

This section describes and compares different results found in our experiments. The obtained results for various models on the original Food-101 dataset are tabulated in Table 1. To generalize our conclusions, we examine the effectiveness of our system for manually captured images in Table 2.

4.1 Food-101 Evaluation

Our system development utilized *Tensorflow* and *PyTorch*, two open-source machine learning platforms. The training process was executed on Google Colaboratory[3], leveraging 12 GB of RAM and an NVIDIA Tesla K80. Different deep learning architectures and training strategies were simulated. The three different strategies described above are indicated as *unfrozen (1 stage)*, *2 stages* and *3 stages*. Classification accuracy and binary cross entropy loss were used as evaluation metrics and they are illustrated in the following table:

Table 1. Training metrics

Model	*Stages*	*Dropout*	*Train Loss*	*Val. Loss*	*Train Acc.*	*Val. Acc.*
InceptionV3	*unfrozen*	*0.5*	*0.0910*	*0.1164*	*96.30%*	*95.89%*
InceptionV3	*3 stages*	*0.5*	*0.0777*	*0.1230*	*96.83%*	*96.16%*
InceptionV3	*2 stages*	*0.75*	*0.0733*	*0.1616*	*97.12%*	*95.46%*
ResNet101	*unfrozen*	*0.6*	*0.1451*	*0.1269*	*93.99%*	*95.68%*
ResNet101	*2 stages*	*0.75*	*0.0776*	*0.2379*	*96.91%*	*94.12%*
VGG16	*unfrozen*	*0.5*	*0.4383*	*0.3475*	*79.10%*	*85.77%*
MobileNet	*unfrozen*	*0.2*	*0.1097*	*0.1309*	*95.63%*	*95.42%*

For a more detailed interpretation of the results, we extracted the confusion matrices and the ROC curves for the validation and training sets of the aforementioned dataset. As has already been discussed, we employed a voting ten-crop strategy to achieve a higher evaluation performance. The measured accuracies were 95.89% and 95.79%, for the validation and the test set, respectively. Those evaluation metrics for the unfrozen InceptionV3 model can be seen in Fig. 4 and Fig. 5.

[3] https://colab.research.google.com/notebooks/intro.ipynb?utm_source=scs-index.

4.2 Real Conditions Evaluation

To evaluate the performance of our model in real food image captures, with challenging light conditions and capture angle, we also created a data collection of 214 real-conditions images. Some examples are depicted in Fig. 6. To evaluate the real-conditions performance, we examined the ten-crop strategy in comparison with the simple prediction method. The highest classification accuracy was obtained for the InceptionV3 unfrozen trained model, while ResNet101 performed also up to the mark. The performances of the different architectures are shown in Table 2. Some examples of predictions are illustrated in Fig. 7.

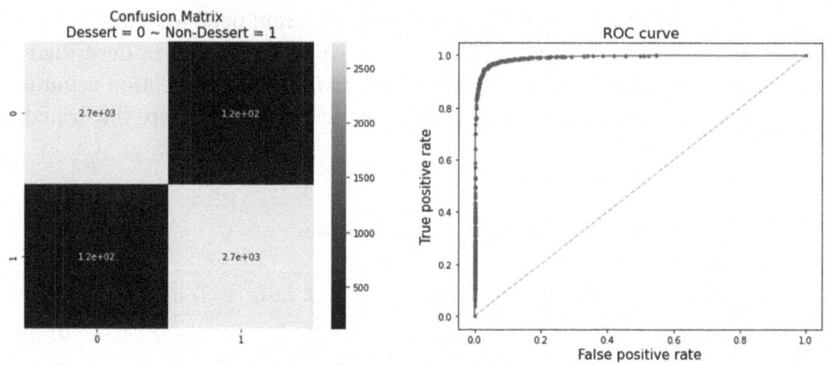

Fig. 4. Confusion matrix and ROC curve for the validation set

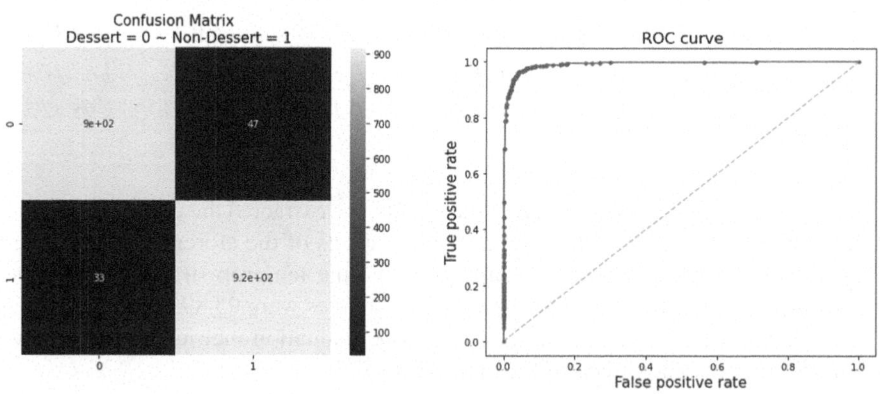

Fig. 5. Confusion matrix and ROC curve for the test set

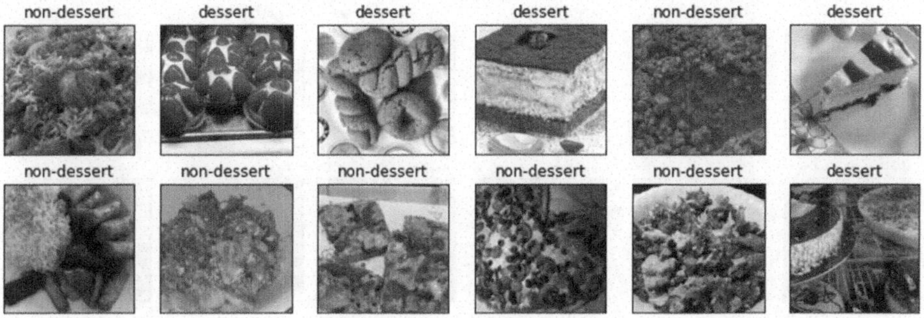

Fig. 6. Real captures examples

Table 2. Real-conditions captures performance

Model	*Training*	*Evaluation Acc. without ten-crop*	*Evaluation Acc. with ten-crop*
InceptionV3	*unfrozen*	*94.86%*	*95.79%*
InceptionV3	*3 stages*	*89.25%*	*92.52%*
ResNet101	*unfrozen*	*89.25%*	*92.99%*
VGG16	*unfrozen*	*85.05%*	*82.24%*
MobileNet	*unfrozen*	*90.65%*	*89.25%*

4.3 Computational Complexity

In the real scene, such systems are usually deployed on mobile devices, which have limited storage and battery capacity. Thus, computational complexity is as important as accuracy of recognition. Computational complexity depends on both the total number of parameters and the prediction time. The prediction time of an image includes the time of image transformation, as well as the time of forward propagation in the model. These metrics for the various models are shown in Figs. 8 and 9, respectively. The lightest and fastest model is MobileNet, while the slowest and most complex is VGG16. In our analysis we chose InceptionV3. This model is twice as slow as MobileNet and requires five times more space to store. Therefore, in applications that require speed or low memory consumption MobileNet could be selected.

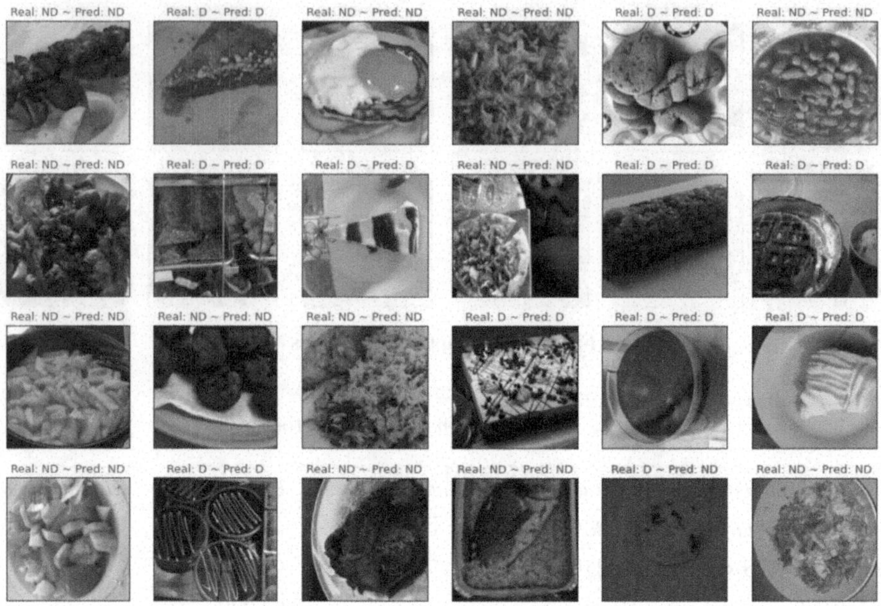

Fig. 7. Real captures predictions

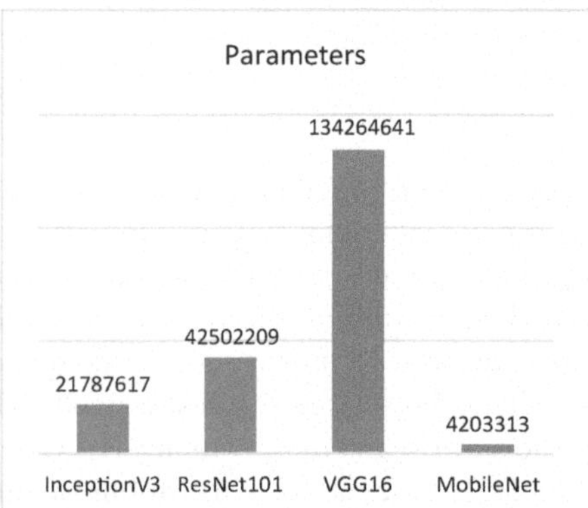

Fig. 8. Parameters of models

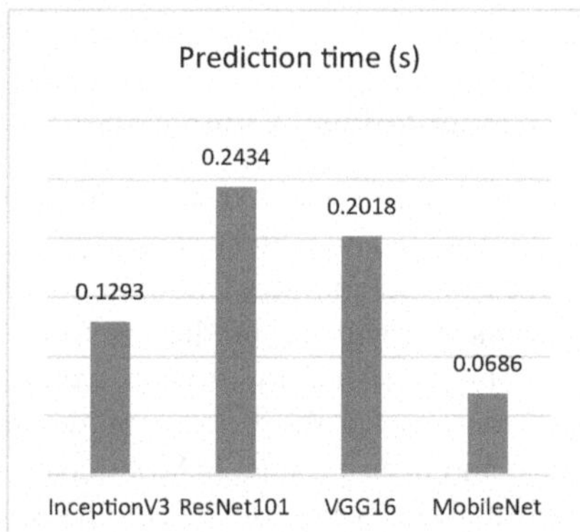

Fig. 9. Prediction time of models

5 Discussion

In the past decade the interest of the scientific community in computer vision was ignited by the challenging task of food recognition. As machine learning approaches require a large range of data, popular large datasets for food classification were presented and the necessity for even richer datasets with specific attributes was emphasized. In this paper, we aimed to solve the urgent problem of recognizing foods containing sugar by leveraging deep learning techniques. We presented the design of a system for automated diet tracking, which was relied on pretrained CNNs. Our model constitutes an autonomous computer vision system aimed at the dietary assessment of obese or diabetic patients. Our objective was to create a system that can be used requiring minimal user interactions, so that it can be used independently from the user's technological literacy.

For the fine tuning of our model, we introduced a new data collection which derived from the original Food-101 dataset. This data collection was split into training, validation and testing sets and the reported evaluation accuracy was 95.89% and 95.79% for the validation and test set, respectively. To demonstrate the adequacy of our system we measured its performance in real conditions. Upon examining the results of the experiments, it is worth mentioning that only InceptionV3 that followed the unfrozen training strategy, managed to cope with this difficult challenge. This shows that with proper training data there are no limitations on the conditions under which a photograph is captured. However, there are restrictions on the identification of types of foods, with which the model has not previously interacted during the training phase.

Future work would involve some optimization on hyperparameters and model components such as which layers to freeze during transfer learning. Due to limited computing resources and time constraints, the choice of the model architecture was made empirically with respect to the measured performance. Nonetheless, a grid-search for the optimization of hyper parameters search would have been more efficient. Furthermore, we contemplate reinforcing the capabilities of our system to recognize different food categories. An automatic calories estimator would provide a crucial assistance in the fight against obesity. Finally, the usability of the system will significantly improve if we integrate it into mobile devices, creating an Android application.

In conclusion, with this work we laid the foundations for the creation of more specific datasets around food and the nutritional value of the individual ingredients. The scope of this research includes the mobilization of technological advances in the direction of combating the scourge of the unhealthy diet. For this reason, the work presented in this paper is a step towards engagement with healthy dietary habits.

Acknowledgments. This project has received funding from the European Union's Horizon 2020 research and innovation programme under grant agreement «GATEKEEPER/857223 Smart Living Homes – Whole Interventions Demonstrator for People at Health and Social Risks» (KOH.021064).

References

1. Shields, M., Tremblay, M.S., Connor Gerber, S., Janssen, I.: Abdominal obesity and cardiovascular disease risk factors within body mass index categories. Heal. Rep. **23**(2), 7–15 (2012)
2. Vucetic, I., Stains, J.P.: Obesity and cancer risk: evidence, mechanisms, and recommendations. Ann. N. Y. Acad. Sci. **1271**(1), 37–43 (2012). https://doi.org/10.1111/j.1749-6632.2012.06750.x
3. Tate, E.B., et al.: mHealth approaches to child obesity prevention: successes, unique challenges, and next directions. Transl. Behav. Med. **3**(4), 406–415 (2013). https://doi.org/10.1007/s13142-013-0222-3
4. Smith, A.J., Skow, A., Bodurtha, J., Kinra, S.: Health information technology in screening and treatment of child obesity: a systematic review. Pediatrics **131**(3), e894–e902 (2013). https://doi.org/10.1542/peds.2012-2011

5. Lau, P.W.C., Lau, E.Y., Wong, D.P., Ransdell, L.: A systematic review of information and communication technology–based interventions for promoting physical activity behavior change in children and adolescents. J. Med. Internet Res. **13**(3), e1533 (2011). https://doi.org/10.2196/jmir.1533
6. Abril, E.P.: Tracking myself: assessing the contribution of mobile technologies for self-trackers of weight, diet, or exercise. J. Health Commun. **21**(6), 638–646 (2016). https://doi.org/10.1080/10810730.2016.1153756
7. O'Mahony, N., et al.: Deep learning vs. Traditional computer vision. In: Arai, K., Kapoor, S. (eds.) Advances in Computer Vision: Proceedings of the 2019 Computer Vision Conference (CVC), Volume 1, pp. 128–144. Springer International Publishing, Cham (2020). https://doi.org/10.1007/978-3-030-17795-9_10
8. Amato, G., Bolettieri, P., de Lira, V.M., Muntean, C.I., Perego, R., Renso, C.: Social media image recognition for food trend analysis. In: SIGIR 2017 Proceedings of the 40th International ACM SIGIR Conference on Research and Development in Information Retrieval (2017)
9. Bossard, L., Guillaumin, M., Van Gool, L.: Food 101 - mining discriminative components with random forests. In: Fleet, D., Pajdla, T., Schiele, B., Tuytelaars, T. (eds) Computer Vision - ECCV 2014. ECCV 2014 Lecture Notes in Computer Science, vol 8694. Springer, Cham, pp 446–461 (2014). https://doi.org/10.1007/978-3-319-10599-4_29
10. Şengür, A. Akbulut, Y. Budakm, Ü.: Food image classification with deep features. In: 2019 International Artificial Intelligence and Data Processing Symposium (IDAP)
11. Attokaren, D., Fernandes, I., Sriram, A., Murthy, Y.V., Koolagudi, S.: Food classification from images using convolutional neural networks. In: Proceeding of the 2017 IEEE Region 10 Conference (TENCON), Malaysia, 5–8 Nov 2017
12. Alexiadis, A., Triantafyllidis, A., Elmas, D., Gerovasilis, G., Votis, K., Tzovaras, D.: A social robot-based platform towards automated diet tracking. In: Proceedings of the Federated Conference on Computer Science and Information Systems, pp. 11–14 (2020)
13. Szegedy, C., Vanhoucke, V., Ioffe, S., Shlens, J., Wojna, Z.: Rethinking the inception architecture for computer vision. In: 2016 IEEE Conference on Computer Vision and Pattern Recognition (CVPR), Las Vegas, pp. 2818–2826 (2016) https://doi.org/10.1109/CVPR.2016.308
14. He, K., Zhang, X., Ren, S., Sun, J.: Deep residual learning for image recognition. IEEE Conf. CVPR **2016**, 770–778 (2016)
15. Simonyan, K., Zisserman, A.: Very deep convolutional networks for large-scale image recognition. In: Published as a Conference Paper at ICLR (2015)
16. Howard, A.G.: MobileNets: efficient convolutional neural networks for mobile vision applications (2017). https://arxiv.org/abs/1704.04861
17. Glorot, X., Bengio, Y.: Understanding the difficulty of training deep feedforward neural networks. J. Mach. Learn. Res. Proc. Track. **9**, 249–256 (2010)

Detection of Epilepsy Seizures Based on Deep Learning with Attention Mechanism

Tuan Nguyen Gia(✉), Ziyu Wang, and Tomi Westerlund

Department of Computing, University of Turku, Turku, Finland
{tunggi,tovewe}@utu.fi

Abstract. Epilepsy cannot be underestimated as it can negatively impact every one of all ages and reduce the quality of life. Epilepsy can lead to sudden tumble and loss of awareness or consciousness, disturbances of movements. Fortunately, epilepsy seizures can be controlled if epilepsy is detected and treated properly. One of the widely used methods for detecting and diagnosing epilepsy is monitoring and analyzing electroencephalogram (EEG) signals. However, the traditional methods of monitoring and analyzing EEG have some challenges such as high costs, requirements of experienced medical experts, non-scalability, or non-support real-time and long-term monitoring. Therefore, in this paper, we present an advanced deep learning neural network approach for the automatic detection of epilepsy seizures. The proposed approach with a customized attention mechanism can be used for a single EEG channel. We evaluate the approach with the Bonn dataset and the CHB-MIT dataset and achieved higher than 98% accuracy, 99% sensitivity, and 98% specificity for a single EEG channel in most of the cases. The results show that the proposed approach is a potential candidate for enhancing automatic epileptic seizure detection systems.

Keywords: Epilepsy · Seizure · Deep learning · Attention mechanism · EEG

1 Introduction

Epilepsy which is a non-communicable neurological disease, is a central nervous system disorder. The brain activity of a person with epilepsy can become abnormal, causing seizures or uncommon physical behaviours [1]. Epilepsy can occur and affect anyone regardless of ages, genders, and human races [1,2]. Although epilepsy is not a contagious disease, epilepsy cannot be underestimated [2,3]. Epilepsy can lead to sudden tumble and loss of awareness or consciousness, disturbances of movements [3]. People with epilepsy have a three-time higher risk of premature death than normal healthy people [3]. For instance, an epilepsy seizure occurring at a certain time can lead to serious consequences such as sudden falling, drowning, and car accidents [1].

X. Gao et al. (Eds.): MobiHealth 2021, LNICST 440, pp. 71–84, 2022.
https://doi.org/10.1007/978-3-031-06368-8_5

Epilepsy can be categorized into sudden and long-term recurrent epilepsy. Sudden epilepsy means that a patient will have seizures unexpectedly in a random interval whilst seizures of recurrent epilepsy occur repeatedly. Therefore, it is more difficult to deal with or diagnose sudden epilepsy than long-term recurrent epilepsy. Both epilepsy types can negatively impact a patient's quality of life. In clinical, epileptic seizures can be categorized into three types including focal onset, generalized onset, and unknown onset depending on the location where the epileptic seizures are activated. Particularly, focal seizures occur on a certain location of a brain and mainly affect one cerebral hemisphere whilst generalized seizures begin in both halves (hemispheres) of the brain at the same time [4]. The unknown onset seizures are the special type in which the beginning of a seizure is unknown. The unknown onset seizures often occur at night and later might be diagnosed as a focal or generalized seizure [5].

Fortunately, epilepsy seizures can be controlled if epilepsy is detected, diagnosed, and treated properly. For instance, it is estimated that more than 70% of the people having epilepsy could avoid seizures if they have used anti-seizure medicines [3]. Currently, the two most common predictors of seizures recurrence are a documented etiology of the seizure and an abnormal electroencephalography [3]. A documented etiology of seizure mainly relies on the medical history collections that have many drawbacks including unreported and missed cases. The method of using Electroencephalogram (EEG) signals seems to be more appropriate as it can overcome the existing limitations of the documented etiology.

Many approaches have been proposed for the automatic detection of epileptic seizures. Among these approaches, systems based on machine learning are widely used as these systems can help achieve a high accuracy level of seizure detection. [6–10]. However, it is still required to have more advanced approaches that can help improve the accuracy of automatic detection of epileptic seizures. Therefore, to achieve the target, this paper proposes an effective and versatile neural network approach based on a customized attention mechanism. The approach uses a single-channel EEG for detecting epilepsy seizures and is evaluated with the Bonn dataset [11] and the CHB-MIT dataset [12] that are open-source and widely used datasets.

The rest of the paper is organized as follows: Sect. 2 reviews the related work. Section 3 introduces the methodology applied in the proposed approach. Section 4 discusses the experimental results and performance evaluation. Section 5 concludes this work and discusses the future work.

2 Related Work

Different approaches are proposed for the automatic detection of epileptic seizures. Many of them have applied traditional machine learning algorithms. For instance, Bajaj *et al.* [13] proposed a EEG classification method based on empirical mode decomposition. The method utilized Hilbert-Huang transform and least squares support vector machine for the seizure classification and its results reach an accuracy of 97.82%. Xie *et al.* [14] introduced a method using a sparse functional linear model based on wavelet to extract EEG features. Then, the authors applied a simple neural network model for classification. Samiee *et al.* [15] proposed a EEG feature extraction method. The collected EEG segments were mapped into an image that was used as an input of a gray level co-occurrence matrix to extract multi-variate features. The results showed that the method achieved sensitivity and specificity of 70.19%, and 97.94%, respectively. Parvez *et al.* [16] used a phase correlation algorithm to detect local features and a relative correlation between adjacent EEG waves. The EEG signals were divided into epochs and arranged in the form of a 2-dimensional matrix. Then, the signals were applied transformation and decomposition methods for extracting features that were finally classified with least squares support vector machines. The results showed that the proposed method could achieve up to 97.32% sensitivity, and 96.68% specificity. Jaiswal *et al.* [17] proposed two feature extraction techniques for classifying EEG signals. The results showed that the proposed techniques with ANN classifier could reach an accuracy of 99% for both cases of normal and epileptic EEG signals. Tzimourta *et al.* [18] introduced a multicenter method based on discrete wavelet transform for automatically detecting seizure. The authors applied decomposition of 5 levels and extracted 5 features. The classification results showed that the presented method could reach 95% accuracy. Mahmoodian *et al.* [19] introduced an approach for epileptic seizure detection using cross-bispectrum of EEG signals. The approach could achieve an accuracy of 96.8% specificity of 96.7%, and sensitivity of 95.6%.

In addition to the above-mentioned approaches, deep learning becomes widely used in EEG analyses, especially self-feature extraction. Ullah *et al.* [20] presented an automated system for epilepsy detection using EEG signals. The system was based on one-dimensional convolutional neural network (P-1D-CNN) models. The system was tested with the University of Bonn dataset and achieve a high level of accuracy of 99% in many test cases. The authors claimed that the system can be customized for other applications detecting other similar disorders. Wang [21] introduced an approach based on deep learning for classifying different classes of EEG involving seizures. The authors applied one-dimensional CNN consisting of three convolution layers and three fully connected layers. The proposed model was tested with the University of Bonn dataset. The results' accuracy was 97.63%–99.52% in the two-class classification, 96.73%–98.06% in the three-class classification and 93.55% in five-class classification. Türk *et al.* [22] applied continuous wavelet transform to achieve two-dimensional frequency-time scalograms which were then fed for a CNN model to learn the properties of the scalograms. The accuracy results were 98.5%–99.5% in the two-class classification, 97.0%–99.0% in the three-class classification and 93.6% in the five-class classification. Acharya *et al.* [23] proposed an approach base on deep convolution neural networks for automated detection and diagnosis of seizure. A 13-layer deep convolution neural network algorithm could achieve 88.67% accuracy, 90% specificity, and 95% sensitivity. Lu *et al.* [24] presented an approach based on a convolution neural network with residual connections for epileptic EEG classification and automated seizure detection. The results showed that their approach could achieve up to 91.8% accuracy when experimenting with the Bern-Barcelona dataset. Asif *et al.* [25] proposed a framework based on multi-spectral deep feature learning for seizure type classification.The framework has experimented with Temple University Hospital (TUH) EEG dataset and achieved a weighted F1 score of 0.98 for seizure type classification.

3 Methodology for Epileptic Seizure Detection Using a Single EEG Channel

In this paper, an approach for epileptic seizures detection using a single EEG channel is proposed. The approach consists of three main stages: feature extraction, classifier training, and classifier evaluation. For feature extraction, a neural network structure based on an attention mechanism is designed. The neural network structure is shown in Fig. 1.

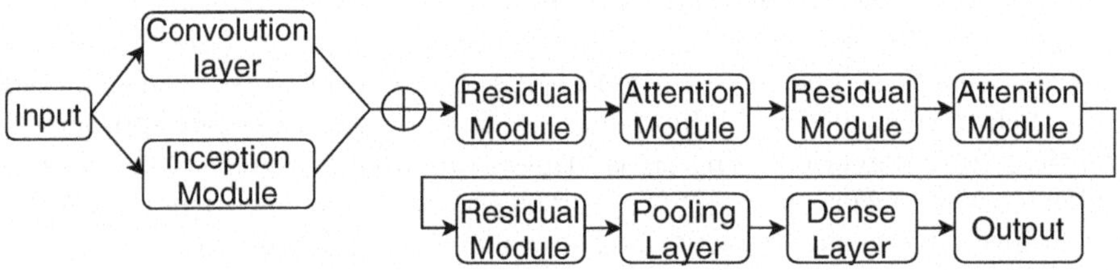

Fig. 1. The proposed neural network structure for a single EEG channel

Before being fed to the structure, raw EEG signals are pre-processed. The pre-processing stage includes data normalization, data fitting, and data re-sampling. In data normalization, raw EEG data having different measurement scales is normalized to have the same scale. We used the standard score method ($Y = \frac{X-\mu}{\sigma}$) which is suitable for distributed data like EEG. In the equation, X and Y are input and output while μ and σ are the mean value and standard deviation, respectively.

It is noticed that raw EEG data from different EEG measurement systems or datasets can be collected by different sampling frequencies. However, the input size should be uniformed. Therefore, data fitting and re-sampling are necessary. First, the B-spline representation [26] of the normalized input is found. Then, the fitted model is re-sampled by a particular frequency. As known that the energy distribution of EEG is mainly between 0.3 Hz and 80 Hz where the frequency components are α wave (8 Hz–13 Hz), β wave (13 Hz–30 Hz), δ wave (0.5 Hz–3.5 Hz), θ wave (4 Hz–8 Hz), γ wave (30 Hz–80 Hz). The effective frequency of EEG signals is not the same but it varies within 0.5 Hz–50 Hz [27]. It would be perfect if the EEG sampling rate is higher than 160 Hz then anti-alias can be achieved without any effort. However, when the neural network structure is too large or deep, the computational time for dealing with the large number of input samples could be very large. In our cases, we would like to develop automatic epileptic seizure detection edge and fog based systems that have limited resources (i.e., computation and memory) comparing to Cloud servers' resources. Therefore, we could not use the original sampling rate of the Bonn EEG dataset (i.e., 173.6 Hz corresponding to 4096 data points in 23.6 s). We had to find out the suitable EEG sampling rate which can achieve reasonable computational time while maintaining a high level of accuracy, sensitivity, and specificity. We tried different sampling rates ranging from 43 Hz to 173.6 Hz from the Bonn EEG dataset by applying moving average filers. Thanks to the cleanness of the EEG signals in the dataset as noises causes by external environments were already removed by experts, results of seizure detection from the applied EEG sampling rates are almost similar in terms of accuracy, sensitivity, and specificity. However, due to our large network, the computational time is dramatically different (e.g., about 4–8 times) between 43 Hz sampling rate and 86 Hz sampling rate. Hence, to reduce computational time and cover most of the characteristic waves (i.e.,α, β, δ, and θ waves) of epilepsy, we decided to apply 43 Hz sampling frequency which corresponds to 1024 points during 23.6 s from the dataset. This selection will be a premise for our future work where some parts of data processing and feature extraction will be run at edge and fog devices. Nevertheless, it is recommended to apply the higher EEG sampling frequency such as 173.6 Hz, or even much higher when Cloud-based systems having powerful computational resources are used. Due to the scope of the paper, edge and fog computing is not discussed in this paper. The detailed information of edge and fog-based systems for health monitoring including requirements and specifications are discussed in detail in [28–30].

Due to the scope of the paper, theoretical information of CNN including the convolution layer, pooling layer, activation function, batch normalization layer, and loss function will not be described in this paper. The detailed information of CNN can be found in [31]. The core of the proposed CNN structure is an attention module based on the attention mechanism that is inspired by an attention mechanism used in computer vision [32]. In general, the attention mechanism helps detect a focused point and enhances the representation of an object at that point. Via our experiments, we found that a neural network structure with the attention mechanism can be a good premise for EEG signal processing. Therefore, the attention mechanism is utilized and customized in the proposed approach for processing EEG signal processing.

In the customized attention mechanism, attention modules shown in Fig. 2 have been designed. Each attention module can be split into an attention trunk and a skip connection. In an attention trunk, the output from the previous module (i.e., residual module) is an input of the trunk. The bottom-up and top-down structures described in [33] are applied to achieve the same size attention mask M(x). This structure imitates the feed-forward and feedback attention procedure which is similar to the feature selection process of a feature pyramid network [33].

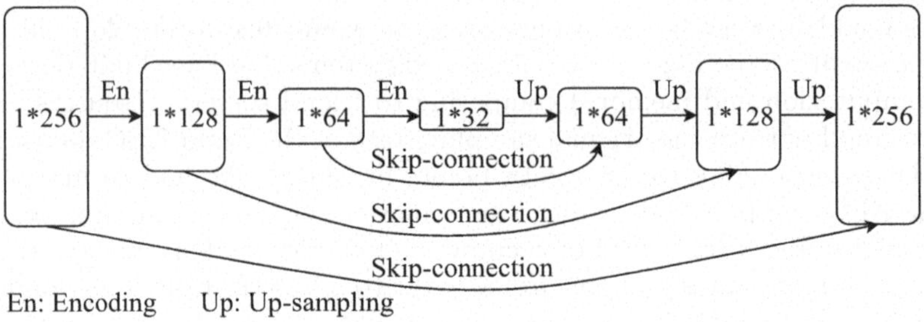

Fig. 2. The proposed attention module for single EEG channel

The output of the attention module is calculated via a formula: $H_{i,c}(X) = M_{i,c}(X) * T_{i,c}(X)$ where i is a range of all the input spatial locations, X is an input vector, $M_{i,c}(X)$ and $T_{i,c}(X)$ are the output of an attention trunk and a skip connection part, respectively. Another important part of the attention mechanism is an attention mask which is used as a feature selector during the feed-forward process and a gradient updater during the backpropagation process.

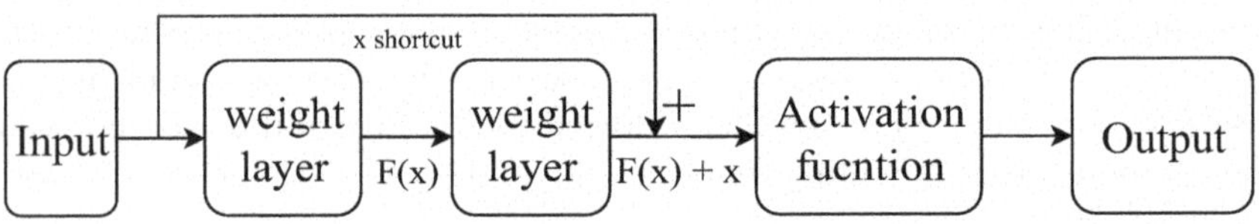

Fig. 3. The basic residual block

The basic residual block of the residual module is shown in Fig. 3 where input and output are vector x and vector y; H(x) and F(x) are the function of the whole residual block and the residual function, respectively. The whole residual block can be represented via the formula: $y = H(x) = F(x) + x$. Since the residual block has two weight layers, the whole residual block can be expressed as by the formula: $y = F(x, M_i) + x$. In our structure, several residual blocks are used to build a residual module which can be seen in Fig. 4.

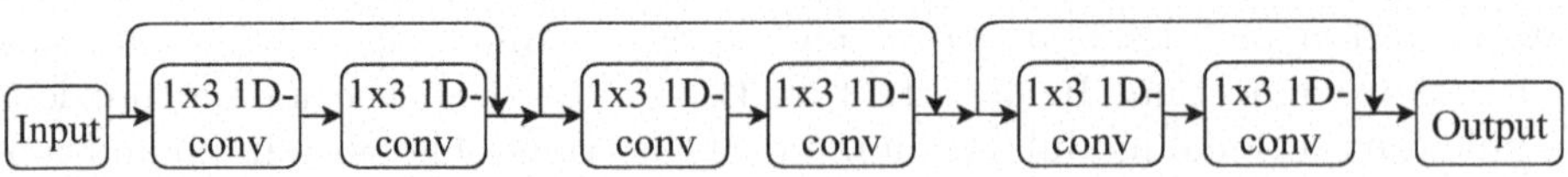

Fig. 4. A three-layer stacked residual module

To extract useful features from EEG, an inception module placing at beginning of the proposed structure was designed based on the inspiration of the design of the inception network [34,35]. In the inception module, several kernels having a size of 1×3, 1×5, and 1×7 are used for the basic convolution layer to avoid patch-alignment issues. Before these kernels are applied, the 1×1 kernel is applied for reducing computation. The result of each convolution is concatenated for forming a multi-dimensional tensor which will be used as an input of other modules. The structure of the inception module is shown Fig. 5.

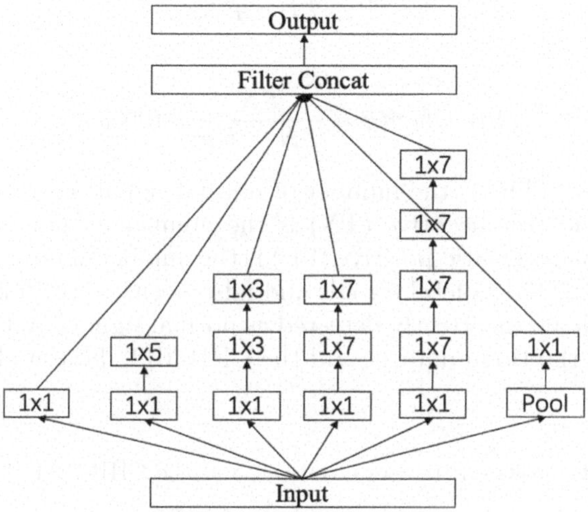

Fig. 5. Inception module structure

4 Experimental Results and Performance Evaluation

We used a cross-validation method and two different datasets such as the Bonn dataset and the Children's Hospital of Boston-Massachusetts Institute of Technology Dataset (the CHB-MIT dataset) to evaluate the proposed neural network structures [11,12]. In the cross-validation method, a small set of data is fed into the structures and the model's performance is estimated when it applies predictions on unseen data. The overall procedure of the cross-validation method with the k-fold described in [36] includes 4 main steps such as (i) randomly shuffling all the data; (ii) randomly selecting data into k categories; (iii) using each category as a testing set to evaluate the model while using all other categories as a training set to train the model, recording the model's performance and iterating the process for k times; (iv) Summing up the performance of all models and concluding the final summary of the proposed neural network structure. In our experiments, the k time value is set to 10, and the accuracy, sensitivity, and specificity are calculated per each test. Then, the average parameters of the final score of each classifier are used on each task. The formulas for calculating accuracy (Acc.), sensitivity (Sen.) and specificity (Spec.) are presented below:

$$Accuracy = \frac{TP + TN}{TP + TN + FP + FN} * 100\%$$

$$Sensitivity = \frac{TP}{TP + FN} * 100\%$$

$$Specificity = \frac{TN}{TN + FP} * 100\%$$

where true-positive (TP) is the number of normal signals correctly identified as normal signals and true-negative (TN) is the number of ictal signals correctly detected as ictal signals; false-positive (FP) is the number of normal signals which are incorrectly detected as ictal signals and false-negative (FN) is the number of ictal signals which are incorrectly detected as normal signals. In the experiments, different tasks in the Bonn dataset and the CHB-MIT dataset shown in Table 1 are evaluated.

Table 1. Tasks on the Bonn dataset and the CHB-MIT dataset

Task	Task meaning	Bonn dataset	CHB-MIT dataset
ZO-S	Normal - Ictal	X	X
NF-S	Interictal - Ictal	X	X
Z-S	Normal with closed eye - Ictal	X	
F-S	Interictal on focal area - Ictal	X	
ZONF-S	Nonictal - Ictal	X	X
ZO-NF-S	Normal - Interictal - Ictal	X	X
Z-F-S	Normal with closed eye - Interictal in focal area - Icta	X	
Z-O-N-F-S	All 5 subclass classification	X	

All the experiments with a single EEG channel in this section are achieved from a computer having an Intel XEON X5675 processor and an NVIDIA GeForce GTX1080Ti GPU that have specifications (e.g., memory and computation) similar to edge and fog devices used by typical health monitoring systems. The deep learning framework is PyTorch [37]. The performance results of the proposed network structure for a single EEG channel are compared with the state-of-the-art approaches including deep-learning-based and traditional algorithm-based approaches. The comparison results are shown in Table 2. The results show that the proposed approach can achieve nearly 100% accuracy in many tasks such as ZO-S, NF-S, Z-S, F-S, ZONF-S, Z-F-S except for the case of all 5 subclass s which have 86.4% accuracy. The reason for a high accuracy rate is that normal signal segments, interictal signal segments, and ictal signal segments are clearly distinguished in the Bonn dataset. One of the reasons causing a lower accuracy rate in the case of 5 subclasses is that the data of cases of "eye open" and "eye closed" is not much different. In some data segments, the data of these cases is almost similar. This issue also affects the results of other state-of-the-art approaches [23, 24].

Table 2. Comparison with state-of-the-art approaches when evaluating on the Bonn dataset

Task	Acharya *et al.* [23]			Lu *et al.* [24]			Tzimourta *et al.* [18]			Our proposed approach		
	Acc.	Sen.	Spec.	Acc.	Sen.	Spec.	Acc.	Sen.	Spec.	Acc.	Sen.	Spec.
ZO-S	0.990	0.970	1.0	0.993	1.0	0.990	-	-	-	**1.0**	**1.0**	**1.0**
NF-S	0.980	0.940	**1.0**	0.979	0.981	0.981	0.981	**0.986**	0.972	**0.986**	0.980	0.99
Z-S	0.990	0.980	1.0	1.0	1.0	1.0	0.999	1.0	0.917	**1.0**	**1.0**	**1.0**
F-S	0.925	0.85	1.0	0.975	0.98	0.97	0.977	0.976	0.979	**0.995**	**0.99**	1.0
ZONF-S	0.992	0.970	0.997	0.993	0.98	**0.997**	0.952	**0.997**	0.974	**0.994**	0.99	0.995
ZO-NF-S	0.887	0.95	0.90	0.976	0.975	**0.979**	0.958	0.960	0.977	**0.978**	**0.978**	0.978
Z-F-S	0.966	0.967	0.969	0.933	0.933	0.941	0.961	0.961	0.980	**0.993**	**0.993**	**0.994**
Z-O-N-F-S	0.418	0.418	NaN	0.795	0.796	0.819	0.822	0.822	**0.950**	**0.864**	**0.864**	0.869

Note: Values in bold text having the best values in their compared category

The comparison results show that the proposed approach is better than other state-of-the-art approaches [18, 23, 24] in terms of accuracy, sensitivity, and specificity in most of the cases. The difference is around from 1% to 8% depending on the case. Although the proposed approach cannot achieve better results in some cases, the difference is around 0.1%–0.2% except for the case of specificity in a 5 subclass task.

In the second experiment, we evaluated the proposed approach on the CHB-MIT dataset and compared it with other state-of-the-art approaches. Four tasks shown in Table 1 are applied for the experiment and their results are shown in Figs. 6, 7, 8 and 9. The collection time of raw EEG data is between 1 to 4 h, with a sampling rate of 256 Hz. Specifically, the EEG signals of each patient contain 23 channels. In this paper, we use the EEG channels of FP1-F7, F7-T7, F8-T8, T8-P8, and FP2-F8 to build the CHB-MIT scalp EEG Dataset.

For the ZO-S task, our proposed approach and state-of-the-art approaches [23] have quite similar results for accuracy, sensitivity, and specificity, except for the case of sensitivity and specificity of the approach [24]. In particular, the proposed approach's results are around 3% less accurate and 4% more accurate than the approach [23] and the approach [24], respectively. For the NF-S task, our results are 4%–15% better than others in terms of accuracy and sensitivity. In the case of the ZONF-S task, we have 3% better accuracy results than others

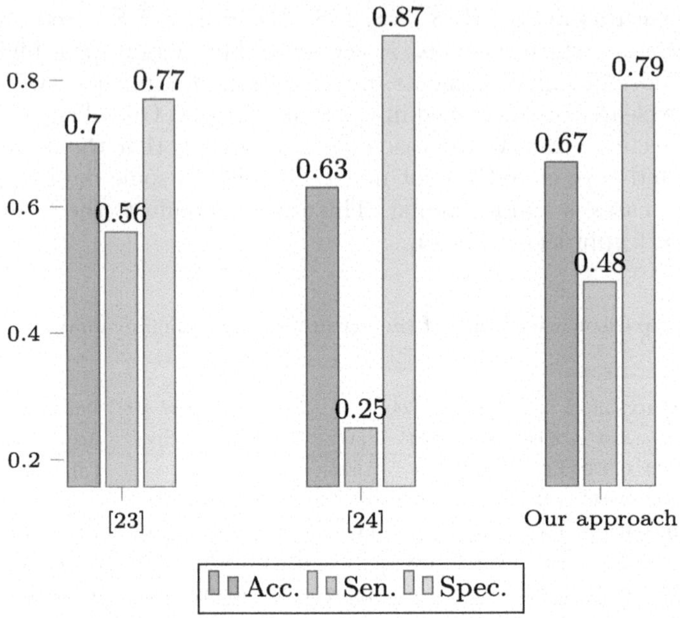

Fig. 6. Results of task ZO-S of CHB-MIT dataset

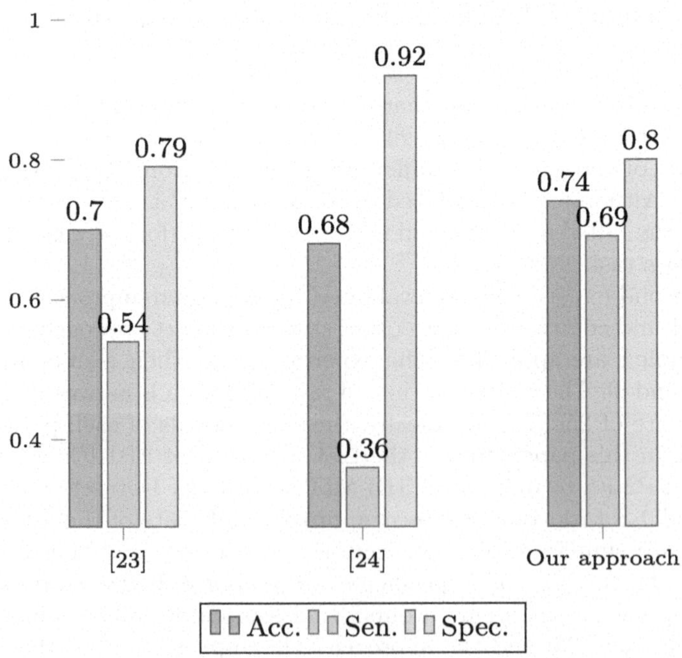

Fig. 7. Results of task NF-S of CHB-MIT dataset

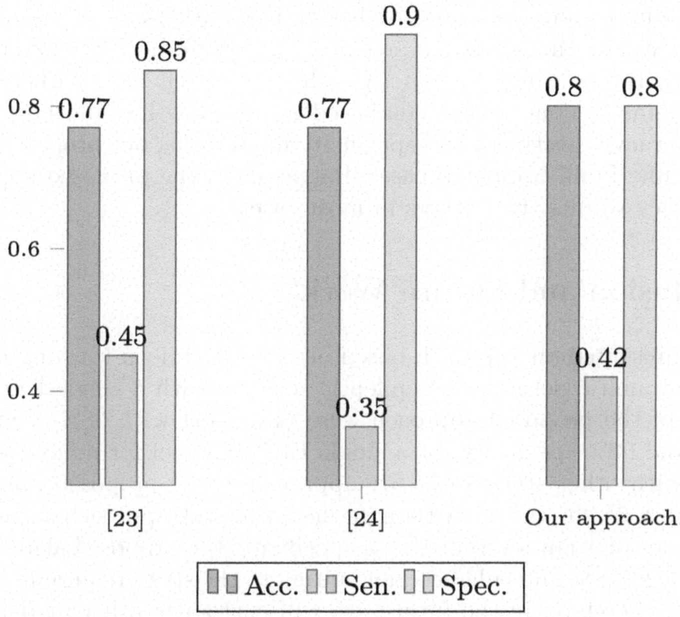

Fig. 8. Results of task ZONF-S of CHB-MIT dataset

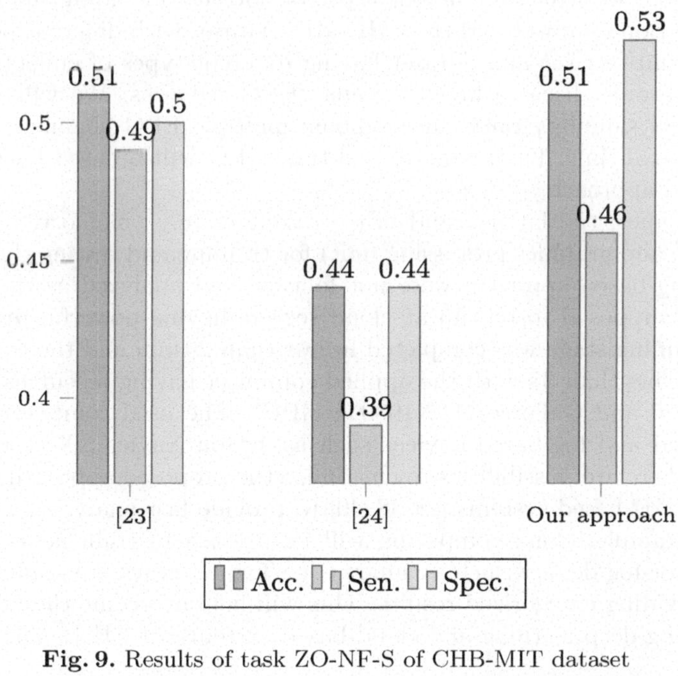

Fig. 9. Results of task ZO-NF-S of CHB-MIT dataset

but our specificity results are around 5%–10% lower than others. For the Z-O-N-F-S task, our results are equal or better than others in terms of accuracy and specificity. For the sensitivity results, our results are 3% lower than the approach [23] but 7% higher than the other approach [24]. Although for the CHB-MIT dataset, none of the compared approaches has the best results in terms of accuracy, sensitivity, and specificity in all tasks, our proposed approach has good results in all compared cases. Particularly, the proposed approach has better accuracy results than others in most cases.

5 Conclusion and Future Work

This paper presented an approach based on advanced deep learning neural networks for automatic detection of epileptic seizures with a single EEG channel. The results of the proposed approach were promising with 98% accuracy, 99% sensitivity and 98% specificity for a single EEG channel for many cases. When comparing with other state-of-the-art approaches, the proposed approach was better in most of the cases. Although the proposed approach achieved good results in terms of accuracy, sensitivity, specificity, the proposed algorithm needs to be more developed and enhanced for suiting to the strict requirements of medical experts. Therefore, in the future, we will customize other models, residual modules and attention modules. The customized modules having skip connections are expected to make the proposed neural networks dynamic to tune the number of layers during training optimally.

In addition, we will use different types of datasets including the one mixed between the Bonn dataset and the CHB-MIT dataset with different percentages of training and test set and dataset having different types of epileptic seizures and other chronic diseases having similar EEG patterns. We will also apply different EEG sampling rates and combine multiple EEG channels from both history and real-time. Furthermore, real-time EEG will be used for evaluating the proposed approach.

In this paper, the latency and usage resources (e.g., memory, central processing unit, and graphics processing unit) for training and testing the proposed deep learning-based approach were not focused and analyzed as the proposed approach is supposed to be run at cloud servers having powerful resources. In fact, the training stage was completed in less than 20 min and the testing stage was done in less than 3 s with the applied computer having resources (i.e., Intel XEON X5675 and GeForce GTX1080Ti GPU). The used computer is similar to edge-based and fog-based devices such as Jetson Xavier NX-based devices. Therefore, there are possibilities to customize the proposed approach for suiting to edge and fog-based systems [28,38–40] to provide fast analysis results at the edge. For example, cloud computing will be utilized to train neural networks whilst edge or fog devices such as smart edge/fog gateways are applied for testing and providing categorized results. This will help overcome the high latency of the existing deep learning and cloud-based systems for EEG analysis.

References

1. Epilepsy. Mayo Clinic (2020). https://www.mayoclinic.org/diseases-conditions/epilepsy/symptoms-causes/syc-20350093. Accessed June 2020
2. Dawda, Y., Ezewuzie, N.: Clinical focus-epilepsy-clinical features and diagnosis. Clin. Pharmacist **2**(3), 86–88 (2010)
3. WHO. Diabetes (2017). http://www.who.int/mediacentre/factsheets/fs312/en/. Accessed Jan 2018
4. Scheffer, I.E., et al.: ILAE classification of the epilepsies: position paper of the ILAE commission for classification and terminology. Epilepsia **58**(4), 512–521 (2017)
5. Type of Seizures. Mayo Clinic (2020). https://www.epilepsy.com/learn/types-seizures. Accessed June 2020
6. Baumgartner, C., Koren, J.P., Rothmayer, M.: Automatic computer-based detection of epileptic seizures. Front. Neurol. **9**, 639 (2018)
7. Ulate-Campos, A., et al.: Automated seizure detection systems and their effectiveness for each type of seizure. Seizure **40**, 88–101 (2016)
8. Osman, A.H., Alzahrani, A.A.: New approach for automated epileptic disease diagnosis using an integrated self-organization map and radial basis function neural network algorithm. IEEE Access **7**, 4741–4747 (2018)
9. Wang, Y., et al.: Automatic detection of epilepsy and seizure using multiclass sparse extreme learning machine classification. Comput. Math. Meth. Medicined, **2017** 2017
10. Wu, J., Zhou, T., Li, T.: Detecting epileptic seizures in EEG signals with complementary ensemble empirical mode decomposition and extreme gradient boosting. Entropy **22**(2), 140 (2020)
11. Andrzejak, R.G., et al.: Indications of nonlinear deterministic and finite-dimensional structures in time series of brain electrical activity: dependence on recording region and brain state. Phys. Rev. E **64**(6), 061907 (2001)
12. Goldberger, A.L., et al.: PhysioBank, PhysioToolkit, and PhysioNet: components of a new research resource for complex physiologic signals. Circulation **101**(23), e215–e220 (2000)
13. Bajaj, V., Pachori, R.B.: Classification of seizure and nonseizure EEG signals using empirical mode decomposition. IEEE Trans. Inf. Technol. Biomed. **16**(6), 1135–1142 (2011)
14. Xie, S., Krishnan, S.: Wavelet-based sparse functional linear model with applications to EEGs seizure detection and epilepsy diagnosis. Med. Biol. Eng. Comput. **51**(1–2), 49–60 (2013). https://doi.org/10.1007/s11517-012-0967-8
15. Samiee, K., et al.: Long-term epileptic EEG classification via 2D mapping and textural features. Expert Syst. Appl. **42**(20), 7175–7185 (2015)
16. Parvez, M.Z., Paul, M.: Epileptic seizure detection by exploiting temporal correlation of electroencephalogram signals. IET Sign. Process. **9**(6), 467–475 (2015)
17. Jaiswal, A.K., Banka, H.: Local pattern transformation based feature extraction techniques for classification of epileptic EEG signals. Biomed. Sign. Process. Control **34**, 81–92 (2017)
18. Tzimourta, K.D., et al.: A robust methodology for classification of epileptic seizures in EEG signals. Health Technol. **9**(2), 135–142 (2018). https://doi.org/10.1007/s12553-018-0265-z
19. Mahmoodian, N., et al.: Epileptic seizure detection using cross-bispectrum of electroencephalogram signal. Seizure **66**, 4–11 (2019)
20. Ullah, I., et al.: An automated system for epilepsy detection using EEG brain signals based on deep learning approach. Expert Syst. Appl. **107**, 61–71 (2018)

21. Zhao, W., et al.: A novel deep neural network for robust detection of seizures using EEG signals. Comput. Math. Methods Med. **2020** (2020)
22. Türk, Ö., Özerdem, M.S.: Epilepsy detection by using scalogram based convolutional neural network from EEG signals. Brain Sci. **9**(5), 115 (2019)
23. Acharya, U.R., et al.: Deep convolutional neural network for the automated detection and diagnosis of seizure using eeg signals. Comput. Biol. Med. **100**, 270–278 (2018)
24. Lu, D., Triesch, J.: Residual deep convolutional neural network for EEG signal classification in epilepsy (2019). arXiv preprint arXiv:1903.08100
25. Asif, U., et al.: Seizurenet: a deep convolutional neural network for accurate seizure type classification and seizure detection (2019). arXiv preprint arXiv:1903.03232
26. Unser, M., Aldroubi, A., Eden, M.: B-spline signal processing. I. Theor. IEEE Trans. Signal Process. **41**(2), 821–833 (1993)
27. Ai, Q., et al.: Advanced Rehabilitative Technology: Neural Interfaces and Devices. Academic Press, Cambridge (2018)
28. Rahmani, A.M., et al.: Exploiting smart e-Health gateways at the edge of healthcare internet-of-things: a fog computing approach. Future Gener. Comput. Syst. **78**, 641–658 (2018)
29. Negash, B., et al.: Leveraging fog computing for healthcare IoT. In: Rahmani, A.M., Liljeberg, P., Preden, J.-S., Jantsch, A. (eds.) Fog Computing in the Internet of Things, pp. 145–169. Springer, Cham (2018). https://doi.org/10.1007/978-3-319-57639-8_8
30. Gia, T.N., et al.: Fog computing in healthcare internet of things: a case study on ecg feature extraction. In 2015 IEEE CIT, pp. 356–363. IEEE (2015)
31. Albawi, S., et al.: Understanding of a convolutional neural network. In 2017 International Conference on Engineering and Technology (ICET), pp. 1–6. IEEE (2017)
32. Yang, X.: An overview of the attention mechanisms in computer vision. J. Phys. Conf. Ser. **1693**, 012173 (2020)
33. Lin, T.Y., et al.: Feature pyramid networks for object detection. In: Proceedings of the IEEE Conference on Computer Vision and Pattern Recognition, pp. 2117–2125 (2017)
34. Szegedy, C., et al.: Going deeper with convolutions. In: Proceedings of the IEEE Conference on Computer Vision and Pattern Recognition, pp. 1–9 (2015)
35. Szegedy, C., et al.: Rethinking the inception architecture for computer vision. In: Proceedings of the IEEE Conference on Computer Vision and Pattern Recognition, pp. 2818–2826 (2016)
36. James, G., Witten, D., Hastie, T., Tibshirani, R.: An Introduction to Statistical Learning. STS, Springer, New York (2021). https://doi.org/10.1007/978-1-0716-1418-1
37. Paszke, A., et al. Pytorch: an imperative style, high-performance deep learning library. In: Wallach, H., et al. (eds.) Advances in Neural Information Processing Systems, vol. 32, pp. 8024–8035. Curran Associates Inc (2019)
38. Gia, T.N., et al.: Low-cost fog-assisted health-care IoT system with energy-efficient sensor nodes. In: Wireless Communications and Mobile Computing Conference (IWCMC), 2017 13th International, pp. 1765–1770. IEEE (2017)
39. Gia, T.N., et al.: Energy efficient fog-assisted IoT system for monitoring diabetic patients with cardiovascular disease. Future Gener. Comput. Syst. **93**, 198–211 (2019)
40. Cheikhrouhou, O., et al.: One-dimensional CNN approach for ECG arrhythmia analysis in fog-cloud environments. IEEE Access **9**, 103513–103523 (2021)

Edge-Computing System Based on Smart Mat for Sleep Posture Recognition in IoMT

Haikang Diao[1(✉)], Chen Chen[2], Xiangyu Liu[3], Amara Amara[4], and Wei Chen[1,2]

[1] Center for Intelligent Medical Electronics, School of Information Science and Technology, Fudan University, Shanghai 200433, China
{19210720023,w_chen}@fudan.edu.cn
[2] Human Phenome Institute, Fudan University, Shanghai 201203, China
chenchen_fd@fudan.edu.cn
[3] College of Communication and Art Design, University of Shanghai for Science and Technology, Shanghai 200093, China
[4] IEEE CASS, Paris, France
amara.amara@tdh.ch

Abstract. Sleep posture has been proven to be a crucial index for sleep monitoring in the Internet of Medical Things (IoMT). In this paper, an edge-computing system based on a smart mat for sleep posture recognition in IoMT is proposed. The system can recognize postures unobtrusively with a dense flexible sensor array. To meet the requirements of embedded system in IoMT, a light-weight algorithm that includes pre-processing, EdgeNet pre-training, model quantization, model deployment is proposed. Finally, the complete algorithm is deployed in embedded systems (STM32) and edge computing for sleep posture monitoring is implement in IoMT. Through a series of short-term and overnight experiments with 21 subjects, results exhibit that the accuracy of the short-term experiment is up to 92.10% and the overnight experiment is up to 75.43%. After quantization, the accuracy of the overnight is up to 74.79%, and the runtime of the complete algorithm is about 65ms in the STM32. Compared with other methods, edge-computing systems have the advantages of low power consumption, low cost, low latency, high reliability, and no risk of privacy leakage. With the promising results, the proposed system is capable of providing sleep posture recognition and can be integrated into IoMT as an edge device.

Keywords: Edge computing · Sleep posture recognition · EdgeNet · Model quantization

1 Introduction

The Internet of Medical Things (IoMT) is a practical application for health care, which combines with the Internet of Things (IoT) devices and MedTech tools [1]. In the field of health care, sleep posture has been proven to be a crucial index for sleep monitoring. Wrong sleep postures may increase the burden of muscles and ligaments and result in

X. Gao et al. (Eds.): MobiHealth 2021, LNICST 440, pp. 85–94, 2022.
https://doi.org/10.1007/978-3-031-06368-8_6

shoulder, neck, or back pain; obstruct the airways to the lung and lead to breathing disorders like sleep apnea; affect the blood circulation, and induce pressure ulcers [2–4]. Therefore, a sleeping posture recognition system that enables long-time sleep posture monitoring and can be integrated into IoMT systems is needed.

Recently, quantities of methods have been proposed to recognize sleep posture. These methods can be classified into three categories. The first is to use video cameras to monitor sleep postures [5], but this method is susceptible to bedsheets and light, and may also produce privacy leaks. The second is to use a variety of wearable sensors to monitor sleep posture [6, 7]. However, with the attached sensors, natural sleep may be disrupted. The third is based on the pressure-sensing smart mat to achieve safe, convenient, comfortable, and non-intrusive sleep posture recognition, which can be applied in hospitals or home scenarios [8, 9]. In our previous study [10], an unobtrusive miniature scale smart mat system based on a dense flexible sensor array along with deep residual networks for sleep posture recognition is proposed. However, all of the methods mentioned above are unable to deploy in embedded systems for edge computing due to the complex algorithms, and therefore cannot be integrated directly into IoMT as an edge device.

In this paper, an edge-computing system based on a smart mat for sleep posture recognition in IoMT is proposed. To meet the requirements of the embedded system, we propose EdgeNet, a highly efficient model, and perform model quantization to significantly compress the model. Finally, the complete algorithm is deployed in embedded systems and edge computing for sleep posture monitoring is implement in IoMT. To verify the feasibility of the proposed system in real scenarios, a series of short-term and overnight experiments and performance evaluations in STM32 were conducted. Compared with other methods, edge-computing systems have the advantages of low power consumption, low cost, low latency, high reliability, and no risk of privacy leakage. The rest of the paper is organized as follows: Sect. 2 describes the system design and implementation. Section 3 presents the algorithm for sleep posture recognition. Section 4 presents the experiment and the results. Section 5 and Section 6 present the discussion and conclusion respectively.

2 System Design and Implementation

The edge computing system is shown in Fig. 1. As introduced in our previous research [10], When a person lies on the mat, the force-sensing mat acquires the voltage in different areas, and then the voltage goes through the signal control and acquisition circuit into the embedded system. Finally, the embedded system is used to convert the voltage signal into a pressure distribution map, and implement the sleep position classification. The electrodes and pins of the mat, the force-sensing resistor, the data acquisition circuit, and the embedded system are shown in Fig. 2.

To implement edge computing, the STM32 system, a cost-effective embedded system, is used as the computing platform. This system is based on STM32F746ZGTx microcontroller with 216 MHz clock speed, 1 Mbyte of Flash memory, and 340 Kbytes of RAM. It provides a lot of peripherals such as serial ports, GPIO, and 12-bit analog-to-digital converter (ADC). Compared to expensive servers, it costs only $5 and can be used as an edge device in IoMT. Meanwhile, it also can run edge algorithms due to its high main frequency and sufficient memory.

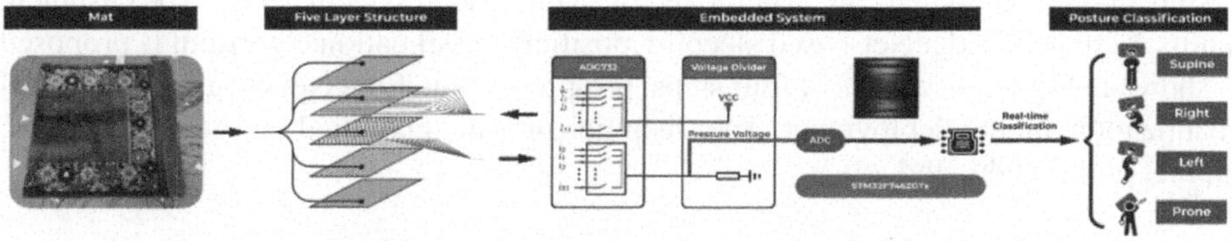

Fig. 1. The structure of the edge computing system.

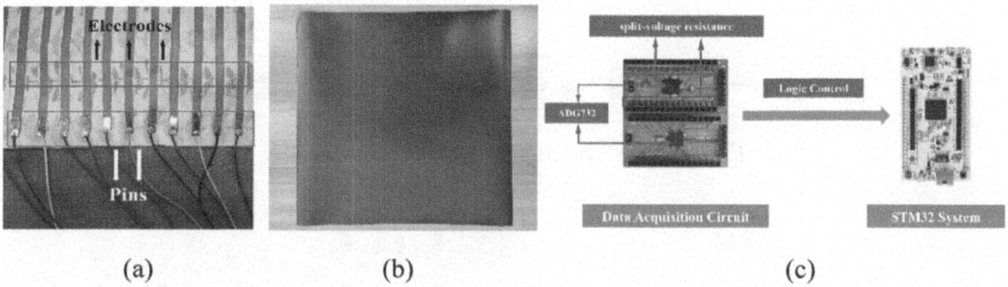

Fig. 2. (a) The electrodes and pins of the mat, (b) the force-sensing resistor, (c) the data acquisition circuit, and the embedded system.

The pressure distribution when one hand is pressed on the mat is shown in Fig. 2. Due to the high sensitivity of the system, the position and contour of the palm and fingers can be detected.

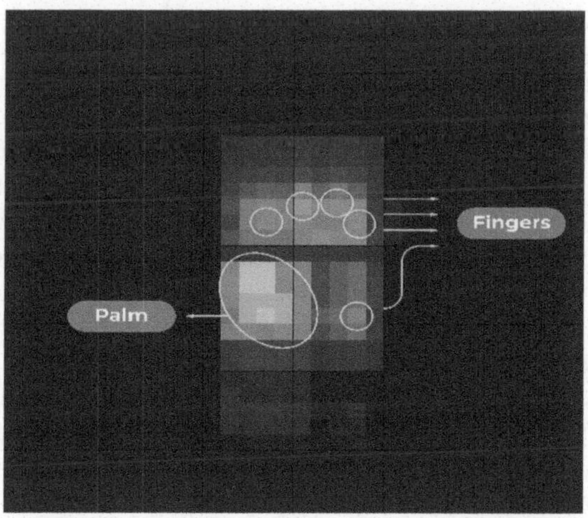

Fig. 3. The pressure distribution when one hand is pressed on the mat.

3 Algorithm Framework

To implement real-time edge computing in IoMT, a light-weight algorithm for sleep posture classification that can be deployed in an embedded system needs to be designed. In this section, an EdgeNet-based sleeping position classification algorithm is proposed as shown in Fig. 3. It consists of four steps: pre-processing, EdgeNet pre-training, model quantization, model deployment. The sleep postures are classified into four categories: supine, prone, right, and left.

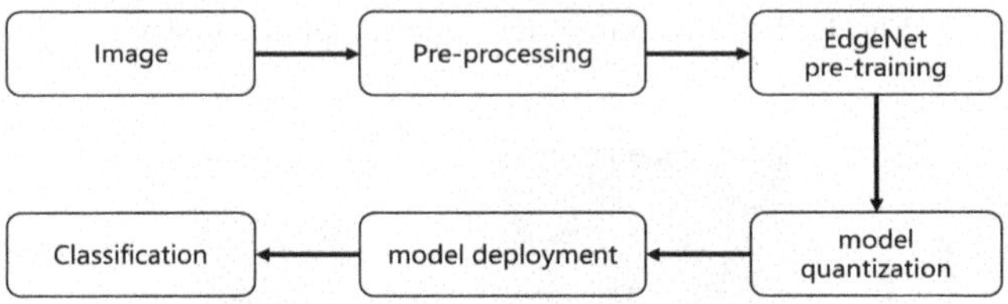

Fig. 4. The overall algorithmic framework.

3.1 Pre-processing

To eliminates the internal noise, high-frequency noise, and redundant information due to the softness and thinness of the pressure sensors embedded in the mat, threshold filtering, Gaussian filtering, and adjacent affected noise removal are used in pre-processing refer to our previous work [10].

3.2 EdgeNet Pre-training

Convolutional Neural Networks (CNN) is a feed-forward neural network, and it has a good effect on image recognition. However, the increase in classification capability comes with another drawback: the size and computational complexity of the model become high and beyond the capabilities of the IoMT system. In this paper, EdgeNet containing 1 Squeeze-and-Excitation block (SE block) [11], 5 bottleneck blocks based on MobileNetV2 [12], and 1 dense layer as shown in Fig. 4. The description of each layer of the network is shown in Table 1: c denotes the number of output channels, s denotes stride, and t denotes expansion factor.

The SE module adaptively reassigns the weights of different feature channels by calculating the interdependencies between channels. MobileNetV2 was proposed by Google Inc in 2018, which is based on the depthwise separable convolutions and inverted residual structure called bottleneck block. The bottleneck block, compare with the normal convolution layer, is more suitable for the embedded system due to the reduction of the FLOPS and parameters.

3.3 Model Quantization

Neural networks are known to be robust to noise and disturbance, and most of the trained weights and activations tend to fall within a small range [13]. Therefore, quantizing the model to reduce the precision requirements for the weights and activations is a convenient and effective way to compress the model. For example, by using 8-bit quantization, we can reduce the size of the model by a factor of 4 with minimum accuracy reduction, which reduces computational complexity, memory consumption, and data access latency.

Table 1. The description of each layer of the network.

Input	Operator	t	c	s
32 × 32 × 1	conv2d	–	16	1
32 × 32 × 16	SE block	–	16	1
32 × 32 × 16	bottleneck	1	8	1
32 × 32 × 8	bottleneck	6	16	2
16 × 16 × 16	bottleneck	6	32	2
8 × 8 × 32	bottleneck	6	64	1
8 × 8 × 64	bottleneck	6	128	2
4 × 4 × 128	avgpool 2 × 2	–	–	–
2 × 2 × 128	FC	–	4	–

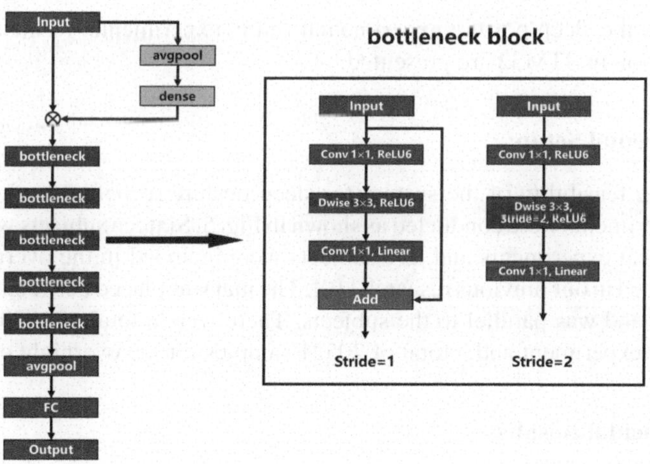

Fig. 5. The structure of the EdgeNet.

In this paper, post-training integer quantization is proposed for model compression after the EdgeNet has been trained. Post-training integer quantization is to convert 32-bit floating-point numbers (such as weights and activation outputs) to the nearest 8-bit fixed-point numbers for the already-trained float model. The operation can be described by the following formula:

$$x_{\text{int}} = \frac{x_f}{s} + z_0 \tag{1}$$

$$s = \frac{f_{\max} - f_{\min}}{2^8 - 1}, z_0 = 255 - \frac{f_{\max}}{s} \tag{2}$$

x_{int} is the quantized value, x_f is the 32-bit value, s denotes the quantized scale and z_0 is the quantized value corresponding to 0.f in a 32-bit value. This is an affine mapping of integers x_{int} to real numbers x_f.

3.4 Model Deployment

The complete sleep posture classification algorithm needs to be deployed to the STM32 to implement edge computing in IoMT. Signal control and pressure data acquisition implemented via the HAL driver library of the STM32. After the neural network model is trained on the TensorFlow platform, it needs to be converted to TF-Lite format before deployment. Then the pre-trained model is converted into an STM32-optimized library by the STM32Cube. AI expansion package. Finally, this STM32-optimized library is integrated into the user project. With this expansion package, neural network models can be inferred in embedded systems instead of on the server.

4 Experiment and Results

In this section, the sleep posture experimental setup, experimental results, and performance evaluation in STM32 are presented.

4.1 Experimental Setup

To evaluate the feasibility of the system for sleep posture recognition, short-term and overnight experiments were conducted as shown in Fig. 5. Sixteen subjects were included in the short-term experiments and five subjects were included in the overnight experiments introduced in our previous research [10]. The mat was placed between the subject's neck and hips and was parallel to the subjects. There were a total of 1059 samples for the short-term experiment and a total of 20521 samples for the overnight experiment.

4.2 Experimental Results

We perform the EdgeNet on the short-term and overnight database respectively. To validate the performance of the EdgeNet, we analyzed the short-term dataset by Leave-One-Person-Out-Cross-Validation. It divides the dataset by subjects, to ensure that the data of the same subject is not included in the training set and validation set at the same time. The overnight database is used as a test set to judge the effectiveness of the proposed algorithm, while the short-term database is used as the training set.

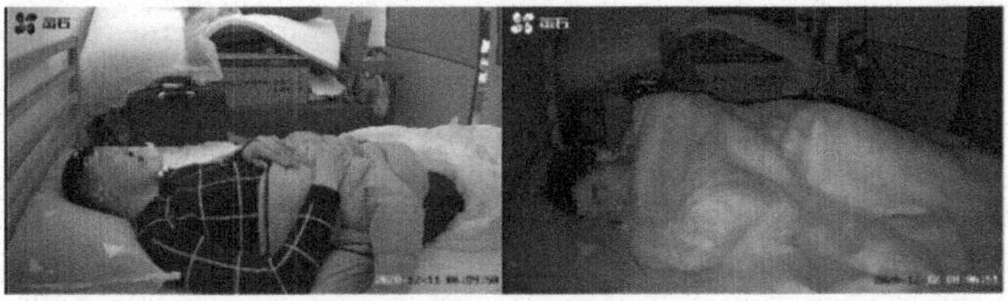

Fig. 6. The video screenshots of the sleep posture collection experiment

For neural network training, the relevant parameters are set as follows: the learning rate is 0.005, the number of iterations for network training is 150, the batch size is 512, the optimization algorithm is adaptive moment estimation (Adam), the loss function is categorical cross-entropy, the momentum is 0.9 and the epsilon is 0.00001 for Batch Normalization.

Table 2 shows the accuracy of the EdgeNet model and other models for sleep posture classification. Compare to other models, the EdgeNet proposed in this paper significantly reduces the size and computational complexity of the model while achieving competitive accuracy. Due to the pre-processing operation, we have simplified the pressure distribution images and removed redundant information, thus achieving high accuracy with the EdgeNet. Meanwhile, by applying the SE module to the input of the network, an attention mechanism is added to the input channels. Thus, the network pays more attention to the channels that are more sensitive to the posture classification task, which improves the efficiency of the model.

Table 2. The model complexity and classification accuracy.

Model	EdgeNet	MobileNet	ResNet10	AlexNet
Short-term	92.10%	93.90%	94.62%	94.90%
Overnight	75.43%	74.82%	77.17%	78.23%
Params	0.11M	2.22M	8.28M	4.37M
Size	0.44 MB	2.49 MB	32.3 MB	17.1 MB
MACC	5.88 M	10.47 M	159.27 M	257.4 M

Table 3. Comparison of EdgeNet before and after quantification

Model	Params	Size	MACC	Overnight
EdgeNet	0.11 M	0.44 MB	5.88 M	75.43%
EdgeNet _Q	0.11 M	0.18 MB	5.94 M	74.79%

It is worth noting that the accuracy of overnight experiments is significantly lower than short-term. First of all, none of the subjects in the overnight sleep experiment had participated in the short-term sleep experiment. Then, to simulate the real sleep situation, subjects may have movements in bed such as turning over as usual. These data are also collected but cannot be effectively identified as to which posture.

Table 3 shows the comparison of the EdgeNet before and after quantization. It can be seen that the size of the model is reduced by 60% after quantization, but the accuracy rate only decreases by 0.64%. This proves that quantization can indeed significantly reduce the model size and computational complexity while ensuring classification accuracy.

4.3 Performance Evaluation in STM32

After the model is quantized, we deploy the EdgeNet in STM32 to evaluate its performance, and for comparison, we also deploy the unquantized EdgeNet in STM32. Table 4 shows the performance and memory usage of the two models in stm32. Since the weights and activation values are quantized from 32 bits to 8 bits, the memory usage, and computational complexity are drastically reduced. Although the MACCs of the two models are similar, the CPU clock cycles required to execute a single operation (Cycle/MACC) are much different. Therefore, the inference time of the quantized model is only 30.7% of that of the unquantized model.

Together with the data acquisition and pre-processing algorithms, the quantized model performs a complete sleep posture acquisition and classification algorithm in less than 65 ms. This proves that the system proposed can be used as an edge device to achieve long-time sleep posture monitoring in IoMT.

Table 4. Performance evaluation in STM32

Model	ROM	RAM	Activations	Runtime	MACC	Cycle/ MACC	Accuracy
EdgeNet	425 KB	228 KB	224 KB	204.58 ms	5.88 M	7.552	75.43%
EdgeNet_Q	111 KB	132KB	128 KB	62.84 ms	5.94 M	2.28	74.79%

5 Discussion

The key index to implement edge computing in IoMT is how to deploy algorithms on small memory, low performance, low power embedded systems, and ensure the utility of the algorithms (low latency and high accuracy). Therefore, the edge algorithm needs to ensure low memory usage and low computational complexity. In our method, compared to the ordinary convolutional layer, bottleneck block can express richer features by expansion factor while reducing memory usage and the number of calculations. Meanwhile, the memory accesses are 28% less than that of the ordinary convolutional layer, which is related to the model runtime.

The mat proposed can still be enhanced by involving the following points. Currently, the model must be trained on the server first and then deployed to the embedded system.

If the model training can be implemented in the embedded system, then the model can be updated and improved according to the usage scenarios. What's more, the respiration rate detection will be included to extend the functionality of the system.

6 Conclusion

In this paper, for offering an edge-computing system for sleep posture recognition in IoMT, a smart mat system based on the EdgeNet is proposed. The algorithmic framework consists of pre-processing, EdgeNet pre-training, model quantization, and model deployment. Experimental results show that the accuracy of the short-term experiment is up to 92.10%, and the accuracy of the overnight is up to 75.43% before quantization. After quantization, the accuracy of the overnight is up to 74.79%, and the runtime of the complete algorithm is about 65ms in the STM32 system, which shows that its ability to provide sleep posture recognition in IoMT. Compare to other methods, our system has the advantages of low cost, low latency, low power consumption, high reliability and no privacy concerns. In the future, the mat system can still be enhanced by integrating embedded network training algorithms and breathing detection.

Acknowledgment. This work was supported in part by the Shanghai Committee of Science and Technology under Grant No.20S31903900, in part by Shanghai Municipal Science and Technology Major Project under Grant No. 2017SHZDZX01, in part by Shanghai Municipal Science and Technology International R&D Collaboration Project (Grant No. 20510710500), and in part by the National Natural Science Foundation of China under Grant No.62001118.

References

1. Ghubaish, A., Salman, T., Zolanvari, M., Unal, D., Al-Ali, A.K., Jain, R.: Recent advances in the internet of medical things (IoMT) systems security. In IEEE Internet Things J. **8**(11), 8707–8718 (2021). https://doi.org/10.1109/JIOT.2020.3045653
2. Parish, J.M.: Sleep-related problems in common medical conditions. Chest **135**(2), 563–572 (2009)
3. Winsky-Sommerer, R., de Oliveira, P., Loomis, S., Wafford, K., Dijk, D.J., Gilmour, G.: Disturbances of sleep quality, timing and structure and their relationship with other neuropsychiatric symptoms in Alzheimer's disease and schizophrenia: insights from studies in patient populations and animal models. Neurosci. Biobehav. Rev. **97**, 112–137 (2019)
4. Soban, L.M., Hempel, S., Munjas, B.A., Miles, J., Rubenstein, L.V.: Preventing pressure ulcers in hospitals: a systematic review of nurse-focused quality improvement interventions. Jt. Comm. J. Qual. Patient Saf. **37**(6), 245-AP16 (2011)
5. Nuksawn, L., Nantajeewarawat, E., Thiemjarus, S.: Real-time sensor- and camera-based logging of sleep postures. In: 2015 International Computer Science and Engineering Conference (ICSEC), pp. 1–6 (2015)
6. Chang, M., et al.: Multimodal sensor system for pressure ulcer wound assessment and care. IEEE Trans. Ind. Inform. **14**(3), 1186–1196 (2018)
7. Jiang, P., Zhu, R.: Dual tri-axis accelerometers for monitoring physiological parameters of human body in sleep. In: 2016 IEEE Sensors, Orlando, pp. 1–3 (2016)

8. Matar, G., Lina, J.-M., Kaddoum, G.: Artificial neural network for in-bed posture classification using bed-sheet pressure sensors. IEEE J. Biomed. Health Inform. **24**(1), 101–110 (2020)
9. Xu, X., Lin, F., Wang, A., Hu, Y., Huang, M.C., Xu, W.: Body-Earth mover's distance: a matching-based approach for sleep posture recognition. IEEE Trans. Biomed. Circuits Syst. **10**(5), 1023–1035 (2016)
10. Diao, H., et al.: Deep residual networks for sleep posture recognition with unobtrusive miniature scale smart mat system. IEEE Trans. Biomed. Circuits Syst. **15**(1), 111–121 (2021). https://doi.org/10.1109/TBCAS.2021.3053602
11. Hu, J., Shen, L., Albanie, S., Sun, G., Wu, E.: Squeeze-and-excitation networks. In: IEEE Transactions on Pattern Analysis and Machine Intelligence, vol. 42, no. 8, pp. 2011–2023, 01 August 2020
12. Sandler, M., Howard, A., Zhu, M., Zhmoginov, A., Chen, L.:MobileNetV2: inverted residuals and linear bottlenecks. In: 2018 IEEE/CVF Conference on Computer Vision and Pattern Recognition, pp. 4510-4520 (2018). https://doi.org/10.1109/CVPR.2018.00474.
13. Jacob, B., et al.: Quantization and training of neural networks for efficient integer-arithmetic-only inference. In: 2018 IEEE/CVF Conference on Computer Vision and Pattern Recognition, Salt Lake City, pp. 2704–2713 (2018)

Retinal Vessel Segmentation Using Multi-scale Generative Adversarial Network with Class Activation Mapping

Minqiang Yang, Yinru Ye, Kai Ye, Xiping Hu(✉), and Bin Hu(✉)

Lanzhou University, Lanzhou 730099, Gansu, China
{yangmq,yeyr18,kye18,huxp,bh}@lzu.edu.cn

Abstract. Retinal vessel segmentation plays a significant role in the accurate diagnosis of retinal diseases. However, existing methods commonly omit micro-vessels in retinal images and generate some false-positive vessels. To alleviate this issue, we propose a multi-scale generative adversarial network with class activation mapping to achieve efficient segmentation. For the problem of small amount of data, we introduce a novel data augmentation method, which can generate multiple samples by cutting pixels from other samples. This method increases the diversity of samples and improve the robustness of the model. We compare our method with previous models with several metrics, and experiments show the superiority and effectiveness of our model.

Keywords: Retinal vessel segmentation · Multi-scale generative adversarial network · Class activation mapping · Data augmentation

1 Introduction

Retinal vessel segmentation has been a longstanding topic in medical image. In the treatment and evaluation of retinal diseases, such as macular degeneration, retinitis pigmentosa [26], the segmentation of retinal vessels in the fundus image is essential. However, traditional medical image processing mainly relies on the personal experience of experts to manually analyze and process images. This manual processing method is inefficient and subjectively affects the analysis results. Therefore, it is imperative for the computer to automatically process the retinal vessel segmentation image.

The methods of retinal segmentation consists of supervised learning and unsupervised learning. Supervised learning requires training through the original fundus images and the images of blood vessels manually labeled by experts. Common supervised learning methods applied to retinal segmentation include support vector machine (SVM) [16], random forest (RF) [30], and multilayer perceptron (MLP) [21]. Unsupervised methods do not require manual label to train the model, such as vessel tracking [36,38], template matching [5,12,31],

X. Gao et al. (Eds.): MobiHealth 2021, LNICST 440, pp. 95–105, 2022.
https://doi.org/10.1007/978-3-031-06368-8_7

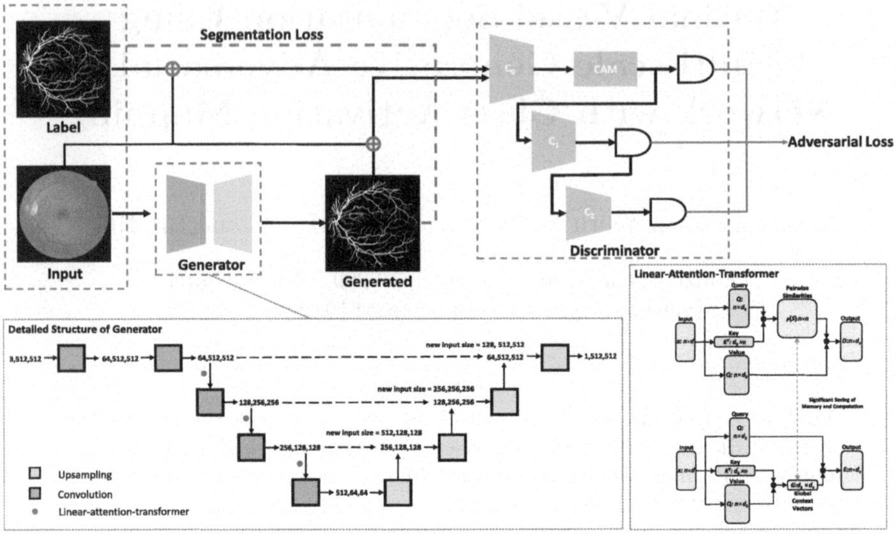

Fig. 1. Structure of our model.

multi-scale analysis [4,15,37], region growth [18]. Olaf et al. proposed U-net methods [14] which has greatly promoted the field of image segmentation, and has achieved great success in this field. However, although the image generated by the existing method has a good value on the metrics, the generated image is full of fragmented blood vessels, which is different from the real blood vessels. For doctors, this is not conducive to auxiliary diagnosis of medical diseases. But it is very challenging to generate images that are almost the same as the real blood vessel distribution, we propose a method that combines generative adversarial network (GAN) and end-to-end network generation. Inspired by locality-aware attention mechanism [22], we add class activation mapping (CAM) to network.

The existing models also have a problem that data collection and labeling of retinal blood vessels are time-consuming and labor-intensive and the amount of data is scarce compared to most tasks. Inspired by data augmentation method proposed by Haocong Rao et al. [23] and Phil Wang [29], we introduce a new data augmentation method called image stitching. this method cut a part of the area but randomly fill in the pixels of other data in the training set. The cropped and filled data can be flipped at a certain angle. Because the location, rotation angle and size of the grafting area are different, only one sample can produce infinite samples. This method increases the diversity of samples and reduces the occurrence of over-fitting.

Finally, we analyze the superiority of our model from a qualitative and quantitative perspective. For quantitative evaluation, we compared the evaluation indicators with other models and showed the changes of the indicators during the training process. For the qualitative point of view, we visualized the attention mechanism and the real classification result.

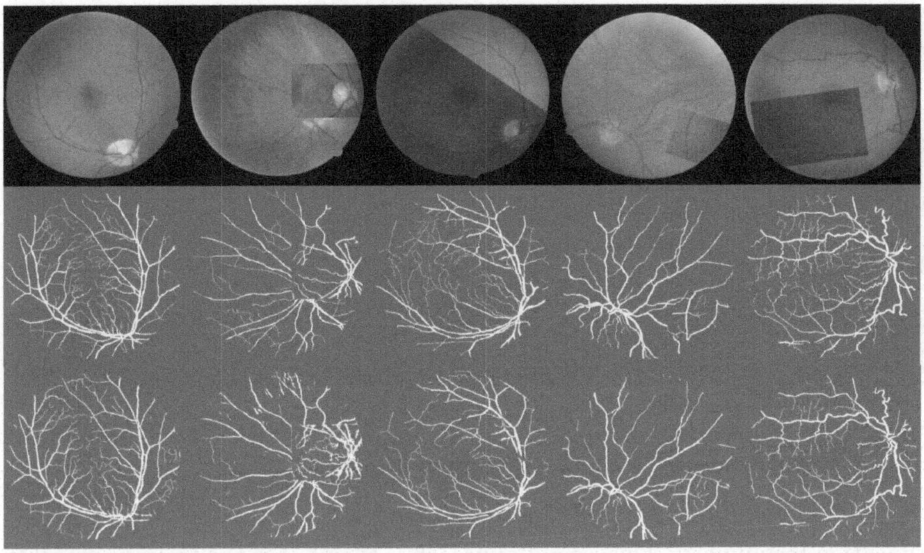

Fig. 2. Image stitching. The top row are eye fundus images after image stitching; the middle row are manual label; the bottom row are results obtained by our method.

2 Related Work

2.1 Image Segmentation

Image segmentation refers to finding the boundary of the region of interest (ROI) in the image, so that the pixels inside and outside the boundary have similar characteristics (intensity, texture, etc.). Medical image segmentation is the basis of other medical image processing. Medical image segmentation is usually used in the following use cases: liver segmentation for computed tomography (CT) images, breast-lesion segmentation, and retinal vessel segmentation. Kumar, S. S. proposed a method which can achieve automatic segmentation of liver and lesion from CT images needed for computer-aided diagnosis of liver [13]. Moi Hoon Yap used convolutional neural networks to detect breast ultrasound lesions automatically [35]. Tiejun Yang finded that SUD-GAN has a good performance in the field of retinal vessel segmentation [19].

2.2 Generative Adversarial Network

GAN [8] has been applied in many fields, such as vessel generation [34], artwork generation [25], and video generation [28]. It can achieve the improvement of image quality [27], image coloring [39]. There are several approaches for GAN to improve the authenticity of generated vessel images from different perspectives. The first one is large-scale training relies on complex calculations(e.g. BIGGAN [3] generated realistic images by increasing batchsize and

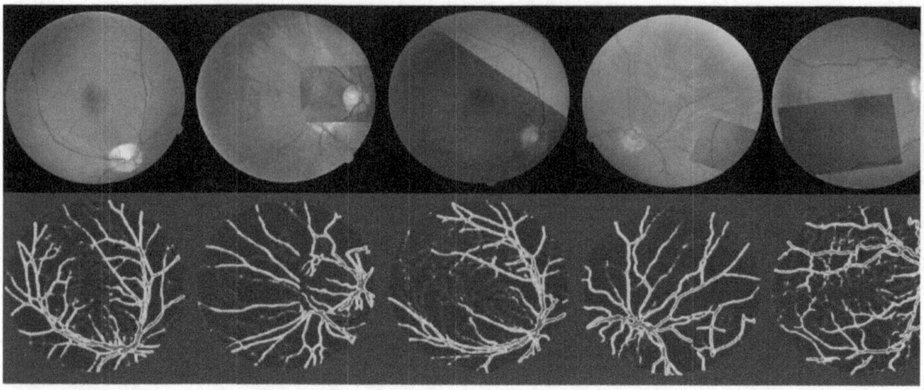

Fig. 3. Class activation mapping. The first row are eye fundus images; the second row are eye fundus images with class activation mapping.

truncation techniques). The second approach is to enhance the training stability (e.g. DCGAN [20] proposed a network structure consisting of stride convolution and transposed convolution to improve training stability). The third one is architectural modifications (e.g. AMCGC-LSTM [33] put spatial attention module into the network).

3 Our Approach

3.1 Discriminator

Compared with the traditional model [10], we use a multi-scale discriminator, which can improve the perceptual ability of the discriminator. It can better distinguish the fine blood vessels and the overall blood vessel distribution. Compared with the previous methods of applying discriminators of different scales to images of different sizes, we present a more direct method to superimpose the input image and segmented images and transmit them to the discriminator. The discriminator passes the input features of different layers to the corresponding size classifier for distinction. As shown in Fig. 1, the discriminator has two components: class activation mapping [41] and classifier. The C1 representation can accept a 128×128 receptive field, and the C2 representation can accept a 256×256 receptive field. The input image and label and the generated segmentation image are respectively used as the input of C0, and then are down-sampled by C1 after passing through CAM [41]. The same is true for C2. For a pair of images (eye fundus images and blood vessel segmentation image), C0, C1, and C2 are all trained to predict the true and false of the image. In addition to the multi-scale effect that is conducive to segmentation, we also use an attention mechanism to allow the model to learn features in the image more efficiently. This attention mechanism was first proposed by CAM. The idea of CAM is to superimpose the weighted linear sum of these visual patterns in different spatial

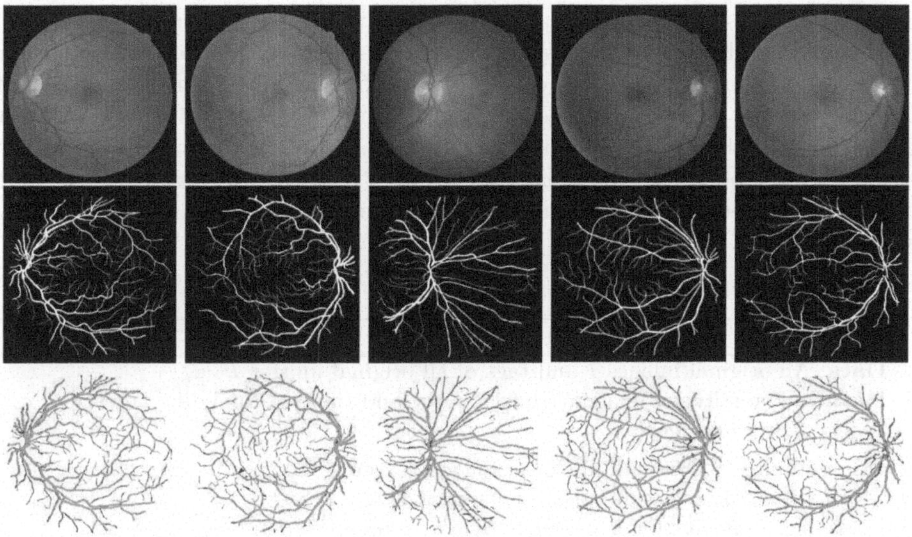

Fig. 4. Segmentation results of an example in the DRIVE dataset. The first row are eye fundus images; the second row are munual lable; the third row are visualization of real classification.

positions and get important information in the image on the input. It enables the model to efficiently focus on the distribution of blood vessels, thereby improving training efficiency.

3.2 Generator

The construction of the generator is inspired by previous work. In the previous work [2], the auto-encoder network constitutes a highly efficient method of dense prediction. Especially U-net can excel in many complex image segmentation tasks. In these image classification networks, basically follow a pattern. The encoder gradually downsamples the input to learn the global features of the input image, and the decoder gradually upsamples to make the output resolution consistent with the input. The two are connected by layer jumps. Data transmission in the same resolution layer can further improve the ability of the network to accurately segment. As shown in Fig. 1, we reconstructed the generator through the residual network, and added linear attention transformation [11] on the original basis. Linear attention transformation can discard information that is irrelevant to blood vessels in the process of downsampling.

3.3 Image Stitching

Since there are often problems in medicine such as small sample size and difficulty in collecting, we propose a data augmentation model to alleviate this problem. Image stitching is a data augmentation method that can increase sample diversity and model robustness. It cuts one picture, embeds it in another picture, and then performs size change, rotation, and mirroring. The details of these processing steps can be seen in Algorithm 1. As shown in Fig. 2, the first row is the data after image stitching, the second row is the real label after image stitching, and the third row is the image after model segmentation. It can be seen that our method can generate a large number of samples, thereby reducing over-simulation.

Algorithm 1: Image stitching

Data: All original images I and tags of all original images L
Result: The stitched image *StitchedImage* and the corresponding label *StitchedLabel*

```
OriginalImage0, OriginalLabel0 ← RandomChoice(I, L);
OriginalImage1, OriginalLabel1 ← RandomChoice(I, L);
StartPoint ← RandomChoice(Image.Height, Image.Width);
EndPoint ← RandomChoice(Image.Height, Image.Width);
StartPoint, EndPoint ← Order(StartPoint, EndPoint);
OriginalImage0 ← Crop(OriginalImage0, StartPoint, EndPoint);
OriginalLabel0 ← Crop(OriginalLabel0, StartPoint, EndPoint);
StitchedImage ← Paste(OriginalImage1, OriginalImage0, StartPoint);
StitchedLabel ← Paste(OriginalLabel1, OriginalLabel0, StartPoint);
Spin ← RandomChoice(360);
Flip ← RandomChoice(1);
StitchedImage ← Rotate(StitchedImage, Spin);
StitchedLabel ← Rotate(StitchedLabel, Spin);
if Flip == True then
    StitchedImage ← Transpose(StitchedImage);
    StitchedLabel ← Transpose(StitchedLabel);
end
```

3.4 Loss Functions

Our model mainly contains two kinds of loss functions in the training process, one is the adversarial loss, and the other is the end-to-end segmentation loss. The specific details are as follows:

Adversarial Loss. The adversarial loss is aim to guide the discriminator to distinguish the generated vessel image and ground truth. The former is generally regarded as the source domain and the latter as the target domain, which have different internal distribution. With the iterative process, it attempts to and make the distribution probability of the output of the generator approach the distribution of the target domain continuously.

$$\min_G \max_D L_{adv}^{x \rightarrow y} = \mathbb{E}_{y \sim \mathcal{Y}}[(D(G(y)))^2] + \mathbb{E}_{x \sim \mathcal{X}}[(1 - D(G(x)))^2]. \tag{1}$$

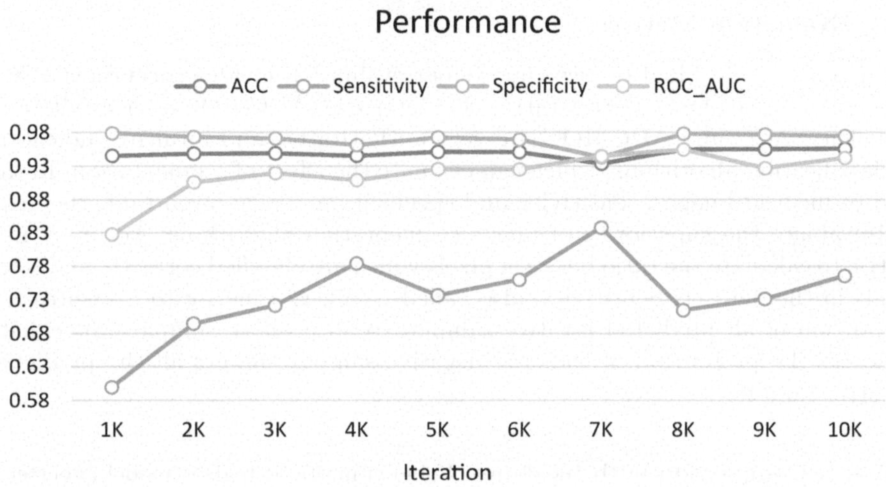

Fig. 5. Iteration performance.

Segmentation Loss. If you only apply the adversarial loss of unsupervised learning, the efficiency is actually low, so we have an additional end-to-end segmentation loss for supervised learning. Because the dataset has unbalanced characteristics and the traditional loss functions will not be able to learn well with features of few samples and difficult samples, we apply focal loss as the segmentation loss.

$$\min_G L_{seg}^{x,y} = \mathbb{E}_{y \sim \mathcal{Y}}[L_{ft}(G(y))]. \quad (2)$$

To prevent an extreme imbalance between background and retinal vessels classes, we apply focal loss to adapt the weight of positive (vessels) and negative (background) samples. For weighting factor $\alpha \in$ [1,0], 1- α refers to as inverse class frequency to balance the significance of positive and negative samples.

$$L_{fl} = \begin{cases} -\alpha(1-\hat{y})^{\gamma} \log \hat{y}, y = 1 \\ -(1-\alpha)\hat{y}^{\gamma} \log(1-\hat{y}), y = 0 \end{cases} \quad (3)$$

4 Experiments

4.1 Dataset

In this article, we use the DRVIE dataset [24] for retinal vessel segmentation. The size of the images and the corresponding labels in the data set is 565 × 584. For data augmentation, all images will be processed by image stitching, rotation, mirroring and other operations, and finally will be cropped to a size of 512 × 512. The data set is divided into two parts for training set and testing set respectively, with a sample size ratio of 20:20. The metrics and results of our model in this article have been iteratively trained 10,000 times.

4.2 Evaluation Metrics

For quantitative evaluation, we choose four evaluation metrics: accuracy(ACC), area under curve of receiver operating characteristic (AUC-ROC), sensitivity and specificity. ACC and AUC-ROC are very authoritative and intuitive indicators in classification algorithms, which can evaluate the effect of segmentation. In the field of medical images, sensitivity and specificity are very important, they can well evaluate the superiority of image segmentation algorithms. Accuracy is a metric to calculate the ratio between pixels which are classfied correctly and total pixels in the dataset. Sensitivity, also called recall, is a metric to measures the proportion of all predicted positive samples to all positive samples. Specificity indicates the proportion of the true negative samples among all the predicted negative samples.

Table 1. Comparison with baselines. Value of metric is higher, model is better.

Methods	DRIVE			
	ACC	Sensitivity	Specificity	AUC - ROC
Odstrcilik et al. [17]	0.9341	0.7847	0.9512	0.9569
Azzopardi et al. [1]	0.9614	0.7655	0.9704	0.9614
YT Zhao et al. [40]	0.9540	0.7420	0.9820	0.8620
C Wu et al. [32]	0.9514	0.7696	0.9780	0.8909
G Azzopardi et al. [1]	0.9442	0.7655	0.9704	0.9614
Y Chen [6]	0.9453	0.7426	0.9735	0.9516
MM Fraz et al. [7]	0.9480	0.7406	0.9807	0.9747
K Hu et al. [9]	0.9521	0.7779	0.9780	0.9782
Ours	0.9559	0.7659	0.9746	0.9424

4.3 Comparisons

As shown in Table 1, we use quantitative analysis to evaluate our model. It can be clearly seen that our model has a good effect on various metrics. The compared model may be more focused on a certain metric, and we can complete the segmentation task while ensuring that the overall metrics are better. Especially for the sensitivity and specificity, from the evaluation results it attests our model can ensure the segmentation of real blood vessels and can be helpful for the auxiliary diagnosis of medical diseases in practical sense.

4.4 Result

In Fig. 5, we can observe the change of each metric as the number of iterations increases. As shown in Fig. 3, we use the CAM, which makes blood vessels be recognized by neural networks, to make the model more efficient to segment blood vessels. Red means that the model pays more attention to this area, and blue means that the model pays less attention to this area. Through the image generated by the attention mechanism in the bottom row, we can clearly see that the attention of model is placed on the blood vessels. And for other irrelevant factors such as background information, our model are not paid much attention to, which allows the generator able to generate better images. For the second row of Fig. 4, it's easily to observe the predicted result of our model. The green blood vessel represents the correctly predicted blood vessel (TP), the red vessel represents the real blood vessel that was not predicted (FN), and the blue vessel represents the non-existent blood vessel generated by the generator (FP). It means our model can clearly identify the main vessels, and there are very few unidentified and incorrectly identified vessels. It proves the superiority of the model.

5 Conclusion

We propose an architecture for retinal vessel segmentation. It can distinguish between global and local perception domains through a multi-scale CAM discriminator, and the generator can also use linear attention to transform more efficient blood vessel segmentation. In addition, we also introduce a data augmentation method called image stitching, so that the model can accept a sufficient variety of images. The evaluation of vision and metrics can show that our model has excellent performance in retinal blood vessel segmentation. It proves that this method achieves fast and accurate blood vessel segmentation.

Acknowledgement. This work was supported in part by the National Key Research and Development Program of China (Grant No. 2019YFA0706200), in part by the National Natural Science Foundation of China (Grant No. 61632014, No. 61627808, No. 61802159), in part by Fundamental Research Funds for Central Universities (lzujbky-2019-26).

References

1. Azzopardi, G., Strisciuglio, N., Vento, M., Petkov, N.: Trainable COSFIRE filters for vessel delineation with application to retinal images. Med. Image Anal. **19**(1), 46–57 (2015)
2. Badrinarayanan, V., Kendall, A., Cipolla, R.: SegNet: a deep convolutional encoder-decoder architecture for image segmentation. IEEE Trans. Pattern Anal. Mach. Intell. **39**(12), 2481–2495 (2017)
3. Brock, A., Donahue, J., Simonyan, K.: Large scale GAN training for high fidelity natural image synthesis. In: ICLR (2019)
4. Budai, A., Bock, R., Maier, A., Hornegger, J., Michelson, G.: Robust vessel segmentation in fundus images. Int. J. Biomed. Imaging (2013)
5. Chaudhuri, S., Chatterjee, S., Katz, N., Nelson, M., Goldbaum, M.: Detection of blood vessels in retinal images using two-dimensional matched filters. IEEE Trans. Med. Imaging **8**(3), 263–269 (1989)
6. Chen, Y.: A labeling-free approach to supervising deep neural networks for retinal blood vessel segmentation. arXiv preprint arXiv:1704.07502 (2017)

7. Fraz, M.M., Remagnino, P., Hoppe, A., Uyyanonvara, B., Rudnicka, A.R., Owen, C.G., Barman, S.A.: An ensemble classification-based approach applied to retinal blood vessel segmentation. IEEE Trans. Biomed. Eng. **59**(9), 2538–2548 (2012)
8. Goodfellow, I.J., et al.: Generative adversarial nets. In: NeurIPS, pp. 2672–2680 (2014)
9. Hu, K., et al.: Retinal vessel segmentation of color fundus images using multi-scale convolutional neural network with an improved cross-entropy loss function. Neurocomputing **309**, 179–191 (2018)
10. Iizuka, S., Simo-Serra, E., Ishikawa, H.: Globally and locally consistent image completion. ACM Trans. Graph. (ToG) **36**(4), 1–14 (2017)
11. Kitaev, N., Kaiser, L., Levskaya, A.: Reformer: the efficient transformer. In: ICLR (2020)
12. Kovács, G., Hajdu, A.: A self-calibrating approach for the segmentation of retinal vessels by template matching and contour reconstruction. Med. Image Anal. **29**, 24–46 (2016)
13. Kumar, S., Moni, R., Rajeesh, J.: Automatic liver and lesion segmentation: a primary step in diagnosis of liver diseases. SIViP **7**(1), 163–172 (2013). https://doi.org/10.1007/s11760-011-0223-y
14. Long, J., Shelhamer, E., Darrell, T.: Fully convolutional networks for semantic segmentation. In: Proceedings of the IEEE Conference on Computer Vision and Pattern Recognition, pp. 3431–3440 (2015)
15. Moghimirad, E., Rezatofighi, S.H., Soltanian-Zadeh, H.: Retinal vessel segmentation using a multi-scale medialness function. Comput. Biol. Med. **42**(1), 50–60 (2012)
16. Noh, K.J., Park, S.J., Lee, S.: Scale-space approximated convolutional neural networks for retinal vessel segmentation. Comput. Methods Programs Biomed. **178**, 237–246 (2019)
17. Owen, C.G., et al.: Measuring retinal vessel tortuosity in 10-year-old children: validation of the computer-assisted image analysis of the retina (CAIAR) program. Invest. Ophthal. Vis. Sci. **50**(5), 2004–2010 (2009)
18. Palomera-Perez, M.A., Martinez-Perez, M.E., Benitez-Perez, H., Ortega-Arjona, J.L.: Parallel multiscale feature extraction and region growing: application in retinal blood vessel detection. IEEE Trans. Inf. Technol. Biomed. **14**(2), 500–506 (2009)
19. Park, K.B., Choi, S.H., Lee, J.Y.: M-GAN: retinal blood vessel segmentation by balancing losses through stacked deep fully convolutional networks. IEEE Access **8**, 146308–146322 (2020)
20. Radford, A., Metz, L., Chintala, S.: Unsupervised representation learning with deep convolutional generative adversarial networks. In: ICLR (2016)
21. Rahebi, J., Hardalaç, F.: Retinal blood vessel segmentation with neural network by using gray-level co-occurrence matrix-based features. J. Med. Syst. **38**(8), 1–12 (2014). https://doi.org/10.1007/s10916-014-0085-2
22. Rao, H., et al.: A self-supervised gait encoding approach with locality-awareness for 3d skeleton based person re-identification. IEEE Trans. Pattern Anal. Mach. Intell. (2021)
23. Rao, H., Xu, S., Hu, X., Cheng, J., Hu, B.: Augmented skeleton based contrastive action learning with momentum LSTM for unsupervised action recognition. Inf. Sci. **569**, 90–109 (2021)
24. Staal, J., Abràmoff, M.D., Niemeijer, M., Viergever, M.A., Van Ginneken, B.: Ridge-based vessel segmentation in color images of the retina. IEEE Trans. Med. Imaging **23**(4), 501–509 (2004)

25. Tan, W.R., Chan, C.S., Aguirre, H.E., Tanaka, K.: ArtGan: artwork synthesis with conditional categorical GANs. In: ICIP, pp. 3760–3764 (2017)
26. Teng, T., Lefley, M., Claremont, D.: Progress towards automated diabetic ocular screening: a review of image analysis and intelligent systems for diabetic retinopathy. Med. Biol. Eng. Compu. **40**(1), 2–13 (2002). https://doi.org/10.1007/BF02347689
27. Tong, T., Li, G., Liu, X., Gao, Q.: Image super-resolution using dense skip connections. In: ICCV, pp. 4809–4817 (2017)
28. Tulyakov, S., Liu, M., Yang, X., Kautz, J.: Mocogan: Decomposing motion and content for video generation. In: CVPR, pp. 1526–1535 (2018)
29. Wang, P.: Linear attention transformer (2020). https://github.com/lucidrains/linear-attention-transformer
30. Wang, S., Yin, Y., Cao, G., Wei, B., Zheng, Y., Yang, G.: Hierarchical retinal blood vessel segmentation based on feature and ensemble learning. Neurocomputing **149**, 708–717 (2015)
31. Wang, Y., Ji, G., Lin, P., Trucco, E.: Retinal vessel segmentation using multiwavelet kernels and multiscale hierarchical decomposition. Pattern Recogn. **46**(8), 2117–2133 (2013)
32. Wu, C., Zou, Y., Yang, Z.: U-Gan: generative adversarial networks with u-net for retinal vessel segmentation. In: 2019 14th International Conference on Computer Science and Education (ICCSE), pp. 642–646. IEEE (2019)
33. Xu, S., et al.: Attention based multi-level co-occurrence graph convolutional LSTM for 3D action recognition. IEEE Internet Things J. (2020)
34. Yang, T., Wu, T., Li, L., Zhu, C.: SUD-GAN: deep convolution generative adversarial network combined with short connection and dense block for retinal vessel segmentation. J. Digit. Imaging **33**(4), 946–957 (2020). https://doi.org/10.1007/s10278-020-00339-9
35. Yap, M.H., et al.: Automated breast ultrasound lesions detection using convolutional neural networks. IEEE J. Biomed. Health Inform. **22**(4), 1218–1226 (2017)
36. Yin, Y., Adel, M., Bourennane, S.: Retinal vessel segmentation using a probabilistic tracking method. Pattern Recogn. **45**(4), 1235–1244 (2012)
37. Yu, H., Barriga, S., Agurto, C., Zamora, G., Bauman, W., Soliz, P.: Fast vessel segmentation in retinal images using multi-scale enhancement and second-order local entropy. In: Medical imaging 2012: computer-aided diagnosis, vol. 8315, p. 83151B. International Society for Optics and Photonics (2012)
38. Zhang, J., Li, H., Nie, Q., Cheng, L.: A retinal vessel boundary tracking method based on Bayesian theory and multi-scale line detection. Comput. Med. Imaging Graph. **38**(6), 517–525 (2014)
39. Zhang, R., Isola, P., Efros, A.A.: Colorful image colorization. In: Leibe, B., Matas, J., Sebe, N., Welling, M. (eds.) ECCV 2016. LNCS, vol. 9907, pp. 649–666. Springer, Cham (2016). https://doi.org/10.1007/978-3-319-46487-9_40
40. Zhao, Y., Rada, L., Chen, K., Harding, S.P., Zheng, Y.: Automated vessel segmentation using infinite perimeter active contour model with hybrid region information with application to retinal images. IEEE Trans. Med. Imaging **34**(9), 1797–1807 (2015)
41. Zhou, B., Khosla, A., Lapedriza, A., Oliva, A., Torralba, A.: Learning deep features for discriminative localization. In: Proceedings of the IEEE Conference on Computer Vision and Pattern Recognition, pp. 2921–2929 (2016)

Robust Intent Classification Using Bayesian LSTM for Clinical Conversational Agents (CAs)

Haris Aftab(✉), Vibhu Gautam, Richard Hawkins, Rob Alexander, and Ibrahim Habli

Department of Computer Science, University of York, York YO10 5GH, UK
haris.aftab@york.ac.uk

Abstract. Conversational Agents (CAs) are software programs that replicate human conversations using machine learning (ML) and natural language processing (NLP). CAs are currently being utilised for diverse clinical applications such as symptom checking, health monitoring, medical triage and diagnosis. Intent classification (IC) is an essential task of understanding user utterance in CAs which makes use of modern deep learning (DL) methods. Because of the inherent model uncertainty associated with those methods, accuracy alone cannot be relied upon in clinical applications where certain errors may compromise patient safety. In this work, we employ Bayesian Long Short-Term Memory Networks (LSTMs) to calculate model uncertainty for IC, with a specific emphasis on symptom checker CAs. This method provides a certainty measure with IC prediction that can be utilised in assuring safe response from CAs. We evaluated our method on in-distribution (ID) and out-of-distribution (OOD) data and found mean uncertainty to be much higher for OOD data. These findings suggest that our method is robust to OOD utterances and can detect non-understanding errors in CAs.

Keywords: Conversational Agents (CAs) · Machine Learning · Model uncertainty · Out-of-distribution (OOD) · Healthcare · Patient safety

1 Introduction

Conversational Agents (CAs) such as Google Home and Amazon Alexa are interactive conversational systems that use Machine Learning (ML) to respond to the user in natural language via voice or text [1]. They can be categorised into two types: task-oriented CAs [2] and chatbots [3]. In healthcare studies, task-oriented CAs are often utilised as they are focused on achieving a task such as booking a consultation or finding a hospital. Chatbots are systems designed for open-ended conversations and mimic unstructured conversations or chats. Common applications of CAs in healthcare include symptom checking [4], chronic disease management [5], health monitoring and medication adherence [6].

CAs employ a pipeline architecture [7] as shown in Fig. 1. The fundamental components in this architecture are Natural Language Understanding (NLU) and Dialog Manager (DM) which enable their understanding and decision making. The user then

X. Gao et al. (Eds.): MobiHealth 2021, LNICST 440, pp. 106–118, 2022.
https://doi.org/10.1007/978-3-031-06368-8_8

receives the response proposed by DM via the Natural Language Generation (NLG) module. In this pipeline architecture, the NLU maps user utterances to intents and slots and has a significant impact on downstream processing. NLU errors may lead to erroneous decision making [8], which can be costly in healthcare because of the risk to human life and ethical issues [9]. Specifically, the NLU in CAs is concerned with the IC and slot-filling (SF) [7]. IC predicts a user's intent from a given utterance, and it is a classification problem of identifying the correct intent label. SF in NLU extracts additional information needed to accomplish the user's task. For example, a user asking a CA *"show me nearby hospitals"* could have *'show_hospital'* as intent and the current user location as the slot value.

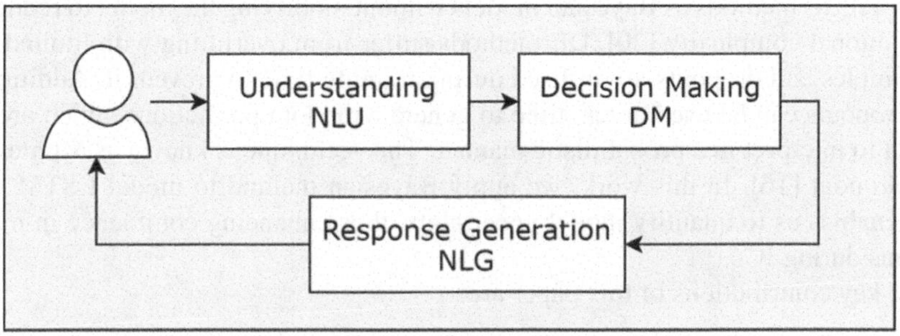

Fig. 1. Conversational Agent (CA) architecture

DL have allowed significant performance enhancements in computer vision and Natural Language Processing (NLP) tasks and their variants such as Recurrent Neural Networks (RNNs) [10, 11] and Long Short-Term Memory Networks (LSTMs) [12] are commonly used for IC in CAs. These networks are able to attain higher accuracy on text classification tasks as they are better suited to model time series data.

Existing state-of-the-art Deep learning (DL) methods are prone to data and model uncertainties [13]. Model uncertainty, also known as epistemic uncertainty, occurs because of the reliance of the model on training data for their prediction. This uncertainty can be reduced by providing enough training data. Estimating model uncertainty is extremely crucial also because of the difficulty to obtain high-quality datasets in healthcare [14]. In addition, it is almost impossible to provide complete data as DL models will always reflect an imperfect representation of the real world [15].

In general, for classification problems, the softmax function is utilised by DL models at the output, resulting in a probability distribution over class labels. The label with the highest probability is then chosen as the prediction. The softmax function calculates relative probabilities between classes but does not provide a measure of the model's uncertainty [16]. The probabilistic nature of softmax output is one of the reasons this score cannot be used as a confidence measure of the model in its prediction. DL models on unseen data tend to make predictions with the high softmax values and thus it is undesirable to use them in safety-critical systems [17].

CAs are vulnerable to failures in understanding user utterance, and non-understanding errors are one of those failures [18]. Non-understanding errors arise when the system is unable to understand user input due to the system's inability to support the requested feature or poorly formatted input. For example, a user asking a COVID symptom checking CA about diabetes symptoms would result in a non-understanding error. Similarly, any unknown or incorrect input would also cause a non-understanding error. A common source of non-understanding errors is out-of-distribution (OOD) data [19]. Non-understanding errors usually result in poor user experience and may not be desirable to have them in safety-critical applications. As described earlier, the way DL models make predictions and are inherently uncertain, the need to detect non-understanding errors is significant in CAs that utilise DL methods.

Bayesian modelling techniques provide a probabilistic representation of model uncertainty but these usually are computationally expensive [16]. It is however possible to interpret DL methods as Bayesian models without modifying the model to reduce this computational complexity [20]. DL methods suffer from overfitting with limited training examples and dropouts are utilised during training time to prevent it. Additionally, these dropouts can be used at test time to generate random predictions which are sampled out to interpret in a probabilistic manner. This technique is known as Monte-Carlo (MC) dropout [16]. In this work, we apply Bayesian method to model LSTM for IC which enables us to quantify model uncertainty, thus enhancing confidence in model's decisions during IC.

The key contributions of this paper are:

1. We utilise Bayesian LSTM with MC dropout for computing uncertainty in IC for CAs.
2. A symptom checking prototype CA is designed to demonstrate the importance of robust IC in CAs and how our method can be utilised for assuring safe response.
3. We evaluate our approach using an OOD evaluation dataset and compare the results to ID data.

2 Related Work

IC methods in CAs range from rule-based to ML approaches, but the state-of-art in IC use DL methods which include RNNs and LSTMs [10, 21]. Westhuizen et al. [22] show the utility of Bayesian LSTMs on medical time series data using MC dropout and concluded their performance enhancements over standard LSTMs. They utilised MC dropout for 100 Bayesian LSTM samples and found that using it during test time enhanced performance on all datasets and provided the added benefit of having a confidence measure alongside the predicted class. Dusenberry et al. [9] investigated several strategies to analyse model uncertainty for electronic health records. In comparison to ensemble RNNs, Bayesian RNNs performed better while only requiring training a single model. These authors concluded that Bayesian RNNs are more efficient, making them better suited for use in medical domain.

Other studies in healthcare involving deep neural networks (DNNs) have employed MC dropout to approximate uncertainty for classification tasks [23, 24]. These, however, make use of image data to estimate uncertainty. This method is also used in other safety-critical domains such as autonomous vehicles (AV), to estimate uncertainty for the AV to make safe decisions such as decelerate to speed limit or brake to stop driving [25].

The use of Bayesian approach, in addition to providing confidence in the decision of the model, enables us to detect non-understanding errors in CAs. As mentioned already, OOD data is one of the sources of these errors. It is critical to correctly identify OOD data in NLU to avoid DM taking an incorrect action [26] which could be catastrophic. Common approaches used for OOD detection rely on a threshold measure, which is subsequently utilised to compute a detection score using various methods. Bayesian models [27], and classifier ensembles [28] are two of these approaches. However, these approaches are computationally expensive, which limits their utility in industrial settings.

Another method for determining OOD detection is to use the highest softmax value as the detection score. However, as recent research has demonstrated [16], the softmax value is not a credible indication of the model's confidence. Other approaches rely on OOD labels with training examples [29], which is not viable since we cannot estimate how many OOD samples are necessary for training a model. A few studies [30, 31] have relied on OOD data creation to boost detection scores. This necessitates the creation of OOD samples for detection and reliance on tagged instances, which is an additional step in OOD detection process.

In [22], MC dropout for classification was utilised using medical data for image and speech datasets. Unlike the work in [22], we employed text data for our classification of medical time series data and analysed the impact of misclassification on patient safety by presenting a use case of symptom checking CA. In addition, we validate our method on an evaluation dataset designed for OOD data [26] which is also used in other studies [31]. We perform a comparison of results of uncertainty estimation between ID and OOD data which is discussed in detail in the Results section.

3 Methods

We employ Bayesian LSTM as part of our RNN architecture for the IC model of NLU. MC dropout [16], which is used at test time is then utilised to evaluate model uncertainty for IC. We designed a use case and implemented a prototype CA that performs symptom checking on medical data. In this use case, we are concerned with how uncertainty estimation in IC in CAs can aid in assuring safe response.

3.1 Bayesian LSTM

Bayesian implementation of LSTM allows us to estimate model uncertainty, which indicates our imperfect understanding of the model's underlying parameters. Dropout at test time allows us to approximate the variational posterior distribution of model parameters (weights and biases). Using random dropout, we can sample different model parameters of this posterior distribution. By introducing a distribution over all model parameters, different functions can be induced. Through the realisation of distinct model parameter values selected from the posterior distribution, these functions lead to varied outcomes. The softmax predictions from each of these sampled parameters are averaged for new data. This allows us to have increased confidence in the softmax prediction. The softmax class prediction is then used to estimate model uncertainty in the form of Shannon entropy [31].

Table 1 shows the architecture of the Bayesian LSTM we utilise for our IC model. We implemented a Bayesian LSTM layer referred to as 'MCLSTM', which allows us to employ the same dropout mask during test time at each time step of recurrent layers of LSTM [20]. A dropout rate of 70% was utilised to estimate model uncertainty. The hyperparameter, dropout, at this percentage produced the best model accuracy and robust model uncertainty. We apply MC dropout after the dense layer allowing us to capture the model uncertainty for the dense layers as well.

Table 1. Recurrent neural network architecture

Layer	Output shape	Parameters
Input Layer	(None, 30)	0
Embedding	(None, 30, 50)	5000000
MCLSTM	(None, 64)	29440
Dense Layer	(None, 256)	16640
Activation	(None, 256)	0
Dropout	(None, 256)	0
Dense Layer	(None, 25)	6425
Activation	(None, 25)	0

3.2 Symptom Checker Use Case

We present a symptom checking CA prototype to highlight the impact of incorrect IC on patient safety and how our method can aid in providing a safe response when the model is uncertain about its prediction. As an example, during the current COVID-19 pandemic, many web and mobile-based applications were developed for the general public to check if they have COVID symptoms [32]. The reliability of the decisions made by these diagnostic systems can not solely rely on their accuracy [9] and this also holds for clinicians making their decisions [33]. From the clinical safety perspective, a calibration of confidence and accuracy is important.

The architecture of our prototype CA is shown in Fig. 2. The input text utterance is provided by the user, which is handled by the NLU and IC is performed using Bayesian LSTM. In the case where the NLU is not certain about the prediction, a safe strategy (asking the user to rephrase or connecting the user to a human clinician) can be utilised before the NLU result is passed to the DM.

We utilise an open-source dataset [34] to train our Bayesian LSTM model for understanding. The dataset contains 6661 text utterances of common medical symptoms like "knee pain", or "headache". The dataset contains 25 distinct intents which are evenly distributed across the dataset as shown in Fig. 3. We pre-process the dataset by performing case normalization and removing punctuations and white spaces. After the pre-processing step, the utterances are padded to be of equal length. To use the data, we

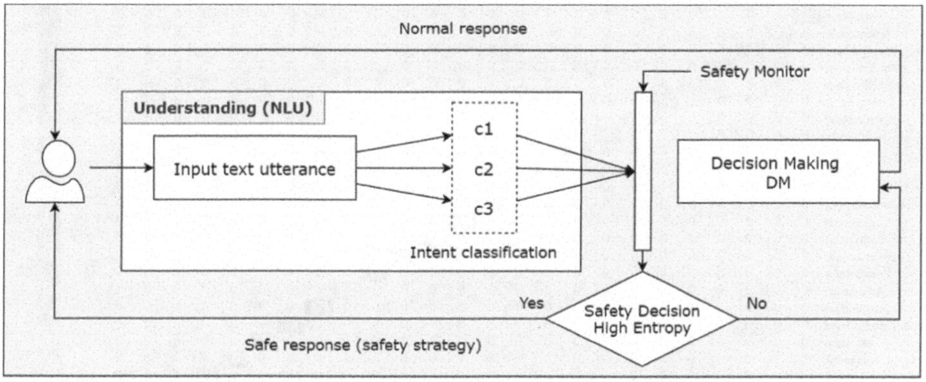

Fig. 2. Symptom checker use case CA architecture diagram

then transform the text utterances to numerical data using one-hot encoding scheme. We use an 85:15 ratio to split the dataset into training and testing, which turns our training size to 5661 and the test size to 1000 utterances.

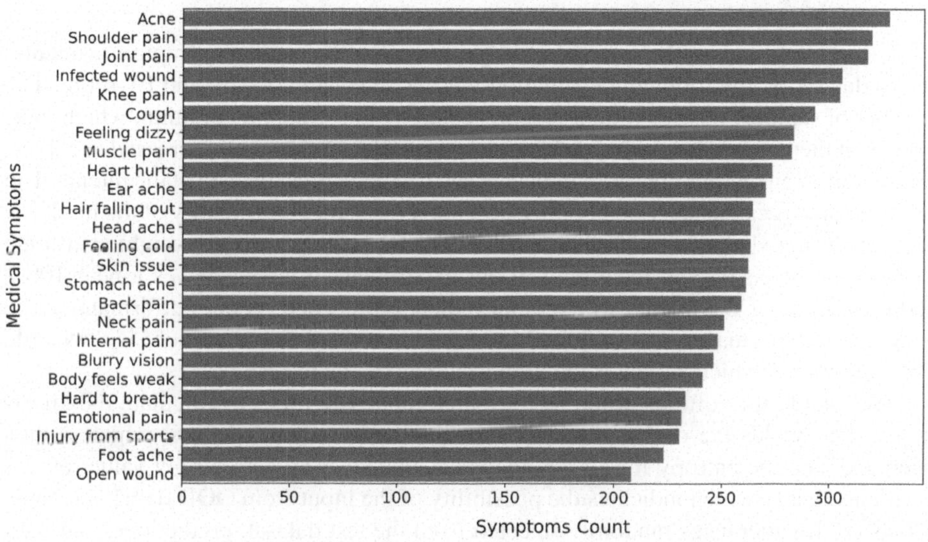

Fig. 3. The distribution of medical symptoms in the dataset

4 Results

Our model utilising Bayesian LSTM achieved an accuracy of 99.4% on the test dataset. Figure 4 shows the confusion matrix which reflects the model's high accuracy. The y-axis lists the actual symptoms, and the x-axis lists the predicted symptoms by the model. Due to the higher accuracy, there are very few misclassifications by the model.

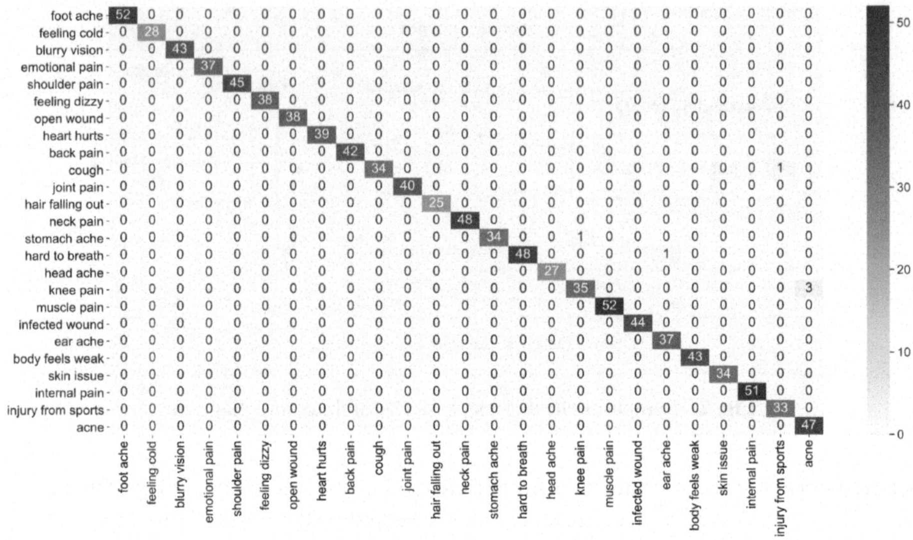

Fig. 4. Confusion matrix of symptoms classification

Table 2 summarises the average findings for each of the medical symptoms (intents) in the dataset by the following evaluation metrics: precision, recall, and F1-score. The number of samples for each intent is represented by the "Support" column, which indicates that there is no class imbalance in the test set. Because of their increased accuracy, these evaluation metrics appear to indicate near-perfect scores for each of the intents. The precision and recall usually do not provide a good measure of the quality of the model as they can be high because of class imbalance. The F1-score provides a weighted average of both the precision and recall and in our experiment, it also achieves a near 100% score for most of the intents which is an indication of good model performance. The average metrics (macro and weighted average) scores indicate that there is very little class imbalance which validates the high accuracy on the test set.

We sample the softmax value for the same input 100 times to calculate the uncertainty. This yields the output posterior distribution for softmax values, which is then averaged, and the entropy for all outputs is calculated. A higher entropy value reflects high uncertainty which indicates the possibility of the input from OOD data [31]. Table 3 lists the ID utterances randomly selected from the test dataset, predictions, and their entropy calculations. The model correctly predicts all the utterances which is due to the higher model accuracy and ID nature of utterances.

Table 2. Average evaluation metrics for medical symptoms

Medical symptoms	Precision	Recall	F1-Score	Support
Acne	1.000	1.000	1.000	52
Back pain	1.000	1.000	1.000	28
Blurry vision	1.000	1.000	1.000	43
Body feels weak	1.000	1.000	1.000	37
Cough	1.000	1.000	1.000	45
Ear ache	1.000	1.000	1.000	38
Emotional pain	1.000	1.000	1.000	38
Feeling cold	1.000	1.000	1.000	39
Feeling dizzy	1.000	1.000	1.000	42
Foot ache	0.971	1.000	0.986	34
Hair falling out	1.000	1.000	1.000	40
Hard to breath	1.000	1.000	1.000	25
Head ache	1.000	1.000	1.000	48
Heart hurts	0.971	1.000	0.986	34
Infected wound	0.980	1.000	0.990	48
Injury from sports	1.000	1.000	1.000	27
Internal pain	0.921	0.972	0.946	36
Joint pain	1.000	1.000	1.000	52
Knee pain	1.000	1.000	1.000	44
Muscle pain	1.000	0.974	0.987	38
Neck pain	1.000	1.000	1.000	43
Open wound	1.000	1.000	1.000	34
Shoulder pain	1.000	1.000	1.000	51
Skin issue	1.000	0.971	0.985	34
Stomach ache	1.000	0.940	0.969	50
Accuracy	0.994	0.994	0.994	0.994
Macro avg	0.994	0.994	0.994	1000
Weighted avg	0.994	0.994	0.994	1000

Table 3. Uncertainty estimation for in-distribution (ID) utterances

Test Utterance (ID)	Prediction	Entropy
My head is so heavy cant think normally	Head ache	0.029
I feel a burning sensation in my shoulder muscle	Muscle pain	0.055
I can hardly breathe	Hard to breath	0.071
I have internal pain whenever I come down with a cold	Internal pain	0.327
When I'm awake in the morning I feel strange and have vertigo	Feeling dizzy	0.507

Table 4. Uncertainty estimation for out of distribution (OOD) utterances

Test Utterance (OOD)	Prediction	Entropy
Am I connected to wifi	Feeling cold	1.057
How much time do I have left on my 0 apr	Shoulder pain	1.110
What casino game has the best odds	Injury from sports	1.862
Please alert me when my iphone battery falls below 30	Neck pain	2.134
What is the warranty on my microwave	Skin issue	2.302

Table 4 shows the five random utterances from OOD dataset [26] with model prediction and entropy calculations. This dataset contains 1000 utterances for evaluation purpose and differs from the dataset on which the IC model is trained. As shown in Fig. 5, the mean entropy for this OOD dataset for an identical number of samples is 2.025 which is substantially higher than the mean entropy of 0.098 for ID utterances. This demonstrates that our method can be utilised to detect non-understanding errors as well as to help assure the safety of CA response in the wake of uncertainty from DL models.

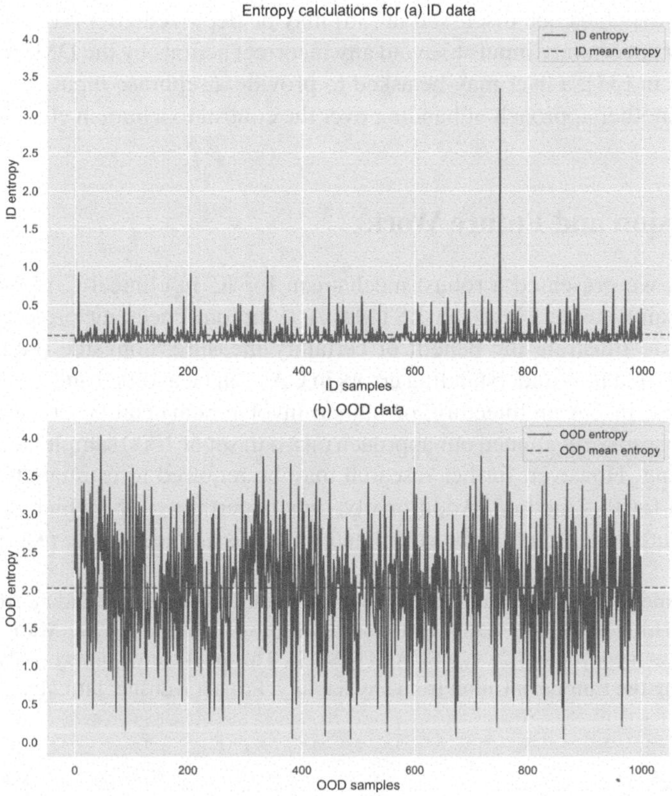

Fig. 5. Entropy calculations for ID (top) and OOD (bottom) data

5 Discussion

Our model based on Bayesian LSTM yielded high accuracy of 99.4% on the test dataset. The training dataset examples contained low class imbalance and we applied dropout during training to improve model performance. The use of MC dropout at test time enabled us to sample multiple outputs and we calculated entropy by averaging out 100 samples from this distribution. It is worth noting that the classifier in this case even having near 100% accuracy cannot be trusted from their prediction alone which we discussed earlier. As seen in Table 4, for all OOD utterances the prediction was incorrect with high uncertainty. The average model entropy for ID data (test dataset) was much lower than the average entropy for OOD data with the same number (1000) of examples. It is yet to be seen if this pattern continues for a very large number of OOD data.

The state-of-art in CAs rely on DL methods [10] which are prone to uncertainties in their decisions [35]. In healthcare, instead of making wrong predictions, these models should be able to say "sorry, I don't know" when they are uncertain. From our findings on OOD of relatively small size (1000 samples), the entropy measure can be utilised to know when a model is uncertain in its decision. We present a use case of symptom checking where this method during IC can be useful for providing a safe response. A safety monitor such as one discussed in [36] may be deployed after NLU output which can filter high uncertainty inputs to avoid any incorrect actions by the DM. Alternatively, as mentioned in [37], a user may be asked to provide a rephrase input. In case of high uncertainty, another approach of handing over the control to a human clinician may also be used [38].

6 Conclusion and Future Work

In this paper, we presented a robust mechanism for IC in clinical CAs by measuring model uncertainty using Bayesian LSTMs. A symptom checking prototype CA was implemented to illustrate the benefit of certainty measure alongside prediction. This method shows that non-understanding errors in CAs can be avoided and a safety strategy (safety monitor in CA architecture, or human involvement) can be utilised to prevent unsafe responses. We evaluated our approach on a dataset of 1000 samples and the results were promising. However, further research may be required to estimate the minimum data required for this method. Additionally, data uncertainty [35] which occurs due to noise in the data may require to be calculated for the assurance of safe response in CAs.

Acknowledgements. The research leading to these results has received funding from the European Union's Horizon 2020 research and innovation programme under the Marie Skłodowska Curie grant agreement No 812.788 (MSCAETN SAS). This publication reflects only the authors' view, exempting the European Union from any liability. Project website: http://etn-sas.eu/.

References

1. Laranjo, L., et al.: Conversational agents in healthcare: a systematic review. J. Am. Med. Inform. Assoc. **25**, 1248–1258 (2018)
2. Gao, J., Galley, M., Li, L.: Neural approaches to conversational AI. In: The 41st International ACM SIGIR Conference on Research & Development in Information Retrieval, pp. 1371–1374 (2018)
3. Harms, J.-G., Kucherbaev, P., Bozzon, A., Houben, G.-J.: Approaches for dialog management in conversational agents. IEEE Internet Comput. **23**, 13–22 (2018)
4. Razzaki, S., et al.: A comparative study of artificial intelligence and human doctors for the purpose of triage and diagnosis, pp. 1–15 (2018)
5. Allen, J., et al.: Chester: towards a personal medication advisor. J. Biomed. Inform. **39**, 500–513 (2006)
6. Fadhil, A.: A conversational interface to improve medication adherence: towards AI support in patient's treatment (2018)
7. Zhang, Z., Takanobu, R., Zhu, Q., Huang, M., Zhu, X.: Recent advances and challenges in task-oriented dialog systems. Sci. China Technol. Sci. **63**(10), 2011–2027 (2020). https://doi.org/10.1007/s11431-020-1692-3
8. Li, X., Chen, Y.-N., Li, L., Gao, J., Celikyilmaz, A.: Investigation of language understanding impact for reinforcement learning based dialogue systems. arXiv Preprint arXiv:1703.07055 (2017)
9. Dusenberry, M.W., et al.: Analyzing the role of model uncertainty for electronic health records. In: Proceedings of the ACM Conference on Health, Inference, and Learning, pp. 204–213 (2020)

10. Louvan, S., Magnini, B.: Recent neural methods on slot filling and intent classification for task-oriented dialogue systems: a survey. arXiv Preprint arXiv:2011.00564 (2020)
11. Yao, K., Zweig, G., Hwang, M.-Y., Shi, Y., Yu, D.: Recurrent neural networks for language understanding. In: Interspeech, pp. 2524–2528 (2013)
12. Yao, K., Peng, B., Zhang, Y., Yu, D., Zweig, G., Shi, Y.: Spoken language understanding using long short-term memory neural networks. In: 2014 IEEE Spoken Language Technology Workshop (SLT), pp. 189–194. IEEE (2014)
13. Gal, Y.: Uncertainty in Deep Learning, 1, 4. University of Cambridge (2016)
14. Challen, R., Denny, J., Pitt, M., Gompels, L., Edwards, T., Tsaneva-Atanasova, K.: Artificial intelligence, bias and clinical safety. BMJ Qual. Saf. **28**, 231–237 (2019)
15. Gauerhof, L., Munk, P., Burton, S.: Structuring validation targets of a machine learning function applied to automated driving. In: Gallina, B., Skavhaug, A., Bitsch, F. (eds.) SAFECOMP 2018. LNCS, vol. 11093, pp. 45–58. Springer, Cham (2018). https://doi.org/10.1007/978-3-319-99130-6_4
16. Gal, Y., Ghahramani, Z.: Dropout as a Bayesian approximation: representing model uncertainty in deep learning. In: International Conference on Machine Learning, pp. 1050–1059. PMLR (2016)
17. Vasudevan, V.T., Sethy, A., Ghias, A.R.: Towards better confidence estimation for neural models. In: 2019 IEEE International Conference on Acoustics, Speech and Signal Processing (ICASSP), ICASSP 2019, pp. 7335–7339. IEEE (2019)
18. Bohus, D., Rudnicky, A.I.: Sorry and I didn't catch that!-an investigation of non-understanding errors and recovery strategies. In: Dybkjær, L., Minker, W. (eds.) Recent Trends in Discourse and Dialogue, vol. 39, pp. 128–143. Springer, Dordrecht (2008). https://doi.org/10.1007/978-1-4020-6821-8_6
19. Aftab, H., Shah, S.H.H., Habli, I.: Classification of failures in the perception of conversational agents (CAs) and their implications on patient safety. Stud. Health Technol. Inform. **281**, 659–663 (2021)
20. Gal, Y., Ghahramani, Z.: A theoretically grounded application of dropout in recurrent neural networks. In: Advances in Neural Information Processing Systems, vol. 29, pp. 1019–1027 (2016)
21. Zhang, L., Zhang, L.: An ensemble deep active learning method for intent classification. In: Proceedings of the 2019 3rd International Conference on Computer Science and Artificial Intelligence, pp. 107–111 (2019)
22. van der Westhuizen, J., Lasenby, J.: Bayesian LSTMs in medicine. arXiv Preprint arXiv:1706.01242 (2017)
23. Camarasa, R., et al.: Quantitative comparison of Monte-Carlo dropout uncertainty measures for multi-class segmentation. In: Sudre, C.H., et al. (eds.) UNSURE/GRAIL 2020. LNCS, vol. 12443, pp. 32–41. Springer, Cham (2020). https://doi.org/10.1007/978-3-030-60365-6_4
24. Ghoshal, B., Tucker, A., Sanghera, B., Wong, W.L.: Estimating uncertainty in deep learning for reporting confidence to clinicians when segmenting nuclei image data. In: 2019 IEEE 32nd International Symposium on Computer-Based Medical Systems (CBMS), pp. 318–324. IEEE (2019)
25. Gautam, V., Gheraibia, Y., Alexander, R., Hawkins, R.D.: Runtime decision making under uncertainty in autonomous vehicles. In: Proceedings of the Workshop on Artificial Intelligence Safety (SafeAI 2021). CEUR Workshop Proceedings (2021)
26. Larson, S., et al.: An evaluation dataset for intent classification and out-of-scope prediction. arXiv Preprint arXiv:1909.02027 (2019)
27. Malinin, A., Gales, M.: Predictive uncertainty estimation via prior networks. Adv. Neural Inf. Process. Syst. **31**, 7047–7058 (2018)

28. Vyas, A., Jammalamadaka, N., Zhu, X., Das, D., Kaul, B., Willke, T.L.: Out-of-distribution detection using an ensemble of self supervised leave-out classifiers. In: Ferrari, V., Hebert, M., Sminchisescu, C., Weiss, Y. (eds.) ECCV 2018. LNCS, vol. 11212, pp. 560–574. Springer, Cham (2018). https://doi.org/10.1007/978-3-030-01237-3_34
29. Kim, J.-K., Kim, Y.-B.: Joint learning of domain classification and out-of-domain detection with dynamic class weighting for satisficing false acceptance rates. arXiv Preprint arXiv: 1807.00072 (2018)
30. Bowman, S.R., Vilnis, L., Vinyals, O., Dai, A.M., Jozefowicz, R., Bengio, S.: Generating sentences from a continuous space. arXiv Preprint arXiv:1511.06349 (2015)
31. Zheng, Y., Chen, G., Huang, M.: Out-of-domain detection for natural language understanding in dialog systems. IEEE/ACM Trans. Audio Speech Lang. Process. **28**, 1198–1209 (2020)
32. Munsch, N., et al.: Diagnostic accuracy of web-based COVID-19 symptom checkers: comparison study. J. Med. Internet Res. **22**, e21299 (2020)
33. Zwaan, L., Hautz, W.E.: Bridging the gap between uncertainty, confidence and diagnostic accuracy: calibration is key (2019)
34. Mooney, P.: Medical Speech, Transcription, and Intent. https://www.kaggle.com/paultimothymooney/medical-speech-transcription-and-intent. Accessed 20 Apr 2021
35. Kendall, A., Gal, Y.: What uncertainties do we need in bayesian deep learning for computer vision? Adv. Neural Inf. Process. Syst. **30** (2017)
36. Machin, M., Guiochet, J., Waeselynck, H., Blanquart, J.P., Roy, M., Masson, L.: SMOF: a safety monitoring framework for autonomous systems. IEEE Trans. Syst. Man Cybern. Syst. **48**, 702–715 (2018)
37. Bickmore, T., Trinh, H., Asadi, R., Olafsson, S.: Safety first: conversational agents for health care. In: Moore, R.J., Szymanski, M.H., Arar, R., Ren, G.-J. (eds.) Studies in Conversational UX Design. HIS, pp. 33–57. Springer, Cham (2018). https://doi.org/10.1007/978-3-319-95579-7_3
38. Sujan, M., et al.: Human factors challenges for the safe use of artificial intelligence in patient care. BMJ Health Care Inform. **26** (2019)

Biomedical and Health Informatics

Me in the Wild: An Exploratory Study Using Smartphones to Detect the Onset of Depression

Kennedy Opoku Asare[1(✉)], Aku Visuri[1], Julio Vega[2], and Denzil Ferreira[1]

[1] Center for Ubiquitous Computing, University of Oulu, Oulu, Finland
{kennedy.opokuasare,aku.visuri,denzil.ferreira}@oulu.fi

[2] Department of Medicine, University of Pittsburgh, Pittsburgh, PA, USA
vegaju@upmc.edu

Abstract. Research on mobile sensing for mental health monitoring has traditionally explored the correlation between smartphone and wearable data with self-reported mental health symptom severity assessments. The effectiveness of predictive techniques to monitor depression is limited, given the idiosyncratic nature of depression symptoms and the limited availability of objectively labelled depression sensor-driven behaviour. In this paper, we investigate the possibility of using unsupervised anomaly detection methods to monitor the fluctuations of mental health and its severity. Informed by literature, we created a mobile application that collects acknowledged data streams that can be indicative of depression. We recruited 11 participants for a 1-month field study. More specifically, we monitored participants' mobility, overall smartphone interactions, and surrounding ambient noise. The participants provided three self-reports: Big five personality traits, sleep and depression. Our results suggest that digital markers, combined with anomaly detection methods are useful to flag changes in human behaviour over time; thus, enabling mobile just-in-time interventions for in-the-wild assistance.

Keywords: Mobile sensing · Mental health · Depression · Anomaly detection

1 Introduction

Today, depression is one of the most prevalent mental disorders. The World Health Organisation (WHO) reports that depression affects 300 million people globally [81]. Individuals afflicted with depression can experience recurrent episodes of sadness, feelings of worthlessness, suicidal ideation, fatigue, sleep disturbance, loss of appetite, cognitive impairments, and are prone to social and physical isolation [55,60,79]. Depression is also known to worsen the outcomes of many medical disorders such as Parkinson's Disease [34], heart failure [51], Alzheimer's Disease and stroke [73]. Depression does not only negatively affect

X. Gao et al. (Eds.): MobiHealth 2021, LNICST 440, pp. 121–145, 2022.
https://doi.org/10.1007/978-3-031-06368-8_9

individuals, but to an extent, those around them also. WHO projects that by 2030 [46], depression will be the single most significant contributor to the global disease burden. In the US alone, the long-term medical care and lost productivity costs add to more than USD 210 billion [31].

Depression is treatable with effective medication and non-pharmaceutical treatments like cognitive behaviour therapy. The challenge, however, is that depression afflicted individuals mostly live unaware or misdiagnosed due to barriers such as social stigma and the scarcity of objective assessment methods. There is the need to extend current clinical diagnosis tools for depression with objective data collected in-the-wild, continuously, and as effortlessly as possible. For the past 30 years, the gold standard for the clinical diagnosis of depression has not changed [24,79] and is based on subjective (self-reported) assessments such as the Patient Health Questionnaire (PHQ-9) [44], Beck Depression Inventory (BDI) [4], and Hamilton Depression Scale (HAMD) [32]. Thresholds are applied to these instruments' scores to classify the severity of depression for each individual. However, the reliability of current clinical diagnosis methods of depression is debated [24,45], mainly owing to their subjectivity, and in some cases, because they were derived from clinical consensus with limited empirical evidence [25]. Lastly, these methods are often employed only a couple of times a year in a controlled laboratory or office setting as they require a professionally trained clinician.

Today, smartphone and wearable devices have become part of our everyday lives, and we can better understand people with them [63,70,78]. Instrumenting smartphones, wearable devices such as Fitbit, and smartwatches with sensor logging software [21,45] have made it possible to passively and unobtrusively collect granular, moment by moment and in-situ datasets outside laboratory confinement. In addition, instrumenting smartphones and wearable devices provide an opportunity to actively collect subjective and self-reported data through the Experience Sampling Method - (ESM) [6,70], instead of paper and pencil diaries or retrospective recollection. Inherent in these time series datasets are human behavioural patterns, i.e., digital biomarkers that are essential in developing interventions for mental health [60,64,70,79].

2 Study Objective

The main objective of this exploratory study is to investigate the feasibility of identifying out of the ordinary human behaviours to enable early detection and monitoring of depression. More specifically, we investigate the feasibility of detecting out of the ordinary behaviours, deterioration of everyday routines, social interactions and mobility, from small datasets of digital biomarkers captured via a smartphone application, using multivariate unsupervised anomaly detection methods. Anomaly detection methods [28] find irregular or nonconforming patterns (outliers) in time series behavioural data, and have been explored in predicting schizophrenia relapses [2,3], abnormal behaviour of the elderly in Smart Homes [50] and detecting depression in imbalanced datasets [26].

The anomaly detection approach differs from predictive analysis, which requires substantial ground truth data for accurate predictions [62,69]. We hypothesise that anomaly detection could be more suited for detecting the early onset and monitoring of depression, given the complex and dynamic nature of depression, the heterogeneity of depression symptoms between individuals [24], and the scarcity of objectively labelled behavioural datasets for depression.

Towards achieving the study objective, we developed an android-based sensing application for smartphones, to passively and unobtrusively collect smartphone sensor data and self-reported surveys. With this application, we collected in-the-wild behavioural data from 11 participants for 4 weeks. We analysed the data to probe deeper into anomalous human behaviours with an ensemble of multivariate anomaly detection algorithms and report our insights into the relationship between the observed anomalous behaviour and depression symptoms.

3 Related Work

Smartphones and wearables (e.g. smartwatches, rings, bracelets) are increasingly accessible to the wider population. These devices are bundled with several sensors to collect and monitor different human activities and their related physiological signals, such as heart rate, sleep quality, body temperature, among others [63]. Lastly and more importantly, most of such devices are, directly or indirectly, connected online [56]. This combination of conditions offers an unprecedented opportunity for a real-time, in-situ understanding of the users' context [22]. The highly personal nature of these devices has driven researchers' interest in investigating the role of Digital Phenotypes/Biomarkers (DPB) in monitoring human behaviour and health conditions [16]. In medicine, phenotypes/biomarkers are physiological, pathological, or anatomical characteristics that are objectively measured and evaluated as an indicator of normal biological, pathological processes or biological responses to therapeutic interventions [12]. Here, we consider a DPB as a multimodal sensory metric, i.e., the outcome of a data analysis that can be compared and measured across individuals using the same combination of data sources.

There are two primary approaches to develop DPBs, e.g., [39]: *active data collection* if a participant is prompted to perform a measurement or provide input (e.g., diaries, self-reports, Experience Sampling Method [6,70]); and *passive data collection* if measurements occur without users' intervention or input (e.g., wrist-worn devices provide estimates of daily steps and calories autonomously, smartphones' sensor data). Active and passive approaches are collected in tandem to correlate the data points, where the source of active data collection is regarded as the ground truth for psychological and subjective measures [56].

For example, in Alzheimer's disease, there is evidence that cognitive, sensory and motor changes occur 10–15 years before their effective diagnosis by a professional with traditional neuropsychological tests [43]. Dexterity and cognitive tasks' performance have been successfully used to monitor cognitive function decline (e.g., working memory, memory, executive function, language) [14].

Parkinson's clinical scales and self-reporting of symptoms also correlated well with smartphone-based sensing: device interactions, motor activities such as going up or downstairs, gait (using smartphone's accelerometer, barometer) and social interaction (e.g., amount of texts and calls) [77]. Actigraphy (i.e., monitoring time sequences of activity vs rest) is useful to predict symptom changes in mood disorders such as bipolar and major depressive behaviour [40]. Geolocation-based digital biomarkers such as distance travelled, the number of locations visited, time spent on location was strongly associated with bipolar disorder and schizophrenia [23,57]. Game-based digital biomarkers such as performance data reflecting cognitive and motor processing and social context such as where, when and with whom a game takes place could predict mental health [54]. More related to our work, in depression symptoms, mobility features such as location variance correlate with depression symptom severity determined by questionnaires such as the PHQ-9 [65].

4 Experiment

4.1 Data Logging Software

We developed an Android-based smartphone sensing application, Me. As a feasibility study and not an intervention study, we aimed at a simple interface and architecture to collect relevant data to explore the use of anomaly detection-based analysis methods to identify potential digital biomarkers for depression.

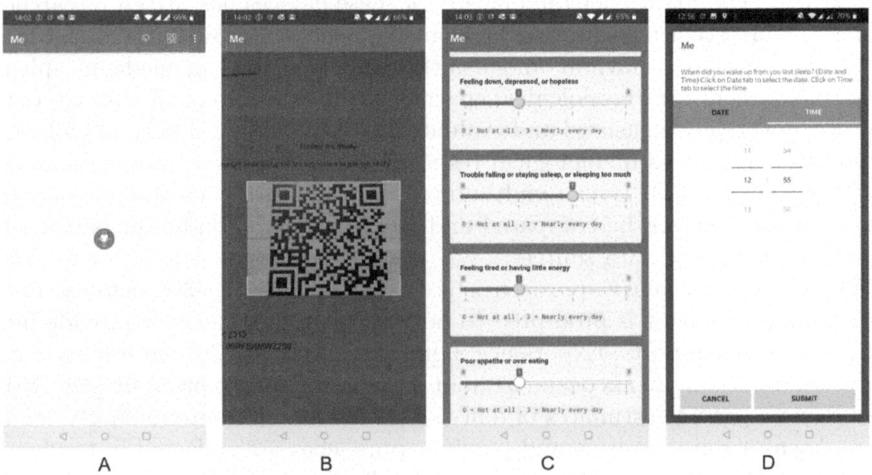

Fig. 1. Four screenshots (A, B, C, D) of the Me application. A is the home screen, B is the QRCode scanner, C and D are screens of self-reported questionnaires.

Smartphone Sensing Application and Online Data Storage: Our application, Me, is compatible with Android 7.0 and above. The application was created using the AWARE Framework [21] Android library. Figure 1 shows different views of Me. Figure 1 A is the initial screen with two top-right menu icons: *on-demand data sync* and a QR-Code scanner. By scanning a study-specific QR Code, as seen in Fig. 1 B, Me connects to the *Online Data Storage*, i.e., our study database, which is a MySQL server instance running on an Amazon EC2 with encryption enabled. All data collected with Me is primarily stored locally on the device. A background data sync service sends the data over a secure encrypted connection to the study's *Online Data Storage* at 30-minute intervals. In other words, the data transmission to the *Online Data Storage* is encrypted with HTTPS. Alternatively, the data sync can be initiated on-demand by tapping on the *on-demand data sync* menu icon. Me also prompts participants to complete scheduled self-reported surveys at specific times using a notification. Participants can click on this notification to open the survey, as shown in Fig. 1 (C and D).

Study Management and Data Analysis: The Study Management dashboard was developed using R Shiny and is used for compliance and data quality monitoring of our participants. The dashboard automatically updates every five minutes with visualisations, including the last time each sensor or survey data was received from each participant. We also developed the *Data Analysis Pipeline* using the R programming language for data pre-processing, visualisation and analysis pipeline for mobile sensing and behavioural analysis.

Data Description and Data Privacy: Me passively collect smartphone sensor data, in addition to self-reported surveys. Based on existing literature [45,64,65,79], several potential digital biomarkers were implemented to detect and monitor mental health. Table 1 details the sensor data that Me collects. In addition to the passively sensed data, Me has built-in self-reported questionnaires for sleep duration, personality traits using the 50-item Big Five personality trait questionnaire [27], and depression assessment using the PHQ-9 [44].

Me inherits AWARE frameworks' privacy-aware features [21]. The study application does not collect any personally identifiable information or sensitive data such as the content of texts, phone calls, visited websites and notifications. We only log metadata such as the time a text was received, the state of the phone screen, i.e., locked or unlocked at a given time. For calls and texts, we anonymise the identity, i.e., *phone number and name* of the other party, into a single alphanumeric trace value, using a one-way SHA-1 hash, on the participant's device. With the one-way SHA-1 hashing method, we retain the same trace value for the same contact and prevent anyone from re-identifying the communicating party. Likewise, Me does not store the actual characters typed using the phone's keyboard, but rather package name, timestamp, and the masked text before and after each keystroke. Text masking is done by replacing all uppercase characters with the letter 'A', lower case characters with the letter 'a', and digits (0,1, ..., 9) with the digit '1'. Finally, the data collected is not tagged with any personally identifiable labels such as name or email. For each new installation of Me on a smartphone, a Universally Unique Identifier (UUID) is randomly

Table 1. A summary of the description, frequency of the data collected with the Me. Each data point is timestamped with the time of the sampling or event.

Sensor data	Frequency	Sensor data description
GPS location	5 min	Latitude, Longitude coordinates
Physical activity		Walking, Running, Biking, and In-Vehicle
Light		Intensity of ambient light
Noise	3-s sample every 5 min	Intensity of ambient noise
Screen	Event-based	Screen locks, unlocks
Touch		Touch interaction type(tap, long tap, scroll)
Battery		Battery level changes, battery charges and discharges
Application		Name of applications that are launched
Notifications		Name of the application that triggered the notification
Calls		Call type (incoming, outgoing, missed), trace of caller
Messages		Message type (received, sent), trace of sender
Keyboard		Masked text before and masked text after a keystroke
Timezone		Device's timezone
Self reports	Frequency	Description
BIG-5	1 per participant at the beginning of the study	50 item personality trait questionnaire
Sleep	1 per day in the morning	Start and end date and time of sleep session
PHQ-9	Beginning of the study and 1 per week	9 item depression test questionnaire

generated on the participant's device and used as the sole identifier of the data from a specific smartphone; thus, all sensor data entries are tagged with this UUID. This UUID is reset if the participant removes and re-installs the app to avoid cross-study matching.

4.2 Recruitment

We conducted a call for participation using a campuswide mailing list, in addition to posting advertisement posters on various faculty and student notice boards. The advertisement had URLs to the study information website that contained a detailed explanation of the purpose of the study, duration, the data collected, participant requirements to be eligible to join the study, and the reward participants would receive after completing the study - a 50 Euro Amazon voucher. A total of 11 participants joined the study, six female and five male, with ages ranging from 19 to 37 years (*Mean: 26.55, Median: 25, SD: 6.02*). Six were undergraduates, three graduate students, and two vocational students. Six out of eleven participants reported a history of clinical diagnosis with depression, anxiety, and other related mental disorders. All participants used a smartphone with Android 8.0 or higher as their primary device. We followed all ethical procedures required by our institution. According to the local ethical board guidelines [75] in the conduct of research, our study is compliant: 1) the study does not deviate from the informed consent; 2) the research does not intervene in the physical integrity of the participants; 3) all our participants are above 15 years old; 4) our study does not expose participants to strong stimuli; 5) there is no intervention, nor there is a foreseeable potential for mental harm to the participants that exceed the limits of participants' normal daily life or those around them.

4.3 Study Protocol

We conducted a 4 weeks study with three stages: *Onboarding*, *Data Collection and Monitoring*, and *Post Study Debriefing and Exit.*

Onboarding: To avoid cross-participant interaction and bias, we invited each participant to a private meeting. At the meeting, we explained the study's purpose, data collection schedule, their right to quit the study at any time and get their data deleted, and the reward for participation. Afterwards, we asked participants to sign a Consent Form and provide their basic demographic information. We then installed the Me application on their Android-based smartphone, and with a short tutorial, we instructed participants how to fill in the study's surveys visible within the app. We showed the participants a snapshot of the actual data that is collected with the application. We configured the Me to bypass the battery optimisation (Doze) feature of the Android OS. This configuration is to allow the Me to run continuously in the background without interference. Next, using Me, the participant joined the study by scanning the enrolment QR Code. Lastly, participants were then asked to fill the baseline questionnaires, that is, the BIG Five personality traits [27] and PHQ-9 [44], also collected in-app. The onboarding meeting took approximately 30 min.

Data Collection and Monitoring: Me (see Fig. 1 A) does not present any visualisations, i.e. feedback to the participants during the data collection period, as we do not want to intervene or influence participant behaviour at this stage. We designed Me to prompt participants with notifications when self-reported surveys are due. However, answering ESMs in longitudinal studies poses a considerable burden for participants [6] mainly because the received EMS prompts may be triggered at inopportune moments, or the prompts may go unnoticed, especially when the device contains numerous notifications pending from other applications. To mitigate these challenges and ensure compliance, we monitor the study using the *Study Management* dashboard. When we observed gaps in the data collected, for instance, because the participant phone is not syncing data to the online study database, the ESM surveys were not answered, or the GPS sensor was turned off, we proactively contacted participants with recommended actions over the phone or by email.

Post Study Debriefing and Exit: During this last stage, we again invited each participant individually for a debriefing meeting. The goal of the debriefing was not to present to the participant an opinion on whether they are depressed or otherwise. This goal was made clear to the participants, and we strictly avoided discussing the participant's depressive state. The goal of the debriefing was to assess with participants whether our algorithms could detect out of the ordinary events that are familiar to participants. At this meeting, we presented participants with statistics and visualisations of out of the ordinary events flagged by our algorithm. Figure 2 shows an example of such visualisation. With a semi-structured interview, we discussed the statistics and visualisations and collected participant's reflections and feedback on the Me application deployment during the study. Finally, we performed a last manual data sync to complete the dataset and uninstalled Me.

5 Analysis Protocol

5.1 Behavioural Analysis

Smartphones are a powerful behavioural observation tool in psychological science [33]. With a focus on finding behaviour indicative of depression, we explore smartphones' sensor data that capture the following behaviours: mobility patterns, daily activities, social interactions [57,59]. Concretely, we investigate how much a participant transit during the day. This analysis provides an overview of mobility, outdoor activities (location accuracy is significantly better for outdoor locations) and the likelihood of social interactions without necessarily exposing visited locations. We also investigate the most used applications (top-10), allowing us to understand whether a participant is socially interacting non-physically and whether sports, music, browsing the internet play a role in someone's daily activities. Lastly, we look into the screen usage length to understand how engaged the participant was with the applications.

5.2 Feature Extraction

We converted the timestamps of each sensor data into a human-readable date and time format using the timezone data of each participant. From the hour of the day, we determined the day segment as follows; *morning* - 06–11 h, *afternoon* - 12–17 h, *evening* - 18–23 h, and *night* - 00–5 h. Except for the Location features, which were computed at a daily level only, we aggregated all other features at the daily and day segment level. The aggregation on the day and day segment level allows for the emphasis of behavioural patterns during specific segments of the day, for example, typing speed and typing error rate at night, and the number of unique applications during the morning.

In addition to the minimum, maximum, mean, median, sum, and standard deviation (SD) aggregation of the computed features, we also captured the degrees of complexity and irregularity of features with Shannon Entropy estimation [67,71] and Normalised Shanon Entropy [65], using the 'entropy' R package [72]. Furthermore, we computed other estimators that are robust to outliers in the computed features, including robust estimator for mean (Huber's M) [38], and variance (VarQn) [13] using the *robustbase* R package [53]. We summarise the features extracted from the sensor data in Table 2. We explain the feature extraction process in more detail next.

Keyboard: We defined a typing session as all keystrokes while the user is using an application. For every two successive keystrokes per typing session, we determine the keystroke transition as *Character-Character* - from a character to a character, *Character-Backspace* - from character to backspace, *Character-Number* - from character to number, *Character-Punctuation* - from character

Table 2. Summary of extracted features from the study dataset. Feature_name* denotes that multiple estimations; sum, minimum, maximum, median, mean, standard deviation, entropy, normalised entropy, robust mean and variance (Huber's M and VarQn) were computed for that feature.

Feature group	Feature metrics
Keyboard	interkey_interval*, count_session, count_keystrokes, speed, pauses_ratio, error_ratio
Location	distance*, speed*, nclusters, location_variance
Call	call_count, distinct_contact, duration*
SMS	sms_count, distinct_contact
Phone usage	unlock_duration, unlock_time_interval*, count_tap, count_long_tap, touch_time_interval*, usage_sec*, usage_count, unique_apps
Ambient noise	episode_sec*, silent_episodes, loud_episodes

to punctuation and *Other*, and also compute *interkey_interval*, i.e. the time difference in seconds between two successive keystrokes. A transition is a *pause* if the *interkey_interval* exceeds the 95th quantile of all *interkey_interval* per the typing session. The quantile method we used does not assume normality for the distribution of the *interkey_interval*. Also, we aggregate all typing sessions as; (1) *count_session*, i.e. count of typing session, (2) count_keystrokes, i.e. count of keystrokes, (3) speed i.e., count_keystrokes divided by sum of the *interkey_interval*, (4) *pauses_ratio*, i.e. count of all pauses divided by count_keystrokes, (5) *error_ratio*, i.e. count of *Character-Backspace* divided by count_keystrokes, and compute additional estimation as shown in Table 2.

Location: We computed the location features [65, 79] at the day level only. First, we computed the Haversine distance and speed between two successive GPS coordinates. Next, with stationary GPS coordinates [65], we apply DBSCAN [19] clustering to identify the *nclusters*, i.e., the number of significant places participants dwell per day. Furthermore, with the stationary GPS coordinates, we also compute the variability [65] in the GPS coordinates as *location_variance*. Aggregating at the day level, we compute additional estimates for distance and speed, as shown in Table 2.

Call and SMS. For each call type; *missed*, *incoming* and *outgoing*, we aggregated the count, i.e.*call_count*, the number of distinct contacts, i.e. *distinct_contact*, and additional estimates of the call duration as shown in Table 2. Likewise, for SMS, for each SMS type; *sent* and *received*, we aggregated the count and number of distinct contact/trace.

Phone Usage. The phone usage features comprise features extracted from the screen interaction, touch interaction and foreground applications. With screen interaction, we defined a screen episode as the time between two screen states (lock, unlock) changes. We used only the screen unlock episodes to compute

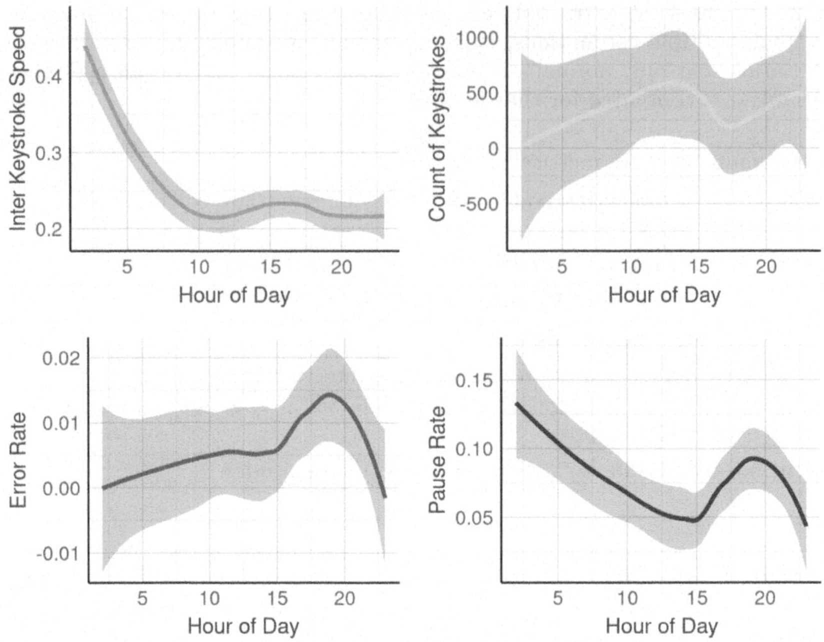

Fig. 2. A visualisation of the typing features of a participant on an anomalous day. The typing speed (top left) gradually declines during morning and evening hours, with a slight increase during afternoon hours. The error rate (bottom left) and pause rate (bottom right) sharply rises and declines between the 15th and 20th h of the day. The participant confirmed during a debriefing session and explained that this typing feature pattern was due to an emotional mental state and fighting period with a friend.

screen episode *duration* and additional estimates, as shown in Table 2, of the time between two successive unlocks, i.e., *unlock_time_interval*. Likewise, for touch interactions, aggregated count of tap, scroll, long tap interactions, and additional estimation, in Table 2, of the time between two successive touch interactions, i.e., *touch-_time_interval*. For features from foreground applications, we added to each app their corresponding category (e.g., social network) based on an external dataset [71] and the Google Play Store [29]. We defined application use episodes as the time during which a particular application is in the foreground. For each application use episode, we computed *usage_sec* as the usage duration in seconds. We then aggregated the *usage_sec*, *usage_count* - count of all application launches, and *unique_apps*- the count of unique application launches at the daily and day segment level for all application categories, and *messaging*, *calling*, *tvvideoapps*, *musicaudioradio*, *email*, *socialnetworks*, *eating*, *healthselfmonitoring*, *datingmating*, and top 1, 2 and 3 used application categories. Furthermore, for *usage_sec*, we computed additional estimates listed in Table 2.

Ambient Noise. We used 50 decibels as a threshold [1,82] to determine the noise state; thus, whether the ambient noise was *silent*- less than or equal to

50 decibels or *loud* otherwise. We determined noise episodes as all intermittent samples until the noise state changes. For each noise episode, we computed the *episode_sec* - total duration of the episodes in seconds after discounting sampling time intervals and maximum, minimum and median decibels. Finally, we aggregate the noise episode features into *silent_episodes* - count of silent episodes, the sum of silent episode_sec, *loud_episodes* - count of loud episodes, sum of loud episode_sec, minimum of all minimum decibels of noise episodes, maximum of maximum decibels of noise episodes, mean of mean decibels of noise episodes, median of median decibels of noise episodes. We also compute additional estimations for *episode_sec*, as shown in Table 2.

5.3 Anomaly Detection

Anomaly detection is a process of finding nonconforming, unexpected or irregular patterns or behaviours in a time series dataset, taking into account only the intrinsic properties of the dataset [28]. Depressive behaviour in an individual may manifest as anomalous - an out of the ordinary behaviour in the context of the individual's routine behaviour [47]. For instance, the depressive behaviours may manifest in unusual sleep changes - inferred from changes in sleep duration, wake up time, screen interactions, touch interactions, and typing during the night or physical and social isolation - inferred from changes in calling, texting, use of social media applications, and reduced physical activity [2,3,55,79]

While different anomaly detection methods exist [28,47], the methods applied in this paper are unsupervised multivariate anomaly detection methods. In contrast to supervised classification methods, unsupervised anomaly detection methods do not need to be trained with labelled datasets of depressive behaviour of the individual, which in practice, may not be available or are scarce at the onset of depression. The applicability of anomaly detection in detecting and monitoring depression is that the growth of anomalous behaviours often translates into critical, significant and actionable information prompting just-in-time interventions. For example, in [3], 71 % higher anomalous behaviour rates were found in the two weeks before relapse of schizophrenia than other times. In healthcare, unsupervised anomaly detection algorithms have been useful to predict health information about smart home residents [48].

We implemented four anomaly detection algorithms; K-Nearest Neighbours (KNN) [7,28], Isolation Forest (ISOFOR) [18,49], Local Outlier Factor (LOF) [10,28,37], and Connectivity-Based Outlier Factor (COF) [28,52,74] to detect anomalies separately in each participant's features (see Table 2), quantified from their 4 weeks dataset. The participant's features computed on the day level and the day segment level were concatenated, into one feature matrix, with each roll representing a particular day. We applied z-score normalisation to the feature matrix before applying the anomaly detection algorithms.

Unlike classification methods that predict a specific class or label, unsupervised anomaly detection algorithms output continuous anomaly scores. Generally for LOF, COF, ISOFOR and KNN, higher anomaly scores indicate a higher likelihood of an anomalous data point [7,18,37,52]. We used the 95th quantile of the anomaly score, without assuming a normal distribution, as a threshold for determining whether the feature matrix point is an anomaly (> the threshold) or non-anomaly otherwise. For each detected participant's anomalous day, we then compute a *weight*; thus, a simple count of the anomalies detected for the day. Figure 3 shows a high-level overview of the anomaly detection process.

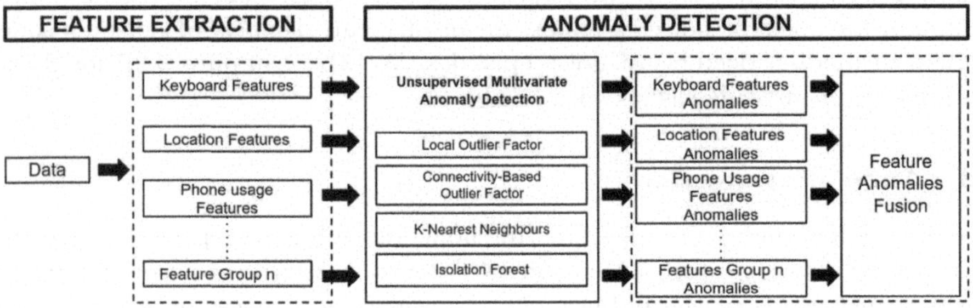

Fig. 3. An overview of the unsupervised multivariate anomaly detection process.

6 Results

6.1 Quantitative Results

We summarise the behavioural data, anomaly detection and self-reported questionnaires collected from 11 participants during our 4 weeks deployment of [OUR-_APP] in Table 1. By applying a threshold [44] on the baseline PHQ-9 responses collected during the *Study Onboarding*, we grouped the participants into *depressed* (PHQ-9 score $\geq$ 10) and *non-depressed* (PHQ-9 score < 10). Out of the 11 participants, 3 participants (**P1**, **P2**, and **P10**) were *depressed* with a mean PHQ-9 score of 16 (*sd* 7.0) at *Study Onboarding*, and 9 participants were *non-depressed* with a mean PHQ-9 at of score 6 (*sd* 2.27) at *Study Onboarding*. Six participants (**P1**, **P4**, **P6**, **P8**, **P9**, **P11**) mentioned they have at some point in their life been clinically diagnosed of depression, anxiety, and other related mental disorders, and we grouped them as *with history*.

Behavioural Analysis: We did not find a statistical difference between our groups. Our participants' sample is modest (N = 11), the groups are not balanced in sufficient numbers. It was incredibly challenging to recruit participants for this pilot. Hence we report our findings using descriptive statistics. As our goal was to pilot the methods and software to assess the usefulness of such in monitoring depression remotely, we conducted this feasibility study with the recruited individuals.

We took the top-10 most used applications and investigated their daily usage patterns (Fig. 4 as an example). This figure shows which app, time of day, and how frequently is the app used at a given time of the day.

Across all the participants, the average application usage time was approximately 8 min. Comparing across groups, the *depressed* and *with history* group

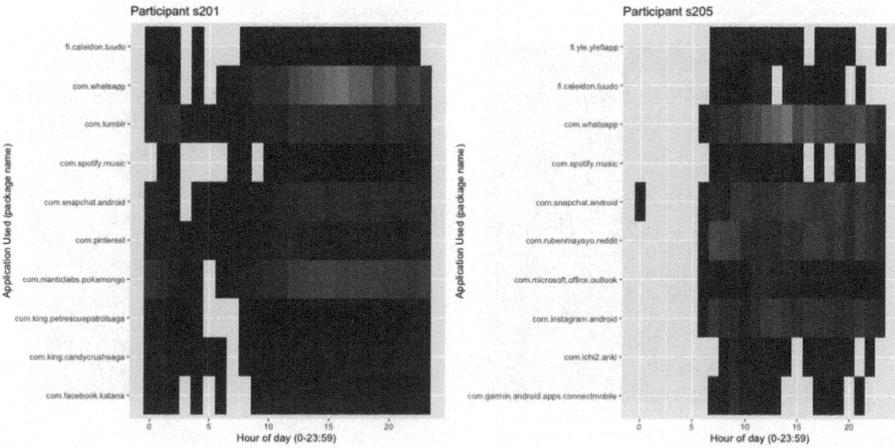

Fig. 4. Example of the most used applications (top-10) for two participants P1 and P5 (depressed and non-depressed, respectively).

had an average application usage time of approximately 9 min. The *non-depressed* group average application usage time was approximately 5 min. In the depressed group, we find application usage reveals a pattern in social application usage (e.g., WhatsApp, Facebook, Snapchat, Tumblr) throughout the day and especially late in the evening (23h00 onward) until the early hours of the day (see Fig. 4, left). The participants in the *depressed* group show more usage of social apps than within the other groups, for longer periods of time – a normalised daily median frequency and app session length: 231 daily sessions, median session length: 12 m 31 s vs 34, 57 daily launches, 5 m 26 s, 7 m 32 s session length in *non-depressed* and *with history*, respectively. We do not find this pattern in the non depressed group, with a clear break in application usage during the early hours (e.g., between 0h and 6h00, Fig. 4, right). We also find the depressed pattern in P11 (*with history*), but not others in the same group.

Next, we investigated engagement with the smartphone using the screen status (being on or off). This allows us to see when the engagement occurs in the day and for how long (in Fig. 5, the longer the engagement the brighter it is).

Across all the participants, the average engagement time was approximately 8 min. Comparing across groups, the *depressed* and *with history* group had an average engagement time of approximately 9 min. The non-depressed group average engagement time was approximately 5 min (see Fig. 5). Following the application usage pattern, the engagement of the depressed group is highlighted in the early hours (see Fig. 5, left). The non-depressed group shows a diluted engagement pattern throughout the day (i.e., more frequent, more brief).

Lastly, we probed the users' daily mobility patterns by the median distance travelled in a given hour (Fig. 6). Across all participants, the median daily total mobility was 7 km. Comparing across groups, the *depressed* and *with history* groups had a median daily total mobility of 7,4 km and 3.6 km, respectively. The

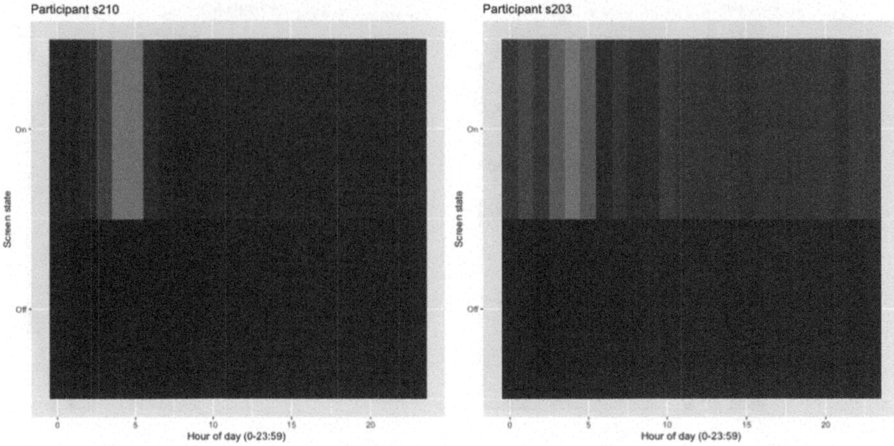

Fig. 5. Example smartphone engagement for two participants P10 and P3 (depressed and non-depressed, respectively).

non-depressed group median daily total mobility was 12 km. Participants in the *depressed* group show a pattern of more mobility in the afternoon hours (11h00 until 18h00, see Fig. 6 left). For the *with history* and *non-depressed* group, the mobility starts earlier in the day, often at 8h00. We also find peaks of mobility for the non-depress-ed group around lunch time (11h00–12h00) (see Fig. 6, right).

Anomaly Detection: We applied four unsupervised multivariate anomaly detection algorithms separately on each participant's data. We computed at least 74 features per participant per day, from the captured behavioural dataset. We did not include features from calls and SMS since the data contained only a few records from 2 participants. Using Spearman's correlation coefficient, we analysed the relationship between the weekly PHQ-9 responses and anomalies detected within two weeks leading to the PHQ-9 survey date.

We found no statistically significant correlation between PHQ-9 scores and anomalies detected. We found pairwise correlations between the individual PHQ-9 question ratings and anomalies detected. However, the correlations were not statistically significant when their *P-values* were adjusted for multiple testing using the Holm-Bonferroni method [35]. We highlight the pairwise correlations where *P-values* < 0.05 for all participants, depressed and non-depressed group.

For all participants, we found a negative correlation ($r = -0.351$, $p = 0.009$) between typing or keyboard feature anomalies and PHQ-9 question seven [*Trouble concentrating on things, such as reading the newspaper or watching television*], a negative correlation ($r = -0.273$, $p = 0.044$) between typing anomalies and PHQ-9 question eight [*Moving or speaking so slowly that other people could have noticed? Or the opposite - being so fidgety or restless that you have been moving around a lot more than usual*]. In addition, we found a negative correlation ($r = -0.283$, $p = 0.037$) between PHQ-9 question eight, and *total anomalies*

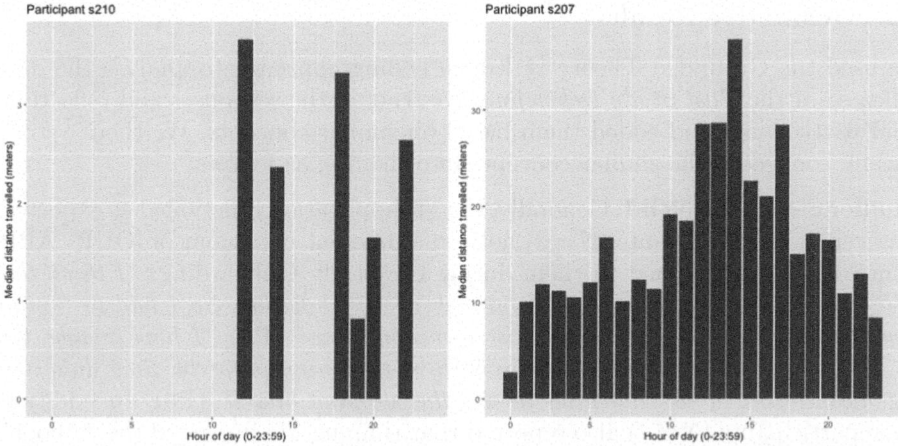

Fig. 6. Example mobility for two participants P10 and P7 (depressed and non-depressed, respectively)

(the sum of anomalies in keyboard, location, phone usage, ambient noise features, see Table 2), *total anomalies* and PHQ-9 question seven ($r = -0.369$, $p = 0.006$). These results suggest that participants with difficulties in concentrating on doing routine activities are more likely to exhibit out of the ordinary and anomalous typing behaviours. Additionally, the results also suggest that participants with restless or fidgety mobility patterns are more likely to exhibit anomalous typing behaviours.

For the *depressed* group, we found a negative correlation ($r = -0.532$, $p = 0.041$) between phone usage feature anomalies and PHQ-9 question three [*Trouble falling or staying asleep, or sleeping too much*], and a negative correlation ($r = -0.545$, $p = 0.036$) between *total anomalies* and PHQ-9 question seven. This suggests that depressed participants experiencing insomnia or hypersomnia at night, are more likely to use their phones (screen interaction, touch interaction and application launches), in an unusual manner compared to other phone usage patterns.

Similarly, for the *non-depressed* group, we found a positive correlation ($r = 0.394$, $p = 0.012$) between phone usage feature anomalies and PHQ-9 question four [*Feeling tired or having little energy*], a positive correlation ($r = 0.356$, $p = 0.024$) between phone usage feature anomalies and PHQ-9 question five [*Poor appetite or overeating*] and a positive correlation ($r = 0.334$, $p = 0.0035$) between ambient noise features anomalies and PHQ-9 question four. This suggests that participants who feel tiredness, stress, poor appetite, and have low energy, are more likely to launch phone applications and interact with their phone through unlocks and scroll in an unusual manner as compared to other phone usage patterns, and might prefer to spend time in low noise environments.

6.2 Qualitative Results

We used the Grounded Theory [11] open coding approach to analyse the data collected at the *Post Study Debriefing.* We read all the responses and reflections from participants and coded them based on similar concepts. We then systematically connected the similar concepts into themes, as follows:

Challenges in the Wild: Generally, the Me application functioned as expected, however some participants (N = 3) noticed a different behaviour of [OUR-_APP] from what was explained to them during the Study Onboarding. *"I think that PHQ-9 questionnaire didn't come through every Thursday. So I had to remind myself to do that. But that was just a minor thing"* (P4) *"I have maybe two or three times where the app was probably not running properly. So I didn't get the notification in the morning to put the sleeping hours"* (P6). In addition, some participants (N = 4) also reported that running Me impacted their phone's storage and battery life. *"I had problem with the flash memory in the device and I'm not sure if it was related to the app or not. Because I was travelling at the time. I took a lot of pictures"* (P6). *"I think the more relevant things I've noticed was the battery because it was going down always."* (P10) *"yeah, the battery drain a bit faster, especially after I got an Oura ring. After that, so, after I stopped using the app, I quickly noticed how my battery lasted longer than usual."* (P4).

Early Feedback: While our research design did not show participants any feedback during the study period, some participants (N = 9) were of the view that early feedback on Me would have been more useful, rather than after 4 weeks. Some participants could not recall what happened, or sounded surprised, when they were asked to reflect on statistics and visualisations of their own data. *"I didn't expect it, for example, like a personal feedback. So that was nice. And also to see, for example, that I make more errors, for example, when I am tired or when I am emotionally in trouble"* (P10). *"7th of November? no I don't remember. I can check, I have my calendar, everything is in there. No I don't have anything here"* (P3) *"Well, it's quite interesting. Maybe it's a bit more apps than I thought it would be. But regarding the number of uses, I'm really wondering what happened on that day"* (P4). *"Well, I think it would be interesting to just look at my own history. What have I done on these days? Because I don't remember right now, what happened during that time?"* (P4).

Plausibility of Detected Anomalies: Whereas some participants could not recall or explain what happened when asked to reflect on visualisations on anomalous behaviours, most participants (N = 6) could quickly explain, relate to and confirm the out of the ordinary behaviours detected by the anomaly detection algorithms. *"I had a party on the 26th and then I remember I really used my phone on the 27th, I was emotional, I've been in a bad mood and yeah, fighting over text"* (P10). *"I don't remember if that was the same day I was travelling. Because if it was, I was in the car as a passenger"*(P4). *"I usually sleep quite well. But some nights I haven't slept so good. And during this period of using the app, I had to change my medication and increase the dosage and that could be the cause"* (P1). *"I've been realising I use my phone the most between*

11 and 12 at night, 10.30 or 11 I'm in my bed, I take the phone, I have the phone for an hour so and then I go to sleep" (P3). *"Maybe some looking out at the game results or something like that. Because I follow Brazilian soccer and then probably looking at the results of the Sunday games. On Mondays because the games are late on Sunday in Brazil, and it's the night here. So on Monday morning, I wake up and check the game scores. And then there are lots of news about it. probably spend some time on that. Yeah."* (P6).

7 Discussion

Our results give us a bulk of smartphone-based user behaviours that may be relevant in monitoring depression unobtrusively. Participants in the *depressed* group went to bed late (i.e., after midnight) - using screen status data - which also provided evidence that it makes it challenging for them to wake up early (first app usage, first time the screen turned on). Moreover, routinely application usage is until late (Fig. 4) and more engaged in the evening/night (Fig. 5), and daily mobility is usually after 10h00 (Fig. 6). The participants in the *depressed* group show more usage of social apps than within the other groups for more extended periods. Participants in the *non-depressed* group followed a device off time night (23h00 onward), picking up the phone at around 8 am. Surprisingly, P11 is a *with history* participant who follows the depressed pattern, but not the others in the same group (they exhibit the non-depressed group pattern). Such information could be beneficial for a mental health professional to investigate further. Participants in the *non-depressed* group are more active (higher daily median mobility) throughout the day, with a peak around lunchtime (11h00–12h00), while others are less mobile.

As depression symptoms are, human behaviour is heterogeneous and varies between individuals. Previous research has established that smartphone usage behaviours and depression varies among different demographics [8,9,61,71]. For example, certain personality traits are associated with compulsive use of YouTube [42], specific application categories can predict personality traits [61], and some applications are more likely to be used at specific hours of the day [8]. Monitoring inherent patterns in these behaviours at the individual level, over time, to detect changes and out-of-the-ordinary behaviours, is helpful in detecting the early onset of depression [2,3,26]. The findings in this study revealed some relationship between anomalous human behaviour and questions 3, 4, 5, 7 and 8 of the PHQ-9 depression scale, which suggests that it is feasible to passively and unobtrusively collect datasets from smartphones, to detect out of the ordinary behaviours related to depression. These findings corroborate the findings of previous studies [3,55,79] with regards to the relationship between biomarkers and depressive symptoms, particularly of typing patterns [55,79], sleep disturbances and fatigue [79], trouble concentrating and psychomotor agitation or retardation [79].

In a hypothetical early detection of depression system, for example, the anomalous behaviour detection system will monitor the increase of detected anomalies in a participants dataset that correlate with depressive symptoms. If a reasonable threshold is exceeded, the system will then prompt the participant to provide a response to a self-reported depression scale such as PHQ-9 [44], Beck Depression Inventory (BDI) [4] and Depression Anxiety and Stress Scales (DASS-21) [58]. The score of the depression scale will determine the requisite course of action.

While it was not the goal of the current study to provide depression interventions to participants, our results suggest that participants expected to see feedback on the study's application. Equally important is the impact of such feedback on participants' behaviour. Previous research [20,45,66] have investigated various feedback mechanisms when providing intervention in mental health systems. Careful design of the feedback mechanism [66] regarding timing, frequency and personalisation is required to prevent a negative impact [20] on the participants' mental health state.

In addition, to prompt actionable feedback [3,66], the feedback should be specific and personalised, interpretable, meaningful to participants. Model interpretability is one advantage anomaly detection methods used in this study have over predictive analysis, whose output interpretation is sometimes challenging [17,68]. Our results suggest that, while some participants could not always recall if something of significance happened on anomalous days, the detected anomalous behaviours (example in Fig. 2) were generally plausible and meaningful to the participants. With prompt and interpretable feedback on detected anomalous behaviours, participants could provide additional context to the dataset by annotating detected behaviours.

Our results also highlighted some application deployment challenges with some participants. In recent years, application distribution platforms such as the Google Play Store [29] have enabled mobile health researchers and application developers to reach millions of people using different smartphone devices and OS versions globally. Not only do these application distribution platforms bring opportunities, they also bring some challenges to application development and deployment [5,36] due to ever evolving device platforms and application deployment guidelines. For instance, recent changes in Google Play Store's application publishing policies [30] restricted the types of applications that can access specific permissions, including SMS and call logging permissions. Consequently, our attempt to publish Me on the Google Play Store was rejected since Me is not a replacement for calls or SMS applications, yet it needs SMS and call permissions to access the call and SMS behaviour data. Consequently, we hosted Me in-house using Jenkins [41]. However, self-hosting applications pose challenges in scaling and updating the application on multiple devices, which are otherwise handled by the application distribution platform. Lastly, Android's Doze and background processing limitations negatively interfere with passive and continuous sensing applications like in Me, justifying why at certain times, the application did not remind the participant.

8 Limitations and Future Work

Notwithstanding the results in this study, the number of participants in the study is limited and were recruited from a general population. With the study being exploratory, evidence of clinical diagnosis with depression was not a recruitment requirement. Secondly, all correlations reported in this study are not statistically significant when their *P values* are adjusted for multiple testing.

In the future work, we replicate the study with a larger cohort drawn from a clinical population to explore further the relationship between out of the ordinary behaviours and depression. With a larger sample size, future research could review the statistically significant relationship between detected anomalies and depression. We could further explore the causal relationship between detected anomalies and depression. Since correlations only reveal linear relationships. In addition, we could investigate both linear and non-linear relationships between depression and detected anomalies, using information theory methods such as Mutual Information (MI) [15]. Additionally, future work could expand the features extracted from the smartphone dataset to include additional measures of routines and variability in human behaviour using methods such as Regularity Index [76,80]. Future work could improve the anomaly detection system with other contextual information such as the Big Five Personality traits, and explore the relationship between anomalous human behaviour and depression using other depression scales such as the BDI [4], DASS-21 [58].

The current study is an exploratory first step towards creating a system for just-in-time depression intervention with anomaly detection methods. As such, the current study does not predict whether an individual is depressed or not. The findings from this study naturally lead to questions such as; how much data will be collected from individuals to constitute a ground truth for their baseline behaviour, how would the system adapt to changing human behaviours such as seasonal changes (e.g. winter and summer), situational changes such as changing jobs, graduating from college, and other environmental changes that may change human behaviour?, how many or what kind of anomalous behaviours will be statistically significant with depression scores, what threshold of detected anomalies will trigger an intervention from the application. These are questions we seek to investigate in future work, ultimately leading to the creation of a system of personalised and labelled datasets of anomalous individual behaviours that are indicative of depression, and personalised models for just-in-time depression interventions.

9 Conclusion

In this study, we investigated the feasibility of using unsupervised multivariate anomaly detection methods to detect at the early onset and monitor the progression of depression. Our quantitative and qualitative findings show that anomalies detected in participants' behaviour collected via smartphone sensing over a 4 weeks period, represented specific and meaningful out of the ordinary behaviour. Our findings also show non statistically significant correlation between the detected anomalous human behaviour and various symptoms of depression under the PHQ-9 depression scale. In spite of our study's limitations, our findings demonstrate a step forward towards detecting and monitoring depression with anomaly detection methods. Further research is needed to replicate these findings in larger population studies, potentially leading to creating just-in-time interventions for depression using anomaly detection methods.

Acknowledgment. The *Me in the Wild* study is supported by the Academy of Finland SENSATE (Grant Nos. 316253, 320089), 6Genesis Flagship (Grant No. 318927), and the Infotech Institute University of Oulu Emerging Project. We thank all the participants of the *Me in the Wild* study.

References

1. I Acoustics: Comparitive Examples of Noise Levels—Industrial Noise Control, January 2020. https://www.industrialnoisecontrol.com/comparative-noise-examples.htm
2. Adler, D.A., et al.: Predicting early warning signs of psychotic relapse from passive sensing data: an approach using encoder-decoder neural networks. JMIR Mhealth Uhealth **8**(8), e19962 (2020). https://doi.org/10.2196/19962
3. Barnett, I., Torous, J., Staples, P., Sandoval, L., Keshavan, M., Onnela, J.P.: Relapse prediction in schizophrenia through digital phenotyping: a pilot study. Neuropsychopharmacology **43**(8), 1660 (2018). 10/gdrks3
4. Beck, A.T., Ward, C.H., Mendelson, M., Mock, J., Erbaugh, J.: An inventory for measuring depression. Arch. Gen. Psychiatry **4**(6), 561–571 (1961). https://doi.org/10.1001/archpsyc.1961.01710120031004
5. Ben-Zeev, D., Schueller, S.M., Begale, M., Duffecy, J., Kane, J.M., Mohr, D.C.: Strategies for mhealth research: lessons from 3 mobile intervention studies. Adm. Policy Mental Health Mental Health Serv. Res. **42**(2), 157–167 (2015)
6. van Berkel, N., Ferreira, D., Kostakos, V.: The experience sampling method on mobile devices. ACM Comput. Surv. **50**(6), 93:1–93:40 (2017). https://doi.org/10.1145/3123988. http://doi.acm.org/10.1145/3123988
7. Beygelzimer, A., Kakadet, S., Langford, J., Arya, S., Mount, D., Li, S.: FNN: Fast Nearest Neighbor Search Algorithms and Applications, February 2019. https://CRAN.R-project.org/package=FNN
8. Böhmer, M., Hecht, B., Schöning, J., Krüger, A., Bauer, G.: Falling asleep with angry birds, Facebook and kindle: a large scale study on mobile application usage. In: Proceedings of the 13th International Conference on Human Computer Interaction with Mobile Devices and Services, pp. 47–56 (2011)
9. Bonful, H.A., Anum, A.: Sociodemographic correlates of depressive symptoms: a cross-sectional analytic study among healthy urban ghanaian women. BMC Public Health **19**(1), 50 (2019)
10. Breunig, M.M., Kriegel, H.P., Ng, R.T., Sander, J.: LOF: identifying density-based local outliers. In: ACM SIGMOD Record, vol. 29, pp. 93–104. ACM (2000)
11. Charmaz, K., Belgrave, L., et al.: Qualitative interviewing and grounded theory analysis. In: The SAGE Handbook of Interview Research: The Complexity of the Craft, vol. 2, pp. 347–365 (2012)

12. Coravos, A., Khozin, S., Mandl, K.D.: Developing and adopting safe and effective digital biomarkers to improve patient outcomes. NPJ Digit. Med. **2**(1), 1–5 (2019). https://doi.org/10.1038/s41746-019-0090-4
13. Croux, C., Rousseeuw, P.J.: Time-efficient algorithms for two highly robust estimators of scale. In: Dodge, Y., Whittaker, J. (eds.) Computational Statistics, pp. 411–428. Springer, Heidelberg (1992). https://doi.org/10.1007/978-3-662-26811-7_58
14. Dagum, P.: Digital biomarkers of cognitive function. NPJ Digit. Med. **1**(1), 1–3 (2018). https://doi.org/10.1038/s41746-018-0018-4
15. Dionisio, A., Menezes, R., Mendes, D.A.: Mutual information: a measure of dependency for nonlinear time series. Physica A **344**(1–2), 326–329 (2004)
16. Dorsey, E.R., Papapetropoulos, S., Xiong, M., Kieburtz, K.: The first frontier: digital biomarkers for neurodegenerative disorders. Digit. Biomarkers **1**(1), 6–13 (2017). https://doi.org/10.1159/000477383
17. Elshawi, R., Al-Mallah, M.H., Sakr, S.: On the interpretability of machine learning-based model for predicting hypertension. BMC Med. Inform. Decis. Mak. **19**(1), 146 (2019)
18. Eric, G.: iForest: Isolation Forest Anomaly Detection, August 2019. https://rdrr.io/github/Zelazny7/isofor/man/iForest.html
19. Ester, M., Kriegel, H.P., Sander, J., Xu, X., et al.: A density-based algorithm for discovering clusters in large spatial databases with noise. In: KDD, vol. 96, pp. 226–231 (1996)
20. Faurholt-Jepsen, M., et al.: Daily electronic self-monitoring in bipolar disorder using smartphones-the Monarca I trial: a randomized, placebo-controlled, single-blind, parallel group trial. Psychol. Med. **45**(13), 2691–2704 (2015)
21. Ferreira, D., Kostakos, V., Dey, A.K.: Aware: mobile context instrumentation framework. Front. ICT **2**, 6 (2015)
22. Ferreira, D., Kostakos, V., Schweizer, I.: Human sensors on the move. In: Loreto, V., et al. (eds.) Participatory Sensing, Opinions and Collective Awareness. UCS, pp. 9–19. Springer, Cham (2017). https://doi.org/10.1007/978-3-319-25658-0_1
23. Fraccaro, P., et al.: Digital biomarkers from geolocation data in bipolar disorder and schizophrenia: a systematic review. J. Am. Med. Inform. Assoc. **26**(11), 1412–1420 (2019). https://doi.org/10.1093/jamia/ocz043
24. Fried, E.I., Nesse, R.M.: Depression is not a consistent syndrome: an investigation of unique symptom patterns in the star* d study. J. Affect. Disord. **172**, 96–102 (2015). https://doi.org/10.1016/j.jad.2014.10.010
25. Fried, E.I., Nesse, R.M.: Depression sum-scores don't add up: why analyzing specific depression symptoms is essential. BMC Med. **13**(1), 72 (2015)
26. Gerych, W., Agu, E., Rundensteiner, E.: Classifying depression in imbalanced datasets using an autoencoder-based anomaly detection approach. In: 2019 IEEE 13th International Conference on Semantic Computing (ICSC), pp. 124–127, January 2019. https://doi.org/10.1109/ICOSC.2019.8665535
27. Goldberg, L.R.: The development of markers for the big-five factor structure. Psychol. Assess. **4**, 26 (1992)
28. Goldstein, M., Uchida, S.: A comparative evaluation of unsupervised anomaly detection algorithms for multivariate data. PLoS ONE **11**(4), e0152173 (2016)
29. Google: Google Play, December 2019. https://play.google.com/store?hl=en%5FGB
30. Google: Use of SMS or Call Log permission groups - Play Console Help, December 2019. https://support.google.com/googleplay/android-developer/answer/9047303?hl=en

31. Greenberg, P.E., Fournier, A.A., Sisitsky, T., Pike, C.T., Kessler, R.C.: The economic burden of adults with major depressive disorder in the united states (2005 and 2010). J. Clin. Psychiatry **76**(2), 155–162 (2015). https://doi.org/10.4088/JCP.14m09298
32. Hamilton, M.: A rating scale for depression. J. Neurol. Neurosurg. Psychiatry **23**(1), 56 (1960)
33. Harari, G.M., Lane, N.D., Wang, R., Crosier, B.S., Campbell, A.T., Gosling, S.D.: Using smartphones to collect behavioral data in psychological science: opportunities, practical considerations, and challenges. Perspect. Psychol. Sci. J. Assoc. Psychol. Sci. **11**(6), 838–854 (2016). https://doi.org/10.1177/1745691616650285
34. Hemmerle, A.M., Herman, J.P., Seroogy, K.B.: Stress, depression and Parkinson's disease. Exp. Neurol. **233**(1), 79–86 (2012). https://doi.org/10.1016/j.expneurol.2011.09.035
35. Holm, S.: A simple sequentially rejective multiple test procedure. Scand. J. Stat. 65–70 (1979)
36. Holzer, A., Ondrus, J.: Mobile application market: a developer's perspective. Telematics Inform. **28**(1), 22–31 (2011)
37. Hu, Y., Murray, W., Shan, Y.: RLOF: R Parallel Implementation of Local Outlier Factor (LOF), September 2015. https://CRAN.R-project.org/package=Rlof
38. Huber, P.J.: Robust Statistics. Springer, Heidelberg (2011)
39. Huckvale, K., Venkatesh, S., Christensen, H.: Toward clinical digital phenotyping: a timely opportunity to consider purpose, quality, and safety. NPJ Digit. Med. **2**(1), 1–11 (2019). https://doi.org/10.1038/s41746-019-0166-1
40. Jacobson, N.C., Weingarden, H., Wilhelm, S.: Digital biomarkers of mood disorders and symptom change. NPJ Digit. Med. **2**(1), 1–3 (2019). https://doi.org/10.1038/s41746-019-0078-0
41. Jenkins.io: Jenkins and Android, January 2019. https://jenkins.io/solutions/android/index.html
42. Klobas, J.E., McGill, T.J., Moghavvemi, S., Paramanathan, T.: Compulsive YouTube usage: a comparison of use motivation and personality effects. Comput. Hum. Behav. **87**, 129–139 (2018)
43. Kourtis, L.C., Regele, O.B., Wright, J.M., Jones, G.B.: Digital biomarkers for Alzheimer's disease: the mobile/wearable devices opportunity. NPJ Digit. Med. **2**(1), 1–9 (2019). https://doi.org/10.1038/s41746-019-0084-2
44. Kroenke, K., Spitzer, R.L., Williams, J.B.: The PHQ-9: validity of a brief depression severity measure. J. Gener. Internal Med. **16**(9), 606–613 (2001). https://doi.org/10.1046/j.1525-1497.2001.016009606.x
45. Lee, J., Lam, M., Chiu, C.: Clara: design of a new system for passive sensing of depression, stress and anxiety in the workplace. In: Cipresso, P., Serino, S., Villani, D. (eds.) MindCare 2019. LNICST, vol. 288, pp. 12–28. Springer, Cham (2019). https://doi.org/10.1007/978-3-030-25872-6_2
46. Lépine, J.P., Briley, M.: The increasing burden of depression. Neuropsychiatr. Dis. Treat. **7**(Suppl. 1), 3 (2011). https://doi.org/10.2147/NDT.S19617
47. Liang, Y., Zheng, X., Zeng, D.D.: A survey on big data-driven digital phenotyping of mental health. Inf. Fusion **52**, 290–307 (2019)
48. Liao, Z., et al.: A visual analytics approach for detecting and understanding anomalous resident behaviors in smart healthcare. Appl. Sci. **7**(3), 254 (2017)
49. Liu, F.T., Ting, K.M., Zhou, Z.H.: Isolation-based anomaly detection. ACM Trans. Knowl. Discov. Data (TKDD) **6**(1), 3 (2012)

50. Lotfi, A., Langensiepen, C., Mahmoud, S.M., Akhlaghinia, M.J.: Smart homes for the elderly dementia sufferers: identification and prediction of abnormal behaviour. J. Ambient. Intell. Humaniz. Comput. **3**(3), 205–218 (2012)
51. Macchia, A., et al.: Depression worsens outcomes in elderly patients with heart failure: an analysis of 48,117 patients in a community setting. Eur. J. Heart Fail. **10**(7), 714–721 (2008)
52. Madsen, J.H.: Connectivity-based Outlier Factor (COF) algorithm in DDoutlier: Distance & Density-Based Outlier Detection, May 2019. https://rdrr.io/cran/DDoutlier/man/COF.html
53. Maechler, M., Rousseeuw, P., Croux, C., Todorov, V., Ruckstuhl, A., Salibian-Barrera, M.: Robustbase: Basic Robust Statistics, May 2019. https://CRAN.R-project.org/package=robustbase
54. Mandryk, R.L., Birk, M.V.: The potential of game-based digital biomarkers for modeling mental health. JMIR Mental Health **6**(4), e13485 (2019). https://doi.org/10.2196/13485
55. Mastoras, R.E., et al.: Touchscreen typing pattern analysis for remote detection of the depressive tendency. Sci. Rep. **9**(1), 1–12 (2019). https://doi.org/10.1038/s41598-019-50002-9
56. Meister, S., Deiters, W., Becker, S.: Digital health and digital biomarkers - enabling value chains on health data. Curr. Dir. Biomed. Eng. **2**(1), 577–581 (2016). https://doi.org/10.1515/cdbme-2016-0128
57. Moshe, I., et al.: Predicting symptoms of depression and anxiety using smartphone and wearable data. Front. Psychiatry **12** (2021). https://doi.org/10.3389/fpsyt.2021.625247
58. Norton, P.J.: Depression anxiety and stress scales (DASS-21): psychometric analysis across four racial groups. Anxiety Stress Coping **20**(3), 253–265 (2007)
59. Opoku Asare, K., Terhorst, Y., Vega, J., Peltonen, E., Lagerspetz, E., Ferreira, D.: Predicting depression from smartphone behavioral markers using machine learning methods, hyperparameter optimization, and feature importance analysis: exploratory study. JMIR Mhealth Uhealth **9**(7), e26540 (2021). https://doi.org/10.2196/26540
60. Opoku Asare, K., Visuri, A., Ferreira, D.S.T.: Towards early detection of depression through smartphone sensing. In: Adjunct Proceedings of the 2019 ACM International Joint Conference on Pervasive and Ubiquitous Computing and Proceedings of the 2019 ACM International Symposium on Wearable Computers, UbiComp/ISWC 2019 Adjunct, pp. 1158–1161. ACM, New York (2019). https://doi.org/10.1145/3341162.3347075
61. Peltonen, E., Sharmila, P., Opoku Asare, K., Visuri, A., Lagerspetz, E., Ferreira, D.: When phones get personal: predicting big five personality traits from application usage. Pervasive Mob. Comput. **69**, 101269 (2020)
62. van der Ploeg, T., Austin, P.C., Steyerberg, E.W.: Modern modelling techniques are data hungry: a simulation study for predicting dichotomous endpoints. BMC Med. Res. Methodol. **14**(1), 137 (2014)
63. Rodarte, C.: Pharmaceutical perspective: how digital biomarkers and contextual data will enable therapeutic environments. Digit. Biomarkers **1**(1), 73–81 (2017). https://doi.org/10.1159/000479951
64. Rohani, D.A., Faurholt-Jepsen, M., Kessing, L.V., Bardram, J.E.: Correlations between objective behavioral features collected from mobile and wearable devices and depressive mood symptoms in patients with affective disorders: systematic review. JMIR Mhealth Uhealth **6**(8), e165 (2018). https://doi.org/10.2196/mhealth.9691

65. Saeb, S., Zhang, M., Kwasny, M., Karr, C.J., Kording, K., Mohr, D.C.: The relationship between clinical, momentary, and sensor-based assessment of depression. In: 2015 9th International Conference on Pervasive Computing Technologies for Healthcare (PervasiveHealth), pp. 229–232. IEEE (2015)
66. Schembre, S.M., et al.: Just-in-time feedback in diet and physical activity interventions: systematic review and practical design framework. J. Med. Internet Res. **20**(3), e106 (2018)
67. Shannon, C.E.: A mathematical theory of communication. Bell Syst. Tech. J. **27**(3), 379–423 (1948)
68. Shmueli, G., Koppius, O.R.: Predictive analytics in information systems research. MIS Q. **35**(3), 553–572 (2011). http://www.jstor.org/stable/23042796
69. Sordo, M., Zeng, Q.: On sample size and classification accuracy: a performance comparison. In: Oliveira, J.L., Maojo, V., Martín-Sánchez, F., Pereira, A.S. (eds.) ISBMDA 2005. LNCS, vol. 3745, pp. 193–201. Springer, Heidelberg (2005). https://doi.org/10.1007/11573067_20
70. Spathis, D., Servia-Rodriguez, S., Farrahi, K., Mascolo, C., Rentfrow, J.: Passive mobile sensing and psychological traits for large scale mood prediction. In: Proceedings of the 13th EAI International Conference on Pervasive Computing Technologies for Healthcare, PervasiveHealth 2019, pp. 272–281. ACM, New York (2019). https://doi.org/10.1145/3329189.3329213
71. Stachl, C., et al.: Predicting personality from patterns of behavior collected with smartphones. Proc. Natl. Acad. Sci. **117**(30) (2020). https://doi.org/10.1073/pnas.1920484117
72. Hausser, J., Strimmer, K.: Entropy: Estimation of Entropy, Mutual Information and Related Quantities, November 2014. https://CRAN.R-project.org/package=entropy
73. Strober, L.B., Arnett, P.A.: Assessment of depression in three medically ill, elderly populations: Alzheimer's disease, Parkinson's disease, and stroke. Clin. Neuropsychol. **23**(2), 205–230 (2009)
74. Tang, J., Chen, Z., Fu, A.W., Cheung, D.W.: Enhancing effectiveness of outlier detections for low density patterns. In: Chen, M.-S., Yu, P.S., Liu, B. (eds.) PAKDD 2002. LNCS (LNAI), vol. 2336, pp. 535–548. Springer, Heidelberg (2002). https://doi.org/10.1007/3-540-47887-6_53
75. TENK: Guidelines for ethical review in human sciences. https://tenk.fi/en/advice-and-materials/guidelines-ethical-review-human-sciences
76. Tseng, V.W.S., et al.: Using behavioral rhythms and multi-task learning to predict fine-grained symptoms of schizophrenia. Sci. Rep. **10**(1), 1–17 (2020)
77. Vega, J., Jay, C., Vigo, M., Harper, S.: Unobtrusive monitoring of Parkinson's disease based on digital biomarkers of human behaviour. In: Proceedings of the 19th International ACM SIGACCESS Conference on Computers and Accessibility, ASSETS 2017, pp. 351–352. Association for Computing Machinery, New York (2017). https://doi.org/10.1145/3132525.3134782
78. Wagner, D.T., Rice, A., Beresford, A.R.: Device analyzer: large-scale mobile data collection. SIGMETRICS Perform. Eval. Rev. **41**(4), 53–56 (2014). https://doi.org/10.1145/2627534.2627553
79. Wang, R., et al.: Tracking depression dynamics in college students using mobile phone and wearable sensing. Proc. ACM Interact. Mob. Wearable Ubiquit. Technol. **2**(1), 43 (2018)
80. Wang, W., et al.: Sensing behavioral change over time: using within-person variability features from mobile sensing to predict personality traits. Proc. ACM Interact. Mob. Wearable Ubiquit. Technol. **2**(3), 1–21 (2018)

81. WHO: Depression, March 2018. https://www.who.int/news-room/fact-sheets/detail/depression
82. Wright, B., Peters, E., Ettinger, U., Kuipers, E., Kumari, V.: Understanding noise stress-induced cognitive impairment in healthy adults and its implications for schizophrenia. Noise Health **16**(70), 166–176 (2014)

An Accurate and Cost-Effective Approach Towards Real-Time Eye Movement Angle Estimation

Yunfeng Zhu[1], Linkai Tao[1,2], Zheng Zeng[1], Hangyu Zhu[1], Chen Chen[3], and Wei Chen[1,3](✉)

[1] Center for Intelligent Medical Electronics, School of Information Science and Technology, Fudan University, Shanghai 200433, China
{20210720162,w_chen}@fudan.edu.cn

[2] Department of Industrial Design, Eindhoven University of Technology, Eindhoven, The Netherlands

[3] Human Phenome Institute, Fudan University, Shanghai 201203, China

Abstract. In this paper, an electrooculography (EOG)-based eye movement angle estimation approach, including signal acquisition, pre-processing, outlier removal and modeling, is proposed. The eye movement angle estimation model is a data-driven approach that using a non-linear polynomial method. It offers a simple, analytical, accurate, and cost-effective solution for real-time and large-space eye movement angle estimation. The feasibility of the proposed model was validated on a realistic scenario across 18 subjects. Experimental results show the horizontal estimation error in angle is less than 3.5°. Compared with most of the existing methods with high computational complexity, the proposed model can provide comparable results with less computational consumption cost in a large-space eye movement angle estimation. Meanwhile, the proposed model can be easily deployed in the embedded platform or mobile device with limited computing power and limited storage space for real-time eye movement angle estimation.

Keywords: Electrooculography · Eye movement angle estimation · Non-linear polynomial model

1 Introduction

Electrooculography (EOG), as a reliable and non-invasive technique, measures the electrical potentials that arise between the cornea and the retina changes when the eyeball rotates. By placing a pair of electrodes either horizontally or vertically around the eyes, these potentials can be recorded. The transitions and magnitude of the obtained potentials are essentially corresponding to the rotation angle of the eyes [1]. Thus, EOG has been widely explored in many health applications, such as wheelchair guidance [2], human-computer interface [3, 4], fatigue detection [5], etc. While, for these applications, eye movement angle estimation is considered to be the fundamental step.

X. Gao et al. (Eds.): MobiHealth 2021, LNICST 440, pp. 146–156, 2022.
https://doi.org/10.1007/978-3-031-06368-8_10

To estimate the eye movement angle, various approaches have been proposed. These approaches can be roughly classified into the physically-driven white box method and the data-driven black-box method. The research idea of the physically-driven white-box model focuses on the EOG eye movement recognition model based on the relationship between the principle of eye movement and gaze location. Under this idea, Barbara et al. [6] proposed an eye movement angle fitting model, by employing the EOG battery model [7] and the spatial geometric relationship between eye movement and the angle of gaze location. However, the model proposed in this work requires a certain amount of trigonometric function operations. Furthermore, the calculation of trigonometric functions mainly relies on the Taylor expansion, which has requirements for computer computing power, or the look-up table method, which has certain requirements for computer storage capacity. As a result, the model training is resource-consuming.

In contrast, the research idea of data-driven black-box focuses on data-driven EOG eye movement angle recognition modeling. Compared with the white-box idea, this technique tends to have higher accuracy. Researches under this idea normally employ data-driven modeling methods and establish regression models between the eye movement angle and the collected EOG signal. According to the type of the proposed regression models, it can be divided into linear models and non-linear models generally. Barbara et al. proposed a linear model in the research to estimate the eye movement angle according to EOG signals [4]. However, other researches show that the eye movement angle within 45° is linear, eye movement angle larger than 45° is non-linear [8–11]. The advantage of the non-linear model is that it has higher accuracy but correspondingly requires higher computing resources to train the model. Although the linear model has a relatively simple model, the requirements for computing resources are correspondingly low, but its accuracy for a larger eye movement angle is not satisfactory. Putting aside the resource usage, focusing only on accuracy and interpretability is not pragmatic enough to apply EOG signals to health application scenarios. The relationship between resource consumption and accuracy is an important issue that is yet to be considered.

To address the above issues, an accurate and cost effective model based on non-linear polynomial regression for eye movement angle estimation is proposed. The model is simple, analytical, fast, and with few parameters. Compared with most of the existing methods with high computational complexity, the proposed model can be easily deployed in the embedded platform or mobile device for real-time eye movement angle estimation. Meanwhile, to verify the feasibility of the proposed method, a series of large-space experiments (range: $-50°$ to $50°$) were conducted. The proposed model provides a favorable accuracy with less computational time.

2 Experiment

2.1 Materials

In this work, EOG signals were recorded from 19 subjects aged 25 ± 4 years (9 males and 10 females), these subjects are healthy adults without strabismus and exophthalmos. All subjects understood and agreed with the experiment process before the experiment. Polysomnography (PSG) with a sampling frequency of 256 Hz, a 0.3–10 Hz band pass filter and a 50 Hz notch filter was applied for the EOG data acquisition.

The electrode configuration was set as shown in Fig. 1, with electrodes placed on the right side of the right eye socket (dot '1') and on the left side of the left eye socket (dot '2'). A reference (dot 'Ref') and a ground (dot 'GND') electrode were also attached to the center of the forehead and on the left mastoid respectively.

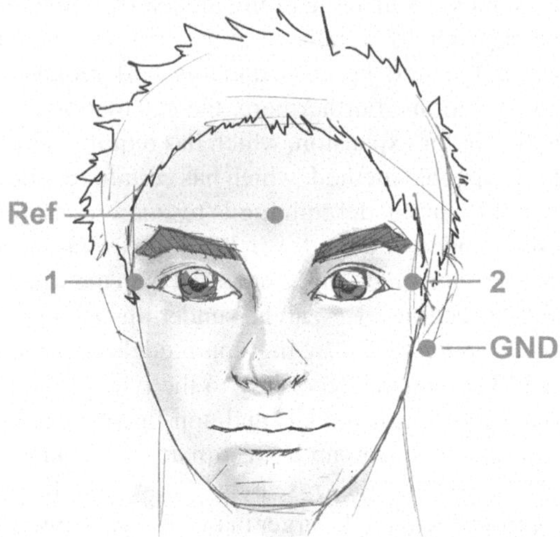

Fig. 1. This is the electrode configuration illustration. The dots mark the placed PSG electrode positions on the face. The dot is on the right side of the right eye socket labeled '1' and on the left side of the left eye socket labeled '2'. A reference (dot 'Ref') and a ground (dot 'GND') electrode are attached to the center of the forehead and on the left mastoid respectively

2.2 Experimental Setup and Procedure

Before the start of the experiment, the subject sat upright in the experimental apparatus in a comfortable position with arms resting on the desk naturally. The face of the subject was cleaned with wet wipes and then connected to conductive gel electrodes. Their head was fixed by a bracket to reduce the impact of head shaking.

The experimenter helped the subject to attach the electrodes. After that, the experimenter configured and tested the PSG (used to acquire EOG signals) and acquisition program (used to guide the experimenter and subject and marked EOG signals). Then, the experimenter ran the EOG acquisition program and prompted the subject to make corresponding saccades according to the experiment requirements. The saccades procedure is shown in Fig. 2. The symbol Θ is the angle between the center point and the target point of saccade. The saccades sequence is $\{0°, 10°, 0°, -10°, 0°, 20°, 0°, -20°, 0°, 30°, 0°, -30°, 0°, 35°, 0°, -35°, 0°, 38°, 0°, -38°, 0°, 40°, 0°, -40°, 0°, 42°, 0°, -42°, 0°, 44°, 0°, -44°, 0°, 46°, 0°, -46°, 0°, 48°, 0°, -48°, 0°, 50°, 0°, -50°, 0°\}$.

Figure 3 shows the experimental paradigm. At the beginning of the saccade procedure, the subject was asked to gaze at the center point (0° point). Then the subject was asked to make a saccade from 0° to 10° according to the audio prompt of the program and keep gazing at the 10° point for 3 s. At the same time, the program marked the saccade signal EOG^1_{0to10} (the potential of electrode 1, saccade from 0° to 10°) and EOG^2_{0to10} (the potential of electrode 1, saccade from 0° to 10°) for subsequent signal processing.

Before proceeding to the next step, the subject can take a short break to relax the eyeballs, blink, etc. The purpose is to reduce the discomfort of the eyes during the experiment and ensure the quality of the data acquired in the experiment. After asking for consent that the subject can continue the experiment, the experiment continues. Then after a short break, the subject was asked to continue to gaze at 10° point to finish the next saccade (from 10° to 0°).

The subject was required to repeat the above process until all saccades sequences had been completed. Finally, we got all saccade EOG signal from one subject (EOG^1_{0to10}, EOG^1_{10to0}, EOG^1_{0to-10}, EOG^1_{-10to0}, …, EOG^1_{0to50}, EOG^1_{50to0}, EOG^1_{0to-50}, EOG^1_{-50to0} and EOG^2_{0to10}, EOG^2_{10to0}, EOG^2_{0to-10}, EOG^2_{-10to0}, …, EOG^2_{0to50}, EOG^2_{50to0}, EOG^2_{0to-50}, EOG^2_{-50to0}).

In addition, another experimenter observed the subject's eye movements and recorded abnormalities (blinks, wrong saccades, etc.) on the experiment log. These abnormalities are excluded when processing these EOG data.

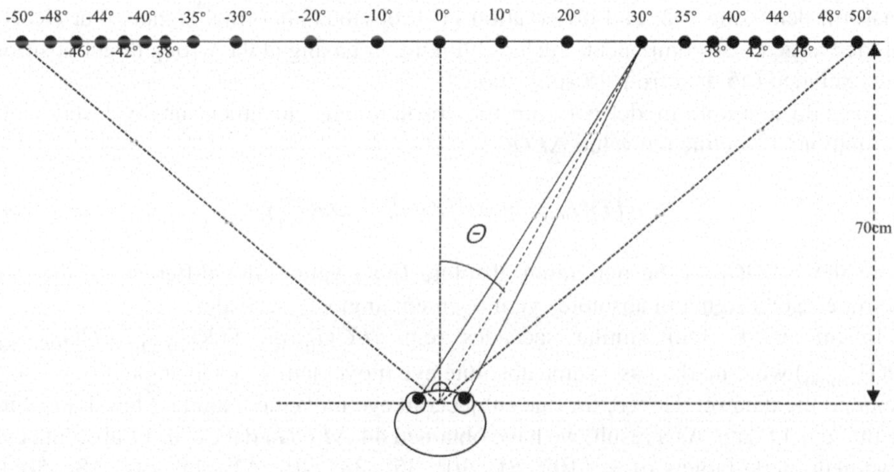

Fig. 2. The illustration of eye saccades experiment. The saccades sequence is {0°, 10°, 0°, −10°, 0°, 20°, 0°, −20°, 0°, 30°, 0°, −30°, 0°, 35°, 0°, −35°, 0°, 38°, 0°, −38°, 0°, 40°, 0°, −40°, 0°, 42°, 0°, −42°, 0°, 44°, 0°, −44°, 0°, 46°, 0°, −46°, 0°, 48°, 0°, −48°, 0°, 50°, 0°, −50°, 0°}.

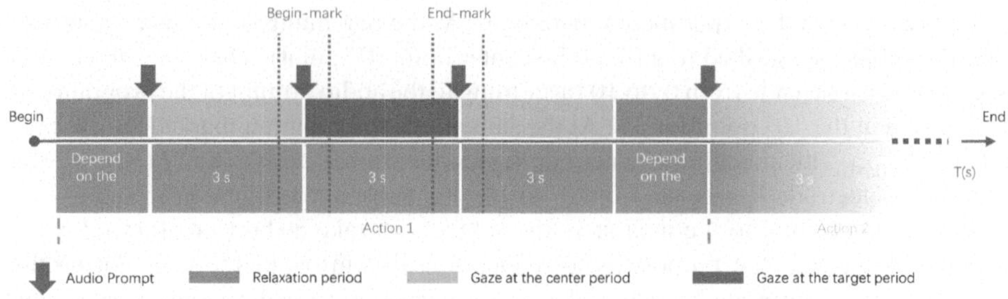

Fig. 3. The illustration of the experimental paradigm.

3 Methodology

3.1 EOG Signal Preprocessing

Before building a model, the raw data need to be preprocessed. The data preprocessing flowchart is shown in Fig. 4. We extracted the data between the begin-mark and the end-mark in the EOG sample as saccade events. Then we excluded the abnormalities according to the experiment log (32 data from 18 subjects and all data from one male subject with completely distorted signal due to bad electrode placement). After the data were captured, the measured EOGs were manually examined, by employing the wavelet transform denoising [12] and observation [13], obvious abnormal signals that clearly included large noise components such as blinking or gazing at the wrong target position were excluded (45 data from 18 subjects).

To build a simple model between the absolute eye movement angle θ and EOG information, we define the value ΔEOG_θ:

$$\Delta EOG_\theta = max(\left|EOG_\theta^1 - EOG_\theta^2\right|) \tag{1}$$

where the ΔEOG_θ is the maximum absolute EOG value after differencing the two electrodes EOG signal in absolute eye movement angle, θ, saccade.

In this work, four similar saccades (e.g., EOG^1_{0to10}, EOG^1_{10to0}, EOG^1_{0to-10}, EOG^1_{-10to0}) were marked as a same absolute eye movement saccade angle θ (e.g., 10°) to extend the data set. Hence, for one subject, an eye movement angle θ has 4 absolute eye movement data. As a result, we have obtained 44 ΔEOG_θ data with 11 absolute eye movement angle targets ($\theta = \{10°, 20°, 30°, 35°, 38°, 40°, 42°, 44°, 46°, 48°, 50°\}$) from 18 subjects.

In real life, due to the activities of humans, some unpredictable situations will happen. It is not enough to exclude the outliers manually, and other non-manual methods are needed to assist in processing the data.

To build a robust model, some outlier excluding methods were applied to the training set before training the model. 3σ criterion (Pauta criterion) [14] and MAD (Median Absolute Deviation) [15] are both the outlier excluding methods. These methods can further ensure that the training data will not deviate too much from the normal value.

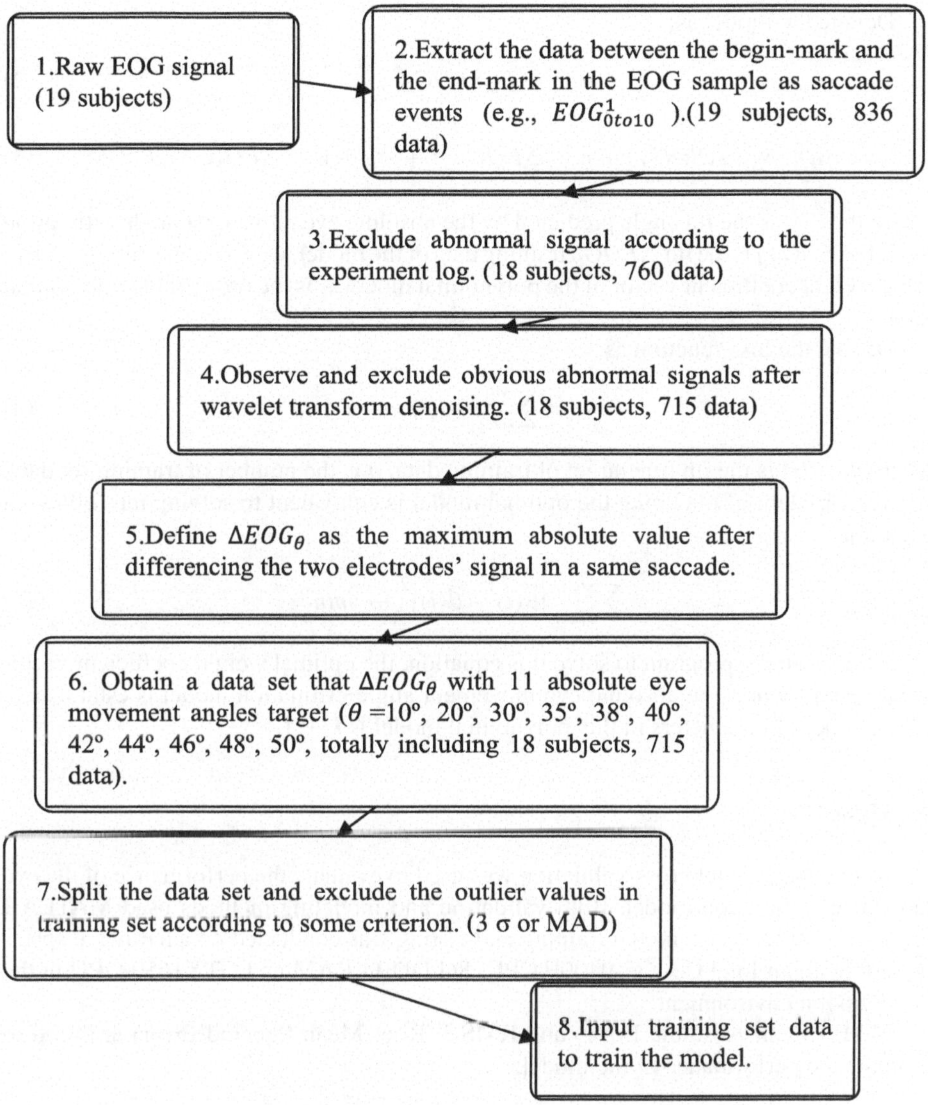

Fig. 4. The flowchart of signal preprocessing.

3.2 Polynomial Fitting Eye Movement Angle Estimation Model

Traditional eye movement angle estimation models consider eye movement angle θ to be a linear relationship with EOG. However, some further studies point out that the relationship between eye movement angle θ and EOG is not completely linear, but approximate linear within a certain range. In this work, we build a polynomial model to represent this incomplete linear relationship.

Denote the model as:

$$\widehat{\theta}(i) = f(\Delta EOG_{\theta,i}, \mathbf{w}) \tag{2}$$

$$= w_0 + w_1 \cdot \Delta EOG_{\theta,i} + w_2 \cdot \Delta EOG_{\theta,i}{}^2 + \cdots + w_k \cdot \Delta EOG_{\theta,i}{}^k, k \in N^+ \tag{3}$$

where the $\widehat{\theta}(i)$ is the ith angle predicted by the absolute eye movement angle estimation model. $\Delta EOG_{\theta,i}$ is the ith ΔEOG_{θ} training data of the model. $\mathbf{w} = [w_0, w_1, w_2, \cdots, w_k]$ is the weight coefficient vector of the polynomial model. k is the order of the polynomial model.

Denote the loss function as:

$$Loss = \sum_{i=1}^{n} [\widehat{\theta}(i) - \theta(i)]^2 \tag{4}$$

where the $\theta(i)$ is the ith true target of training data. n is the number of training set data.

The problem of obtaining the optimal model is equivalent to solving the following equation:

$$\sum_{i=1}^{n} [\widehat{\theta}(i) - \theta(i)]^2 \rightarrow min \tag{5}$$

After coding a program to solve this equation, the optimal weight coefficient vector $\mathbf{w}$ has been found. The absolute eye movement angle estimation model is established. The number of parameters in this polynomial model is $k + 1$.

4 Results

Leave-one-subject out cross-validation was used to evaluate the performance of the eye movement estimation model. Both validation and modeling methods used MATLAB R2021a software. Each model training and testing was conducted on a hardware specification with an Intel Core i5-9400F CPU, 8G DDR4 RAM and GTX1650 GPU in the Win10-64bit environment.

MAE (Mean Absolute Error) and RMSE (Root Mean Squared Error) are used to evaluate the performance of the model.

$$MAE = \frac{1}{n} \sum_{i=1}^{n} \left| \widehat{\theta}(i) - \theta(i) \right| \tag{6}$$

$$RMSE = \sqrt{\frac{1}{n} \sum_{i=1}^{n} (\widehat{\theta}(i) - \theta(i))^2} \tag{7}$$

where n is the number of test sample, $\widehat{\theta}(i)$ is the ith predict absolute eye movement angle value of the model in test set, $\theta(i)$ is the ith true target in the test set.

4.1 The Result of the Proposed Method

In this method, all ΔEOG data with angle target are separated according to each subject (totally 18 subjects). For all subjects, leave one of all subjects as the test set in turn, and all the others as the training set.

Figure 5 shows the performance change of the polynomial model from 1-order to 9-order. The performance increases significantly with the increase in number of orders before the 3rd order and reaches the best around 3rd or 4th order. The performance doesn't improve with the order increasing, but the computational resource consumption and parameters continue to increase.

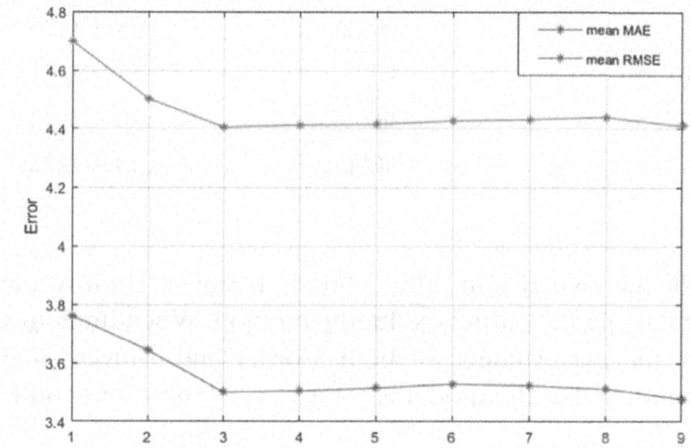

(a)

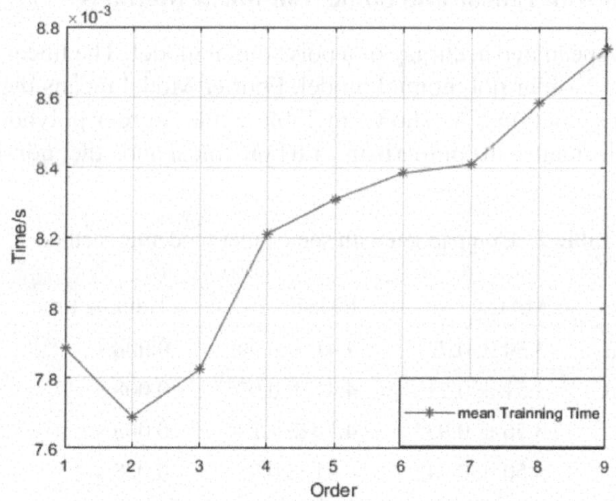

(b)

Fig. 5. The performance and running-time change of the polynomial model from 1-order to 9-order. Figure (a) shows the mean MAE and RMSE values of different orders. Figure (b) shows the training time of different orders.

The following Table 1 shows the best result of leave-one-subject method. The model is best when the order of the polynomial is 3 and 4. Parameters of the model are 4 and 5 respectively. To accurately evaluate the model and reduce the interference of random errors, here the mean and standard deviation of 18 subjects' results are provided.

Table 1. The results of the eye movement angle estimation model

Model	Model parameters	Outlier excluding	MAE	RMSE
3-order polynomial	4	–	$3.50 \pm 0.72°$	$4.41 \pm 0.99°$
	4	3σ	$3.50 \pm 0.74°$	$4.41 \pm 1.01°$
	4	MAD	$3.48 \pm 0.76°$	$4.40 \pm 1.03°$
4-order polynomial	5	–	$3.51 \pm 0.71°$	$4.41 \pm 0.97°$
	5	3σ	$3.50 \pm 0.73°$	$4.42 \pm 0.99°$
	5	MAD	$3.49 \pm 0.75°$	$4.41 \pm 1.01°$

Compared with the two results, the 3-order model is slightly better than the 4-order model without using the outlier excluding method. When implementing the outlier excluding method, the performance of both 3-order and 4-order models are slightly enhanced. It also implies that the model is robust even when some outliers exist.

4.2 Comparison with Linear and Some Non-linear Methods

Table 2 shows the speed and accuracy of a polynomial model. The linear model can also be considered as a 1-order polynomial model. Fourier Model means the model is fitted by cosine and sine functions. As shown in Table 2, the 3-order polynomial model can achieve better performance in comparison with both linear and other non-linear methods.

Table 2. Comparison with some other modeling methods

Model	MAE	RMSE	Training time	Multiples
3-order polynomial	**3.50** $\pm$ 0.72°	**4.41** $\pm$ 0.99°	**0.008 s**	**1.0**
4-order polynomial	$3.51 \pm 0.71°$	$4.41 \pm 0.97°$	0.008 s	1.0
Linear	$3.76 \pm 0.93°$	4.70 ± 1.24	0.008 s	1.0
Fourier	$3.50 \pm 0.71°$	$4.41 \pm 0.98°$	0.028 s	3.5

4.3 Compared with the Existing Works

Barbara et al. proposed a physically-driven, white-box and explicit electrical battery model of the eye movement angle estimation [6]. $2.42 \pm 0.91°$ is the MAE of angle estimated by Barbara's model. The accuracy of the model is better than ours (3.50 ± 0.72°). Compared with our model, this battery model is subject-dependent because it requires the distance between the subject's face-plane and the target-plane while we don't. Barea et al. proposed an electrooculographic eye model based on wavelet transform and neural networks with an error of less than 2° during long periods of use [16]. But there is a 250 ms lag between the eye movement and confirmation of the same. In this paper, the model we proposed is designed to deploy in embedded platforms or mobile devices with limited computing power limited storage space.

5 Conclusion

In this paper, a non-linear polynomial eye movement angle estimation model is proposed. With the optimal 3-order of the model, the estimation error in angle is less than 3.5° within a large-space from −50° to 50°. The model is simple, analytical, fast, and with less than 5 parameters. For single model training, the minimum time is about 0.008 s with an Intel Core i5-9400F CPU, 8G DDR4 RAM, and GTX1650 GPU. Experimental results in realistic scenarios across 18 subjects exhibit that the proposed model can achieve favorable performance in terms of accuracy and consumption cost. Consequently, the model can be easily deployed in the embedded platform or mobile device with limited computing power and limited storage space for real-time eye movement angle estimation. The proposed model is expected to be integrated with mobile devices to realize real-time eye movement angle estimation for EOG-related healthcare applications. However, it is also worth noticing that this paper is preliminary research that offers a novel and accurate model for eye movement angle estimation. Currently, only horizontal eye movement angle was estimated. In further research, experiments to collect both horizontal and vertical eye movement data for building a comprehensive eye movement angle estimation model will be explored. Meanwhile, to further verify the model, we will deploy it in a hardware system for realizing real-time estimation.

Acknowledgment. This work was supported in part by Shanghai Municipal Science and Technology International R&D Collaboration Project (Grant No. 20510710500) in part by the National Natural Science Foundation of China under Grant No. 62001118, and in part by the Shanghai Committee of Science and Technology under Grant No. 20S31903900.

References

1. Heide, W., et al.: Electrooculography: technical standards and applications. The international federation of clinical neurophysiology. Electroencephalogr. Clin. Neurophysiol. Suppl. **52**, 223–240 (1999)
2. Barea, R., et al.: Wheelchair guidance strategies using EOG. J. Intell. Robot. Syst. **34**(3), 279–299 (2002)
3. Deng, L.Y., et al.: EOG-based human–computer interface system development. Expert Syst. Appl. **37**(4), 3337–3343 (2010)
4. Barbara, N., Camilleri, T.A., Camilleri, K.P.: EOG-based eye movement detection and gaze estimation for an asynchronous virtual keyboard. Biomed. Signal Process. Control **47**, 159–167 (2019)

5. Zhang, Y.-F., et al.: A novel approach to driving fatigue detection using forehead EOG. In: 2015 7th International IEEE/EMBS Conference on Neural Engineering (NER). IEEE (2015)
6. Barbara, N., Camilleri, T.A., Camilleri, K.P.: Eog-based gaze angle estimation using a battery model of the eye. In: 2019 41st Annual International Conference of the IEEE Engineering in Medicine and Biology Society (EMBC). IEEE (2019)
7. Shinomiya, K., Shiota, H., Ohgi, Y., et al.: Analysis of the characteristics of electrooculogram applied a battery model to the eyeball. In: 2006 International Conference on Biomedical and Pharmaceutical Engineering, pp. 428–431. IEEE (2006)
8. Kumar, D., Poole, E.: Classification of EOG for human computer interface. In: Proceedings of the Second Joint 24th Annual Conference and the Annual Fall Meeting of the Biomedical Engineering Society Engineering in Medicine and Biology, vol. 1. IEEE (2002)
9. Manabe, H., Fukumoto, M., Yagi, T.: Automatic drift calibration for EOG-based gaze input interface. In: 2013 35th Annual International Conference of the IEEE Engineering in Medicine and Biology Society (EMBC). IEEE (2013)
10. Naga, R., et al.: Denoising EOG signal using stationary wavelet transform. Measur. Sci. Rev. **12**(2), 46 (2012)
11. Sadasivan, P.K., Narayana Dutt, D.: A non-linear estimation model for adaptive minimization of EOG artefacts from EEG signals. Int. J. Bio-Med. Comput. **36**(3), 199–207 (1994). https://doi.org/10.1016/0020-7101(94)90055-8
12. Bulling, A., et al.: Eye movement analysis for activity recognition using electrooculography. IEEE Trans. Pattern Anal. Mach. Intell. **33**(4), 741–753 (2011)
13. Manabe, H., Fukumoto, M., Yagi, T.: Direct gaze estimation based on nonlinearity of EOG. IEEE Trans. Biomed. Eng. **62**(6), 1553–1562 (2015)
14. Li, L., Wen, Z., Wang, Z.: Outlier detection and correction during the process of groundwater lever monitoring base on Pauta criterion with self-learning and smooth processing. In: Zhang, L., Song, X., Wu, Y. (eds.) AsiaSim/SCS AutumnSim 2016. CCIS, vol. 643, pp. 497–503. Springer, Singapore (2016). https://doi.org/10.1007/978-981-10-2663-8_51
15. Leys, C., et al.: Detecting outliers: do not use standard deviation around the mean, use absolute deviation around the median. J. Exp. Soc. Psychol. **49**(4), 764–766 (2013). https://doi.org/10.1016/j.jesp.2013.03.013
16. Barea, R., et al.: EOG-based eye movements codification for human computer interaction. Expert Syst. Appl. **39**(3), 2677–2683 (2012). https://doi.org/10.1016/j.eswa.2011.08.123

Adaptive Distance Sensing in Contact Tracing Applications Through Indoor/Outdoor Detection

Zaccaria Essaid, Dario Lorenzoni, Niccolò Scatena, Riccardo Xefraj, and Alessio Vecchio(✉)

University of Pisa, Pisa, Italy
alessio.vecchio@unipi.it

Abstract. Physical distancing is one of the most effective measures for limiting the spreading of the COVID-19 disease. Smartphones, being carried by their owners most of the time, are particularly appealing for increasing the awareness of people about their closeness to other individuals. Sensing the distance using communications technologies like Bluetooth is known to be affected by the surrounding environment. In this paper, we study the benefits that can be achieved by automatically recognizing if the user is indoor or outdoor and then defining a customized threshold for improving the accuracy of social distancing applications.

Keywords: Smartphone sensors · Distance estimation · Social distancing

1 Introduction

The COVID-19 disease is more likely to spread in crowded places, close-contact settings, and in confined spaces with poor ventilation [20]. The main suggestion from the World Health Organization is to maintain a minimum distance of 1 m between people, in order to reduce the probability of getting infected. Many works focused on the use of smartphones as a means to fight the spread of the virus: being personal devices that are almost always carried by their owners, smartphones are able to detect a wide range of unsafe behaviors. A well-known example is represented by the Exposure Notification (EN) service, a joint effort by Google and Apple to detect close interaction between users. EN relies on Bluetooth Low Energy (BLE). Many apps produced by health authorities include the EN service for tracing the contacts of infected users [3]. One of the key elements of a social distancing app is the capability of correctly estimating the distance between users. This is generally achieved using BLE, as it is a widely available technology and its energy requirements are compatible with prolonged use. In particular, the distance between two devices can be estimated, at the receiver, using the Received Signal Strength Indicator (RSSI), which is related to the distance as follows:

X. Gao et al. (Eds.): MobiHealth 2021, LNICST 440, pp. 157–165, 2022.
https://doi.org/10.1007/978-3-031-06368-8_11

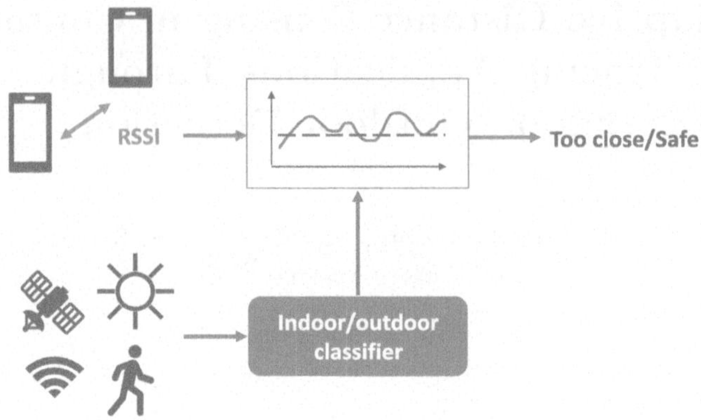

Fig. 1. Overview of the method.

$$RSSI = P_{tx} + G_{tx} + G_{rx} + 20log(\frac{c}{4\pi f}) - 10nlog(d) \tag{1}$$

where P_{tx} is the transmission power, G_{tx} and G_{rx} are the two antenna gains, c is the speed of light, f is the frequency, n is the path-loss coefficient, and d is the distance. Several positioning systems have been based on BLE [1,19]. Unfortunately, estimating the distance with great accuracy is difficult, mostly because of the impact of the surrounding environment (obstacles, walls, furniture, and other physical elements have an impact on the value of n). In this paper, we use the sensors available on common smartphones to automatically detect if the user is indoors or outdoors. This information is then used to recognize users that are too close (< 1 m) or at safe distance (> 1 m) with improved accuracy compared to an environment-unaware approach.

2 Method

Overall, the approach is summarized in Fig. 1: information produced by the sensors available on common smartphones is processed to produce a feature vector; the feature vector is given as input to a previously trained classifier, based on Machine Learning (ML) techniques, which detects the current environment of the user (only two classes are considered: indoor and outdoor); RSSI values are compared to a threshold (S) to understand if the transmitter device, carried by another user, is at safe distance or not. The threshold, used for understanding if the distance between the two devices is safe or not, is set to a value that depends on the current environment: S_{IN} and S_{OUT}, for indoor and outdoor settings respectively.

Indoor/Outdoor Detection. To understand if the user is indoors or outdoors, we use only the information produced by smartphone sensors. In other words, we

Table 1. Features extracted from the Android sensors.

Current luminosity
Mean luminosity (last 30 s)
Mean luminosity (last 30 s before proximity sensor is covered)
Last luminosity value before the proximity sensor is covered
Current proximity
Time elapsed since the last time the proximity sensor was uncovered
Number of Wi-Fi access points currently visible
Number of Bluetooth devices currently visible
Number of GPS satellites in line of sight
Number of fixed GPS satellites
Time elapsed since the last GPS fix
Daylight (night, twilight, daylight)
User's activity (running, walking, still, vehicle, bicycle, on foot, tilting)

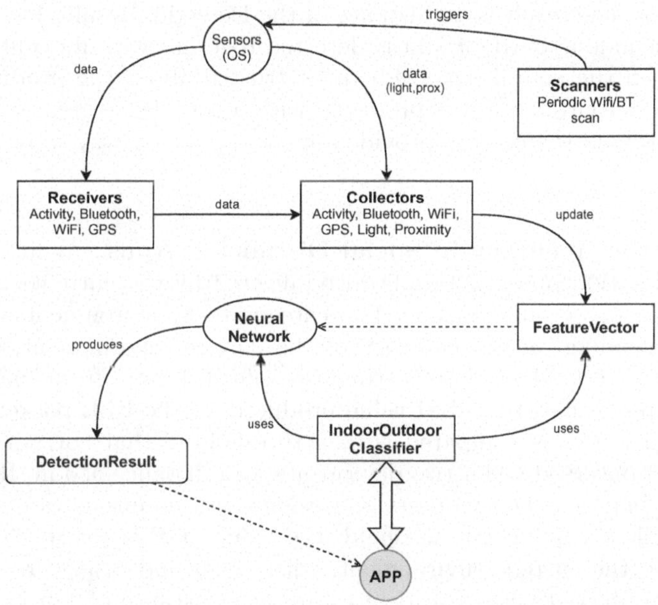

Fig. 2. Structure of the indoor/outdoor detection library.

do not rely on any infrastructure deployed in buildings, streets, etc. The classifier receives as input a vector of 21 elements extracted from the following sensors and communication technologies: light, proximity, GPS, Wi-Fi, Bluetooth. The light sensor is relevant as during daytime outdoor environments are generally characterized by higher values of luminosity. The proximity sensor can be useful to understand if the device is in a pocket or in a backpack. The GPS signals are shielded by buildings, and so they are typically less intense indoors compared to outdoors. Similarly, Wi-Fi access points and Bluetooth devices are generally more abundant indoor compared to outdoor. To foster its reuse, the mechanisms for detecting the current indoor/outdoor scenario have been implemented as an Android library. The library uses a TensorFlow Lite model [8], trained with Python scripts. The model also takes as input the activity of the user as detected by the software sensor included in the Android OS. The features extracted from the information sources are summarized in Table 1. The first 11 features do not need any specific encoding. The last two features, daylight and user's activity, are categorical features and they have been one-hot encoded, increasing the size of the feature vector to 21 elements. The high-level structure of the library is shown in Fig. 2. The receiver classes listen for data produced by sensors (with the exception of luminosity and proximity that are received directly by the collectors). Scanners are used to periodically scan for Wi-Fi AP and Bluetooth devices. The collectors prepare a FeatureVector instance. The IndoorOutdoorClassifier is the main entry point for the applications that want to use the library, and it is responsible for periodically running the neural network with the latest feature vector. The result is an instance of the DetectionResult class which contains the last indoor/outdoor status detected together with its confidence level (i.e. how much the neural network can be trusted about the produced value). The last indoor/outdoor status produced with a confidence greater than a configurable threshold is stored to provide apps with an easy way to retrieve recent information.

Improving the Accuracy in Social Distancing Apps. As mentioned, the distance estimation phase is significantly affected by the current environment. In our approach, we only consider two categories of environments: indoor and outdoor. Depending on the category of the current environment, as detected via ML, the threshold used to distinguish safe distances from unsafe ones is changed. In particular, the RSSI value produced by the BLE packets transmitted by another user is compared with a threshold S that corresponds to the average RSSI observed when two devices are at a distance of 1 m. If RSSI $> S$, the distance between the two users is considered to be unsafe (and vice-versa). Instead of using a universal threshold, the value of S is set to S_{IN} or S_{OUT} depending on the current environment, where S_{IN} and S_{OUT} are the average RSSI values observed when two devices are at a distance of 1 m in indoor and outdoor environments respectively. This is done to improve the accuracy of the system, as the RSSI is known to be influenced by the surrounding environment.

3 Exerimental Evaluation

Collection of Data. An auxiliary app was developed to log the abovementioned data and create an indoor/outdoor dataset. The app was used for two consecutive days by four volunteers. During the data collection phase, the users only had to manually trigger the transitions between indoor and outdoor

Table 2. Indoor/outdoor dataset.

	Indoor	Outdoor
Training set	68190	68190
Test set	1050	1050

settings in order to collect the ground-truth label. Due to the presence of time periods without movements, some repeated values were collected. To limit the bias in the training set, the adjacent duplicates have been discarded. A test set made of completely new data has been collected to evaluate the performance of the classifier. The size of the dataset obtained during the collection phase is reported in Table 2. The trained model was evaluated on the test set, and we obtained 59.4% of accuracy. This non-excellent result is due to the fact that the training set was built using the data collected by three volunteers, whereas the test set was made with the data collected by the fourth volunteer. To better understand the phenomenon, we repeated the training phase now including also 25% of the data collected by the fourth volunteer. The system trained in this way was able to obtain an accuracy of 92.83%. An important lesson can be learned from these results: indoor/outdoor detection can be carried out with high accuracy (~93%), but only when the training phase includes information about the specific environment where the system is going to operate. While a more diverse and large training set can improve the capacity of the system to generalize beyond the environments provided during the training phase, these preliminary results seem to highlight the benefits of customizing the model according to the specific environment.

Benefits of Adaptation in Social Distancing Applications. We collected 100 RSSI samples using two devices placed at the following distances: 0.5, 0.75, 1.0, 1.25, and 1.5 m. The collection has been carried out in an indoor environment and in an outdoor one. The devices involved in the collection were an iPhone SE 2, used as the transmitter, and a Samsung Galaxy J5, used as the receiver. The empirical pdfs of the RSSI values are shown in Fig. 3. The samples at 1 m distance were used to compute the thresholds S_{IN} and S_{OUT}, represented as dashed lines in the two graphs. As can be noticed, the RSSI values are influenced by the environment where the collection took place. We define the accuracy of the system as the percentage of samples collected at a distance < 1 m that are characterized by an RSSI value higher than S. The same was done for the samples collected at a distance greater than 1 m, but in this case RSSI had to be lower than S. Let's suppose that a single threshold is used for both the indoor and outdoor scenarios and that such threshold has been computed indoor (i.e., $S = S_{IN}$). In this case, the accuracy is equal to 91% for the indoor experiment and 72% for the outdoor one. On the other hand, when using S_{OUT} for the two environments (i.e., $S = S_{OUT}$) the accuracy values for the two environments are equal to 79% and 93%. Obviously, if the S_{IN} threshold is used for the indoor

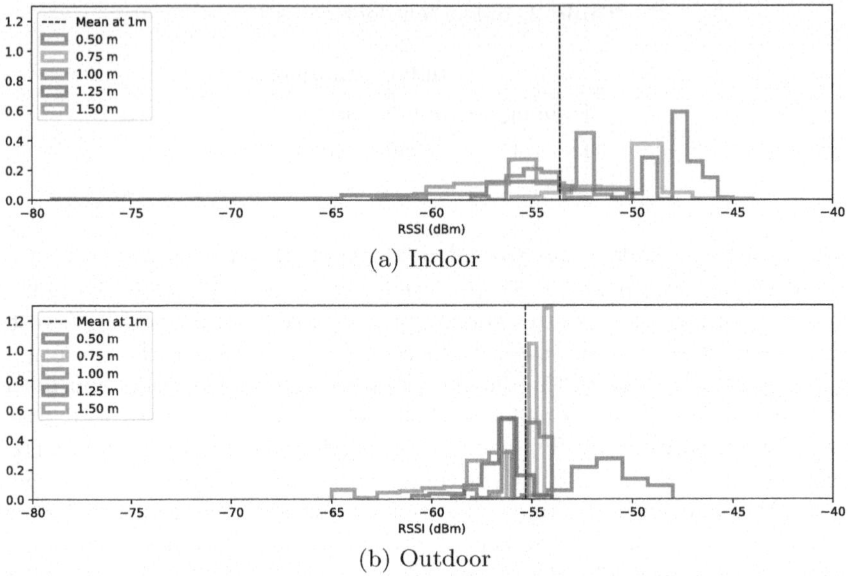

Fig. 3. RSSI values collected at different distances for the indoor and outdoor settings; S_{IN} and S_{OUT} are represented as dashed lines.

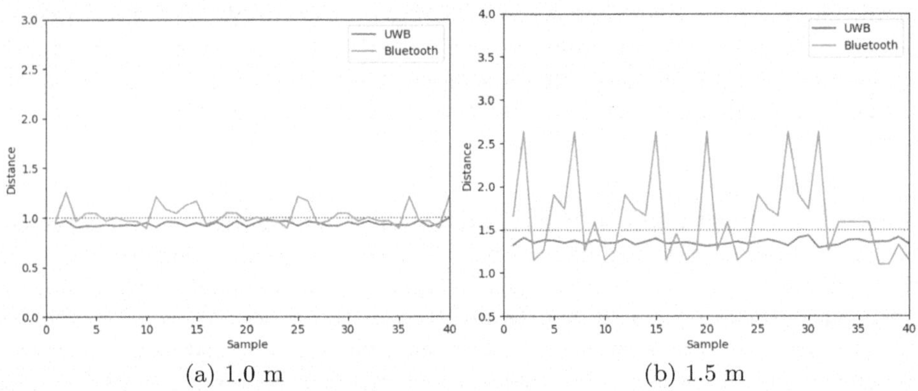

Fig. 4. Distance estimation using BLE vs UWB. On the x-axis the sample number is reported, whereas on the y-axis the estimated distance.

environment and S_{OUT} is used for the outdoor one, the accuracy values are equal to 91% and 93% respectively.

Overall, a threshold that is environment-specific improves the accuracy of 7–9%, and the technique should be considered for being included in social distancing or contact tracing applications.

Comparison with UWB. UltraWideBand (UWB) is a communication technology increasingly adopted in smartphones. UWB proved to be particularly effective in several applications involving human sensing [4,5,16–18], thanks to its capacity to estimate the distance between a transmitter and a receiver with good accuracy. We carried out a small experimental comparison of distance estimation using BLE vs UWB. For UWB experiments, we used the prototyping boards of a Decawave MDEK1001 kit [6]. For both technologies, we estimated the distance between a couple of nodes in an indoor environment, with four different target distances (0.5, 1.0, 1.5, and 2.0 m). For BLE, we assumed that environment-detection methods allow determining the best n value to be used in the RSSI-to-distance conversion process (Eq. 1). The distances estimated from the two technologies are quite similar for small distances (in the range of 0.5m and 1m). As the distance increases the UWB has a better and more stable estimation accuracy. The results obtained at two of the four considered distances are shown in Fig. 4 (the other results are similar).

4 Related Work

This work lies at the intersection of [11] and [2]. In the former, Liu et al. used Bluetooth for detecting face-to-face interaction between users, as a way to quantitatively assess social relationships. The study, carried out on a campus, highlighted that the sensors commonly available on smartphones, could be used for improving the detection of face-to-face interaction, for instance by recognizing that the device was in a backpack. In the latter ([2]), the authors devised a technique for improving the detection of indoor/outdoor environments. The problem of indoor/outdoor detection was also studied in [13] for logging the life of users, in [14] where the moving direction of the user was included for improving the detection accuracy, and in [10] using just magnetic sensors, light sensors, and cell tower signals. Indoor/outdoor detection for improving the recognition of the activities of daily living was proposed in [15].

5 Conclusion

BLE is a popular communication technology and one of the most convenient means for estimating the distance between people in contact tracing applications, as it works across different vendors and requires a limited energy budget. Unfortunately, its accuracy in estimating the distance between devices, and thus between people, is not particularly accurate [7,9,12]. Methods for automatically recognizing the environment where the users are located (indoor vs outdoor) can help in increasing the accuracy of RSSI-based distance estimation. The detection capability of the current setting (indoor vs outdoor) can also be useful for adapting the allowed physical distance between users. For instance, indoor the safe distance can be set to 2 m because of the poor ventilation, while outdoor a distance of 1 m could be sufficient.

Acknowledgment. This work is partially funded by the Italian Ministry of Education and Research (MIUR) in the framework of the CrossLab project (Departments of Excellence). The views expressed are solely those of the authors.

References

1. Alsmadi, L., Kong, X., Sandrasegaran, K., Fang, G.: An improved indoor positioning accuracy using filtered RSSI and beacon weight. IEEE Sens. J. **21**(16), 18205–18213 (2021). https://doi.org/10.1109/JSEN.2021.3085323
2. Anagnostopoulos, T., Garcia, J.C., Goncalves, J., Ferreira, D., Hosio, S., Kostakos, V.: Environmental exposure assessment using indoor/outdoor detection on smartphones. Pers. Ubiquit. Comp. **21**(4), 761–773 (2017). https://doi.org/10.1007/s00779-017-1028-y
3. Apple: https://covid19.apple.com/contacttracing
4. Bonsignori, C., et al.: Estimation of user's orientation via wearable UWB. In: 2020 16th International Conference on Intelligent Environments (IE), pp. 80–83 (2020). https://doi.org/10.1109/IE49459.2020.9154983
5. Brombin, L., et al.: User's authentication using information collected by smart-shoes. In: Mucchi, L., Hämäläinen, M., Jayousi, S., Morosi, S. (eds.) BODYNETS 2019. LNICST, vol. 297, pp. 266–277. Springer, Cham (2019). https://doi.org/10.1007/978-3-030-34833-5_21
6. Decawave: https://www.decawave.com/product/mdek1001-deployment-kit/
7. Giovanelli, D., Farella, E.: Rssi or time-of-flight for bluetooth low energy based localization? an experimental evaluation. In: 2018 11th IFIP Wireless and Mobile Networking Conference (WMNC), pp. 1–8 (2018). https://doi.org/10.23919/WMNC.2018.8480847
8. Google: https://www.tensorflow.org/lite/
9. Li, G., Geng, E., Ye, Z., Xu, Y., Lin, J., Pang, Y.: Indoor positioning algorithm based on the improved rssi distance model. Sensors **18**(9) (2018). https://doi.org/10.3390/s18092820, https://www.mdpi.com/1424-8220/18/9/2820
10. Li, M., Zhou, P., Zheng, Y., Li, Z., Shen, G.: Iodetector: a generic service for indoor/outdoor detection. ACM Trans. Sen. Netw., **11**(2) (2014). https://doi.org/10.1145/2659466
11. Liu, S., Jiang, Y., Striegel, A.: Face-to-face proximity estimationusing bluetooth on smartphones. IEEE Trans. Mob. Comp. **13**(4), 811–823 (2014). https://doi.org/10.1109/TMC.2013.44
12. Maratea, A., Salvi, G., Gaglione, S.: Bagging to improve the calibration of RSSI signals in bluetooth low energy (BLE) indoor distance estimation. In: 2019 15th International Conference on Signal-Image Technology Internet-Based Systems (SITIS), pp. 657–662 (2019). https://doi.org/10.1109/SITIS.2019.00107
13. Mizuno, H., Sasaki, K., Hosaka, H.: Indoor-outdoor positioning and lifelog experiment with mobile phones. In: Proceedings of the 2007 Workshop on Multimodal Interfaces in Semantic Interaction, pp. 55–57. WMISI '07, Association for Computing Machinery, New York, NY, USA (2007). https://doi.org/10.1145/1330572.1330582
14. Okamoto, M., Chen, C.: Improving GPS-based indoor-outdoor detection with moving direction information from smartphone. In: Adjunct Proceedings of the 2015 ACM International Joint Conference on Pervasive and Ubiquitous Computing and Proceedings of the 2015 ACM International Symposium on Wearable Computers,

pp. 257–260. UbiComp/ISWC'15 Adjunct, Association for Computing Machinery, New York, NY, USA (2015). https://doi.org/10.1145/2800835.2800939
15. Ouchi, K., Doi, M.: Indoor-outdoor activity recognition by a smartphone. In: Proceedings of the 2012 ACM Conference on Ubiquitous Computing, p. 537. UbiComp '12, Association for Computing Machinery, New York, NY, USA (2012). https://doi.org/10.1145/2370216.2370297
16. Vecchio, A., Cola, G.: Fall detection using ultra-wideband positioning. In: 2016 IEEE Sensors, pp. 1–3 (2016). https://doi.org/10.1109/ICSENS.2016.7808527
17. Vecchio, A., Cola, G.: Method based on UWB for user identification during gait periods. Healthc. Technol. Lett., **6**, 121–125 (2019). https://digital-library.theiet.org/content/journals/10.1049/htl.2018.5050
18. Vecchio, A., Mulas, F., Cola, G.: Posture recognition using the interdistances between wearable devices. IEEE Sens. Lett. **1**(4), 1–4 (2017). https://doi.org/10.1109/LSENS.2017.2726759
19. Viswanathan, S., Srinivasan, S.: Improved path loss prediction model for short range indoor positioning using bluetooth low energy. In: 2015 IEEE Sensors, pp. 1–4 (2015). https://doi.org/10.1109/ICSENS.2015.7370397
20. World Health Organization: https://www.who.int/news-room/q-a-detail/coronavirus-disease-covid-19-how-is-it-transmitted

Development and Validation of Algorithms for Sleep Stage Classification and Sleep Apnea/Hypopnea Event Detection Using a Medical-Grade Wearable Physiological Monitoring System

Zhao Wang[1], Zhicheng Yang[2], Ke Lan[3], Peiyao Li[4], Yanli Hao[3], Ying Duan[5], Yingjia She[6], Yuzhu Li[6](✉), and Zhengbo Zhang[7](✉)

[1] Medical School of Chinese PLA, Beijing, China
[2] PAII Inc., Palo Alto, Santa Clara, CA, USA
[3] Beijing SensEcho Science and Technology Co., Ltd., Beijing, China
[4] Department of Computer Science and Technology, Tsinghua University, Beijing, China
[5] Sleep Medicine Division, Airforce Medical Center, Beijing, China
[6] Department of Respiratory Medicine, Chinese PLA General Hospital, Beijing, China
lyz301@163.com
[7] Center for Artificial Intelligence in Medicine, Chinese PLA General Hospital, Beijing, China
zhengbozhang@126.com

Abstract. Sleep is critical to the overall health of humans. Polysomnography (PSG) is the current gold standard for measuring sleep and diagnosing sleep-related breathing disorders. However, this method is labor-intensive, time-consuming, and confined to a sleep laboratory. In this paper, we leverage algorithms for sleep stage classification and sleep apnea/hypopnea event detection by using signals from single-lead electrocardiograph (ECG) and respiration. To validate the accuracy of the above two algorithms, two independent validation studies were conducted using a medical-grade wearable monitoring system to collect physiological data from patients in both clinical and home settings. In the validation study of sleep stage classification, the average accuracy of our four-class stage classification using the bi-directional long short-term memory (BLSTM) method is 77.83% on our in-house dataset of 30 enrolled patients. In the experiments of sleep apnea screening, the two-level apnea-hypopnea index (AHI) classification reports the overall accuracies of 96.67% and 91.43% in clinical and home environments,

Zhao Wang and Zhicheng Yang equally contributed to this work.
This work was done during Zhicheng Yang's internship at Beijing SensEcho Science & Technology Co., Ltd., Beijing, China, when he was a Ph.D. candidate at University of California, Davis, CA, USA.

X. Gao et al. (Eds.): MobiHealth 2021, LNICST 440, pp. 166–185, 2022.
https://doi.org/10.1007/978-3-031-06368-8_12

respectively. The results showed that the sleep analysis algorithms presented in this paper have good performance in both sleep stage classification and sleep event detection, either in clinical scenario and home settings, indicating that our device can be used along with the two algorithms for sleep analysis.

Keywords: Sleep stage classification · Sleep apnea/hypopnea event · Apnea-hypopnea index · Physiological monitoring · Wearable system · Polysomnography

1 Introduction

Sleep is critical to one's mood, cognition, physiological internal environmental balance and resilience [5,9]. To appropriately present one's sleep condition, sleep is commonly classified into multiple stages in which physiological signals have different patterns that indicate various physiological functions. According to the American Association of Sleep Medicine (AASM), sleep is divided into five stages: wake, rapid eye movement (REM) and three levels of non-rapid eye movement sleep (including N1, N2, N3) [1]. Among the numerous criteria for sleep stage classification, the four-class sleep stage criterion (W-N1/N2-N3-REM) is more commonly adopted for its adequacy in sleep architecture assessment than two-class (W-N1/N2/N3/REM) and three-class (W-N1/N2/N3-REM) classification [14,23,42]. In recent years, the prevalence of sleep disorders has been globally increasing and attracted more attention [18]. Compared with the other types of sleep disorders, sleep apnea/hypopnea is a potentially serious one that is likely to lead to sudden and severe medical conditions [4,39]. Accurate classification of sleep stages and detection of sleep apnea/hypopnea events are essential to the analysis of sleep architecture and identification of various sleep-related disorders.

For a typical sleep analysis, polysomnography (PSG) test is the gold standard, which involves the electroencephalogram (EEG), electrooculogram (EOG), electromyogram (EMG), electrocardiogram (ECG), respiratory effort signals, and other measurements. However, subjects have to wear manifold attachments which cause extra mental and physical burdens during the test, and this procedure is also time-consuming as well as labor-intensive for clinical specialists [27,29]. To overcome the above drawbacks, researchers are searching for methods to automatically analyze sleep based on cardiopulmonary physiological signals that can be relatively easily acquired by low-cost wearable devices. Studies have shown that ECG and respiratory signals can be used for sleep staging and apnea/hypopnea event detection. Pedro Fonseca et al. extracted 142 features from ECG and thoracic respiratory signal of 25 subjects, and applied a linear discriminant classifier with an accuracy of 69% for four-class sleep staging on a 30-second epoch basis [8]. Magnusdottir et al. used two algorithms (cardiopulmonary coupling and heart rate cyclic variation) to identify sleep apnea based on automated analysis of single-lead ECG data. The results showed that the algorithms were as accurate as the automated scoring software for identifying patients with moderate to severe sleep apnea [15]. Recently, deep learning methods have become a center of attention in sleep analysis due to their advantages in handling time series over traditional machine learning methods. A long short-term memory (LSTM) network was applied to find out about sleep architecture by extracting 132 hand-engineering HRV features based on a comprehensive dataset (SIESTA [11]), and a five-fold cross-validation was performed on this dataset with satisfactory accuracy ($77.00 \pm 8.90\%$) [23]. Iwasaki A et al. adopted LSTM to distinguish patients with moderate-to-severe sleep apnea syndromes and from healthy subjects and achieved a sensitivity of 100% and specificity of 100% based on a threshold of apnea-hypopnea index (AHI) ≥ 15 events/h [10]. Despite the large number of sleep stage classification and event detection algorithms that have been developed, most of them are based on internal validation of the dataset itself, and the performance of these algorithms needs to be further validated with data collected from real clinical settings.

There have been some researches on validating commercial wearable devices in clinical scenarios. Pigeon et al. recruited 27 healthy adult subjects to validate their wrist-worn sleep monitoring actigraphy for sleep-wake scores with another commercially available actigraphy during a one-night PSG test [19]. GDL Pinheiro et al. proposed the validation of a wireless wearable oximeter on 58 patients for the diagnosis of obstructive sleep apnea (OSA) compared to the PSG test [20]. However, those wrist-based wearable devices are considered somewhat unreliable for clinical purposes. Xu et al. enrolled 80 subjects to validate the performance of a portable monitor (Nox-T3) to diagnose OSA in both laboratory and home settings [38]. Pion-Massicotte et al. validated the three-class (W-N1/N2/N3-REM) sleep stage classification of biometric shirts based on 2 nights of sleep lab recordings from 20 healthy adults, with a mean agreement rate of 77.4% when compared with PSG [21]. These validation studies are necessary if algorithms or systems are to achieve robust sleep monitoring for medical purposes.

In this paper, we developed sleep analysis algorithms focusing on four-class sleep stage classification and apnea/hypopnea event detection. To validate the accuracy of the algorithms, two independent validation studies were conducted using a medical-grade wearable physiological monitoring system to collect physiological data from patients in both clinical and home settings. Our key contributions were summarized as follows:

1. For the sleep stage classification algorithm, 152 features were extracted from ECG and respiratory signals, in which three new features were proposed to effectively detect abrupt changes in the RR intervals. Then, the bi-directional long short-term memory (BLSTM) network was leveraged for four-class sleep stage classification, because the bi-directional architecture of BLSTM was able to learn from past and future information. This advantage was suitable for our proposed sleep stage classification task in which the valuable "context" of sleep stage can be leveraged by BLSTM well. As for the sleep event detection algorithm, a new method was established to automatically detect sleep apnea and hypopnea by thoracic and abdominal respiratory movements.

2. Unlike many previous studies, sleep analysis algorithms proposed in this study were first trained and validated on a large public dataset before external validation was performed with data collected both from clinical (in a sleep laboratory) and home settings.
3. Compared with existing literature based on a single type of sleep analysis algorithm only, our study included both types of sleep analytics, empowering us to achieve a holistic and robust analysis.
4. We adopted a medical-grade wearable physiological monitoring system *SensEcho* [13,35–37,40,41], to collect physiological data. Both the performance of the algorithm and the system was validated in real clinical and home settings. The preliminary study showed that the system equipped with the algorithm can be used for sleep measurement and analysis.

2 Material and Methods

2.1 Algorithm Design

Sleep Stage Classification Algorithm. We used a public sleep database, Sleep Heart Health Study (SHHS) for model training [22], which consisted of the PSG monitoring of 6,600 patients in the U.S., including the records of sleep stage classification (Wake, N1, N2, N3, N4 or REM) for each subject manually determined by clinical specialists using modified Rechtschaffen & Kales (R&K) criteria [6]. N3 and N4 were combined into a single N3 label to align with AASM. First-time admissions patients (SHHS1) were screened with high-quality ECG and respiratory signals. Finally, 4887 subjects were selected to construct the dataset from the SHHS1. To align our four-class sleep stage classification, we converted sleep stage data to four-class (Wake-Light sleep(N1/N2)-Deep sleep(N3/N4)-REM).

Our feature extraction was processed on either one 30-second epoch or a larger window consisting of several consecutive epochs. The moving step size was set at one epoch. When multiple consecutive epochs (a larger sliding window) were used, the number of epochs was odd so that the calculated features could be associated with the central epoch. A total of 152 features were extracted from RR intervals (including time-domain features (features commonly used for the HRV analysis, and conventional statistical features on RR intervals, such as the mean, and quantiles, we also extracted 6 non-linear features including sample entropy, zero-crossing analysis.) [8,24,34], frequency domain features(21 features of the frequency domain were extracted, such as the mean, spectrum power, entropy.) [34]), respiratory signals (We extracted 25 statistical features. For example, in the time domain, the mean and standard deviance of respiratory peak sequence, kurtosis and skewness were extracted; features in the frequency domain included the dominant peak and energy.) [8,24], and cardiopulmonary coupling (CPC) effect [33]. We also designed three novel features for RR intervals as follows:

$$f_1 = \overline{I_n^{\mathrm{mid}}} - \overline{I_n} \tag{1}$$

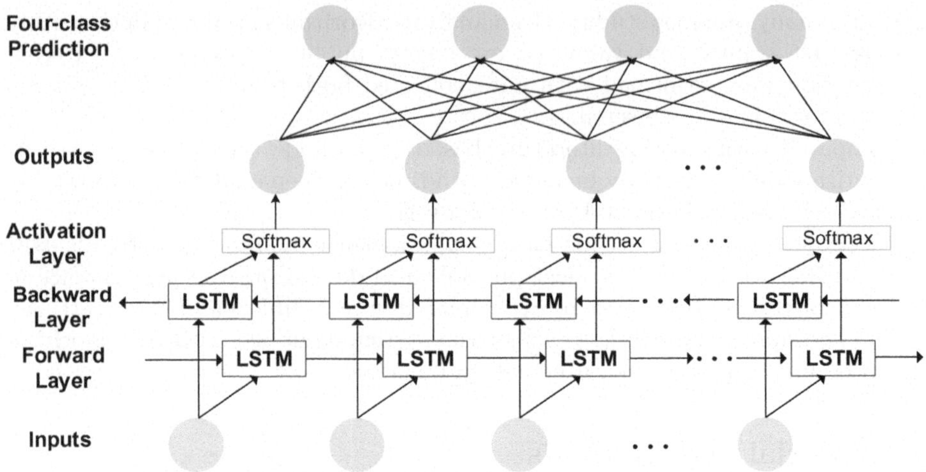

Fig. 1. Architecture of the BLSTM.

$$f_2 = \overline{I_n^{\text{mid}}} - \widetilde{I_n} \tag{2}$$

$$f_3 = \sqrt{\frac{1}{n}\sum_{k=1}^{n}\left(\overline{I_n^k} - \overline{I_n}\right)^2} \tag{3}$$

where I_n referred to raw RR intervals in the consecutive n epochs; I_n^k denoted the k-th epoch of I_n; I_n^{mid} was the middle epoch of I_n; $\overline{I_n}$ represented the average value of I_n; $\widetilde{I_n}$ denoted the median value of I_n. The three features investigated the impact of sudden variation of RR intervals in one epoch over the longtime series.

Unlike other conventional machine learning methods, the effectiveness of the LSTM approach has been proved in many studies for time series problems, because LSTM is able to effectively learn latent patterns from previous related information in a time series. Furthermore, the BLSTM is able to learn from past and future information. This advantage can facilitate our proposed sleep stage classification in which the valuable "context" of the sleep stage could be leveraged by BLSTM well. The structure of the BLSTM was illustrated in Fig. 1.

We randomly split the dataset into a training set and a validation set at a ratio of 4:1. No subject from the training set appeared in the validation set. All the feature vectors were fed into two 16-unit BLSTM layers and one fully connected layer with 4-unit outputs corresponding to the four sleep stage classes. The categorical cross-entropy loss was used as a loss function. In the process of training, the base learning rate was set at 1×10^{-3}, and the overall amount of training epochs was 5,000. The learning rate decay factor was 1×10^{-2}, and the minimum learning rate was 1×10^{-5}. The Adam optimizer was used. The networks were trained with a batch size of 256, and the dropout was 0.2. Five-fold cross-validation was performed to test our model in the training phase with an average accuracy of 78.84% (±0.08) and a kappa coefficient of 0.67 (±0.13). The optimal model was selected to further validate the performance on our in-house dataset.

Sleep Apnea/Hypopnea Event Detection Algorithm. A sleep event detection algorithm was used to determine sleep apnea/hypopnea through thoracic and abdominal respiratory movements. In the signal pre-processing step, we apply a median filter to the collected respiratory signals to remove outliers, remove the wavelet variation from the baseline of the respiratory signals, and adopt a band-pass filter with the frequency of 0.1∼0.5 Hz to remove noise. The denoised thoracic and abdominal respiratory signals are used to calculate relative tidal volume. Based on the detected peaks and troughs of relative tidal volume, we calculate the amplitude of respiration series and eliminate pseudo-peaks (the amplitude of respiration ≤ 0.15). The processed amplitude of respiration series is used to generate our key value *baseline respiratory amplitude*, which was defined as the median of the second to fourth highest respiratory amplitude within the first two minutes. The respective thresholds for apnea θ_a and hypopnea θ_h were then defined below:

$$\theta_a = A_{\text{base}} \times \alpha_a \tag{4}$$

$$\theta_h = A_{\text{base}} \times \alpha_h \tag{5}$$

where A_{base} denotes the baseline respiratory amplitude, α_a and α_h represent the scale factors for apnea and hypopnea thresholds, respectively. In our cases, we set α_a as 0.35 and α_h as 0.70. The following criteria were used to determine sleep apnea/hypopnea events:

- Central sleep apnea: (i) The interval between the two peaks exceeds 10 s and there is no respiratory movement in either thoracic or abdominal; (ii) The amplitude of respiration less than θ_a for more than 10 s with no peaks detected, or the interval between the two peaks is more than 10 s.
- Obstructive sleep apnea: (i) The interval between the two peaks exceeds 10 s and at least one of the thoracic and abdominal respiratory movements shows respiratory effort; (ii) The amplitude of respiration less than θ_a for more than 10 s and more than 6 peaks are detected, or no more than 6 peaks are detected, and the interval between peaks is not more than 10 s.
- Mixed sleep apnea: If the above two criteria are satisfied at the same time, and the central sleep apnea appears before the obstructive sleep apnea.
- Hypopnea: The amplitude of respiration less than θ_h but greater than θ_a signal for more than 10 s, accompanied by a decrease in oxygen saturation of more than 4%.

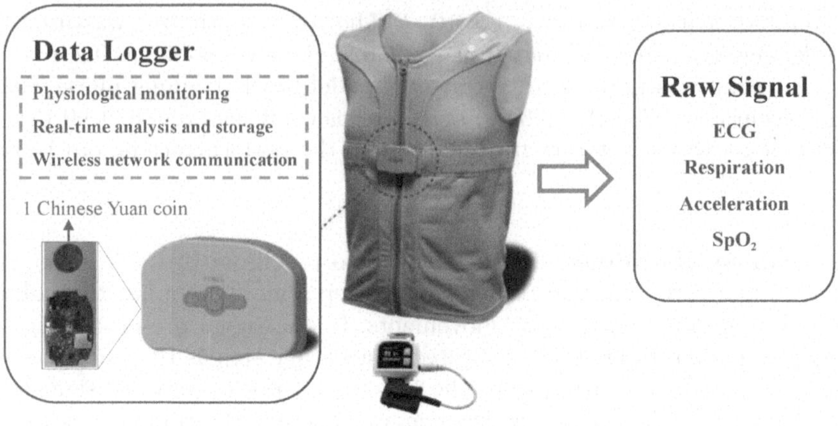

Fig. 2. Hardware and signal acquisition of SensEcho.

To evaluate the algorithm performance, 600 subjects were randomly selected from the SHHS database. There were 300 cases each with AHI < 5 (normal) and AHI ≥ 5. The accuracy for the two-class AHI classification was 92.18%.

2.2 Wearable Device Used in Validation Studies

Our medical-grade wearable device *SensEcho* is a wearable vest embedded with multiple biosensors to monitor various vital signs [13,35–37,40,41]. The system consists of three parts, including the monitoring terminal of accompanying physiological parameters, wireless networking and data transmission, and the central monitoring system. It has three comfortable electrode patches to capture the single-lead ECG signals at a sampling rate 200 Hz. Two sensing bands are embedded at the locations of the thorax and abdomen for monitoring the two types of breathing behaviors (thoracic and abdominal respiratory movements) at 25 Hz sampling rate. The error of heart rate and respiratory rate measurement is ± 2 and ± 0.15 beats per minute, respectively. SensEcho also has an ultra-low-power, 3-axis accelerometer MMA7260 (Freescale Inc., TX, USA) that is integrated into a data acquisition unit to capture posture and motility information. The accuracy of the 3-axis accelerometer measurement is 8 mg/LSB (Least Significant Bit). The main control chip of the system is ultra-low power ARM cortex-m3 MCU (EFM32GG330, Silicon Labs, USA). The power consumption of SensEcho is 100 mW. The device and its mainboard are shown in Fig. 2. Additionally, a wrist oximeter communicates with SensEcho via Bluetooth, whose sampling rate 1 Hz. SensEcho also provides local and cloud data storage options. When the cloud storage is neither stable nor available, the local storage can be activated to save the raw data in a 2-GB integrated flash drive.

The quality of acquired signals in wearable devices is very important for further data analyses and applications. SensEcho's signal quality can be mainly

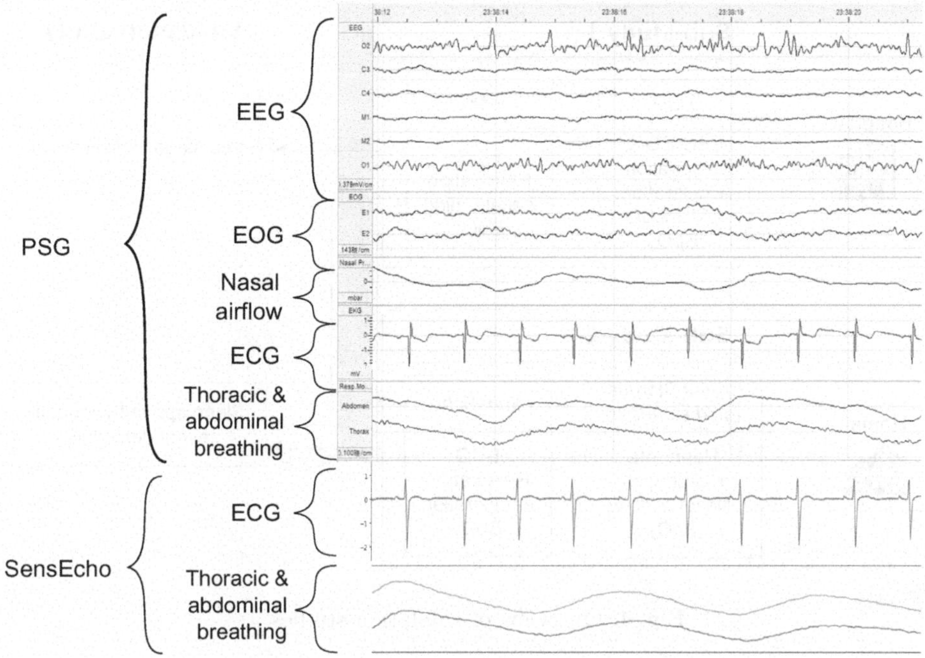

Fig. 3. A comparison of acquired signals between PSG and SensEcho.

interpreted in terms of device signal acquisition and wireless signal communication.

- Device signal acquisition: A comparison of signals of SensEcho and PSG records during an example period is depicted in Fig. 3. We can see that the consistency of the ECG signal and amplitude is higher between SensEcho and PSG, and the respiratory signal is also highly consistent with the PSG device. Compared with the gold standard, SensEcho can acquire signals with few errors.
- Wireless signal communication: The wireless physiological signal transmission unit is a network system based on Wi-Fi technology, including an ultra-low-power Wi-Fi module and WLAN system, which is capable of mobile monitoring, wireless network and roaming data transmission of multiple patients in the ward. The average packet loss rate between SensEcho and access points between 17 wards in our hospital was less than 0.1% for 16 months. The successful re-transmission rate was 100%. The data can be also successfully re-transmitted after the device is powered on next time, thus ensuring data integrity.

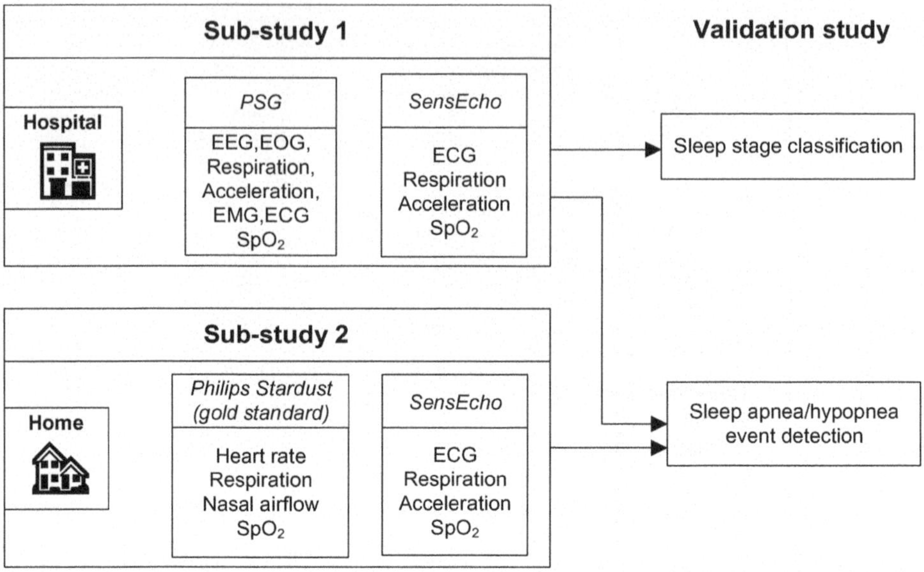

Fig. 4. Overview of validation studies.

2.3 Validation Study Design

Our study consisted of two independent sub-studies to validate sleep stage classification and sleep apnea/hypopnea event detection in clinical and home settings, respectively. Sub-study 1 was conducted in the sleep lab of Chinese PLA General Hospital, Beijing, China. All the research participants enrolled in this study wore both SensEcho and PSG. Aside from a well-controlled clinical laboratory environment, we also conducted another sub-study 2 in the home environment. All enrolled participants were asked to wear SensEcho and a CFDA-approved device (as the gold standard) for sleep apnea/hypopnea event detection due to the unavailability of PSG outside the hospital. An overview of two sub-studies was illustrated in Fig. 4. Every participant in both sub-studies complied with the protocol approved by the IRB review board (IRB number: S2018-095-01) and signed the written informed consent, and this study was conducted in accordance with the Declaration of Helsinki. Demographic information was collected by a questionnaire survey, including age, gender, weight and height.

Sub-study 1: SensEcho Compared with PSG for Sleep Stage Classification and Sleep Apnea/Hypopnea Event Detection. A total of 30 participants, who were suspected of sleep apnea in a respiratory clinic and met

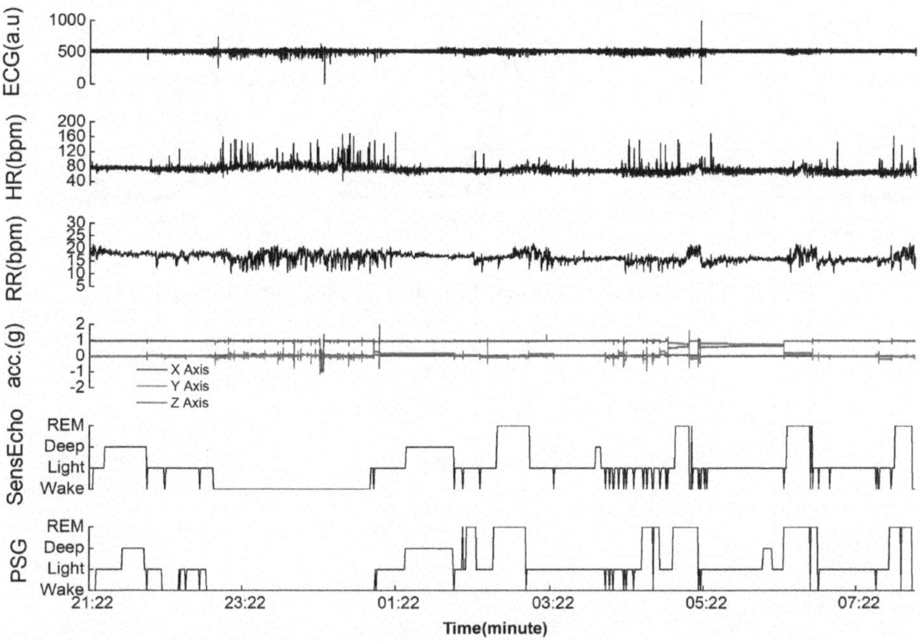

Fig. 5. Example raw ECG, heart rate, respiratory rate, acceleration of SensEcho, sleep stage classification of SensEcho and PSG for one night. "acc" stands for acceleration.

the inclusion and exclusion criteria, were enrolled in sub-study 1. The inclusion criteria included: (1) 18 years of age and over [17,19]; (2) willingness to cooperate with clinicians and to provide informed consent as determined. The exclusion criteria included: (1) current pregnancy; (2) recent healthy history of major psychiatric disorders or drug dependency or history of schizophrenia. Such criteria were endorsed by clinicians according to the recommendation of previous research [19]. PSG recordings of each subject were collected by Embla N7000 [16] The device settings and the electrode placement followed the regulation of the AASM [2]. The time-series data in a PSG test was segmented into 30-second epochs, and each epoch was scored by several certified sleep specialists' consent following the commonly adopted guideline [2]. During the PSG test, each participant wore SensEcho under the guidance of doctors. SensEcho synchronously collected his/her physiological data of ECG, respiration, posture/activities, and SpO_2 for one night depending on the actual sleep time. The configuration of SensEcho strictly followed the product's manual. Figure 8a showed the actual set-up of a participant who had signed written informed consent for use of his image in sub-study 1.

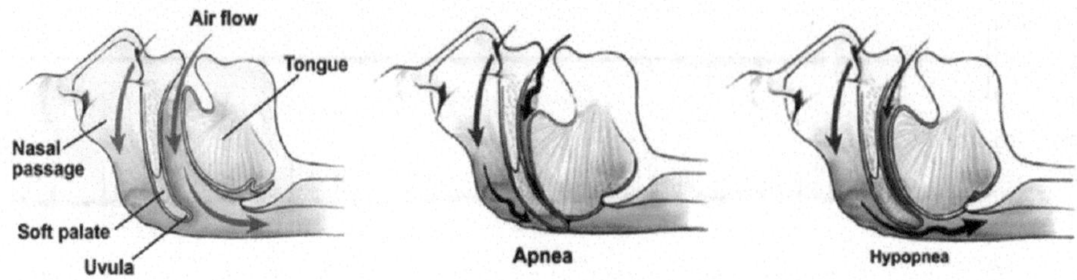

Fig. 6. The airways of normal breathing, apnea, and hypopnea.

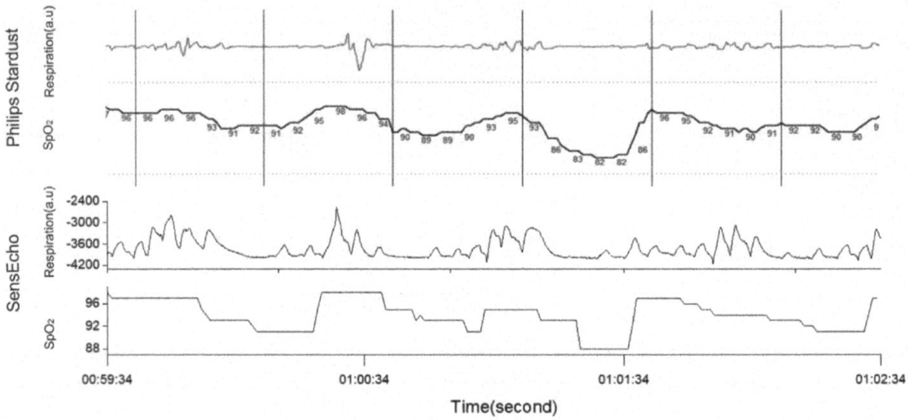

Fig. 7. An episode of sleep events lasting 3 min extracted from SensEcho recordings from one participant.

Before further analysis, clinicians first determined the sleep and awake points from the PSG data to extract the valid sleep duration. Every 30-s epoch of the sleep duration was then manually classified by clinicians into four categories (Wake-Light sleep(N1/N2)-Deep sleep(N3)-REM). The acquired physiological signals and the calculated vital signs by SensEcho of a subject and his four-class sleep stage classification are presented in Fig. 5.

Apart from sleep stage classification, we also compared sleep apnea/hypopnea event detection by SensEcho with PSG (shown in Fig. 3). Among various sleep disorder symptoms, we focused on apnea and hypopnea, which were the two most common ones [25,30]. Apneas were defined as more than 90% reduction in airflow from baseline for at least 10 s. Hypopneas referred to a decrease in airflow greater than 30% of baseline for at least 10 s duration accompanied by a decrease in blood oxygen saturation more than 3% and/or arousal, or a decrease in airflow greater than 30% of baseline for at least 10 s duration associated with more than 4% oxygen desaturation. Figure 6 shows the airways of normal breathing, apnea, and hypopnea(re-organized from Fig. 1 in the article [28]). We here leveraged the metric of AHI (the average number of apnea and hypopnea

Table 1. Participant characteristics.

Participants	In-house dataset in Sub-study 1 (sleep stage and apnea/hypopnea event detection)	In-house dataset in Sub-study 2 (apnea/ hypopnea event detection)
Number	30	35
Sex (F/M)	8/22	6/29
Night (number)	30	35
Age (year)		
Mean (std)	66.10 ± 12.85	43.74 ± 10.03
Maximum	90	64
Minimum	42	20
BMI (kg/m^2)		
Mean (std)	29.64 ± 4.74	26.89 ± 3.67
Maximum	41.15	34.40
Minimum	23.29	18.73
AHI		
< 5	5	6
≥ 5	25	29

events per hour) to detect apnea/hypopnea events. A cutoff of AHI = 5 events/h was used as a threshold in clinical practice for determining whether a subject had sleep apnea/hypopnea (AHI ≥ 5) or not (AHI < 5) [25].

Sub-study 2: SensEcho Compared with a CFDA-approved Device for Sleep Apnea/Hypopnea Event Detection. A total of 35 patients who met the eligibility criteria of our hospital's respiratory department were enrolled in the study. The inclusion criteria included: (1) 18 years old and over; (2) patients with suspected symptoms of sleep apnea. The exclusion criteria were the same as in sub-study 1.

All participants were required to wear SensEcho and a CFDA-approved device, Philips Stardust (PS), simultaneously for one-night sleep apnea/hypopnea event detection at home. The heart rate, respiratory effort, nasal airflow, and SpO_2 readings were recorded in PS, while the ECG signals, respiratory effort, body movements, SpO_2 data of SensEcho were collected. Figure 7 depicts the example signals of PS and SensEcho of a subject suspected of OSA. The process of wearing SensEcho was identical to that in sub-study 1. The AHI values of SensEcho and PS were compared to validate SensEcho's sleep apnea/hypopnea event detection performance, which was presented in the result.

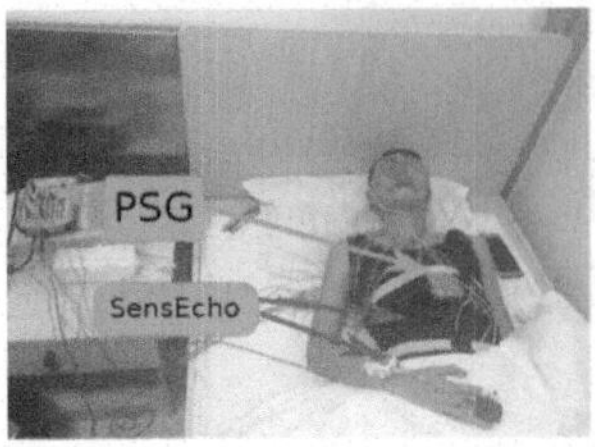

(a) A subject wore SensEcho during a PSG test to record his sleep behavior

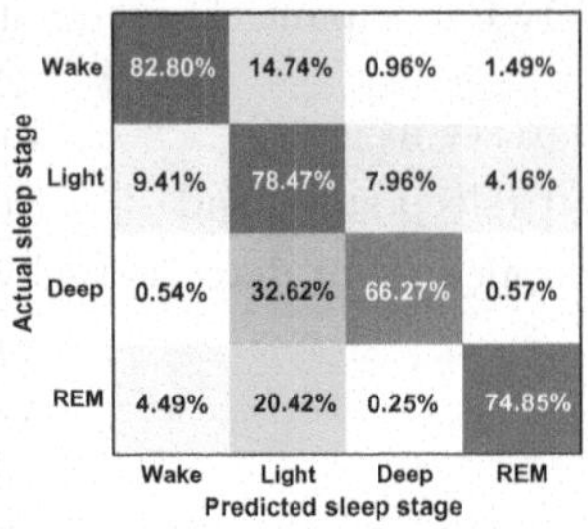

(b) Confusion matrix

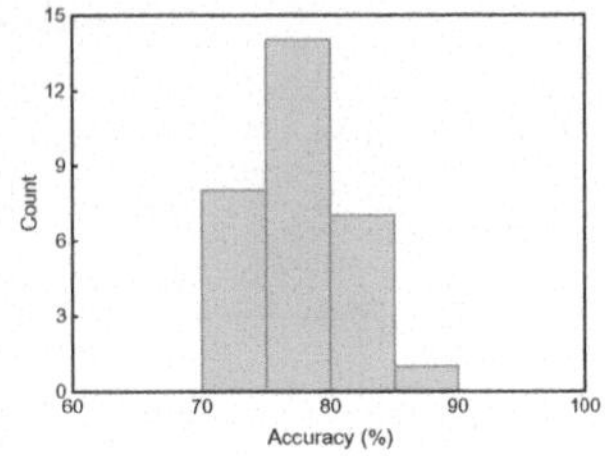

(c) Histogram of the accuracy distribution of all participants

Fig. 8. 4-class sleep stage classification on our in-house dataset in sub-study 1.

3 Experiment Results

Throughout our study, no unexpected incidents or study withdrawals were reported. All collected data were qualified for analysis: a total of 30 participants with 27,669 scored epochs in sub-study 1, and 35 participants with complete night data of SensEcho and PS in sub-study 2. Participant characteristics of the entire samples in both sub-studies are provided in Table 1.

3.1 Sub-study 1: SensEcho Compared with PSG for Sleep Stage Classification and Sleep Apnea/Hypopnea Event Detection

Results of Sleep Stage Classification. The average accuracy of BLSTM was 77.83% (±0.04%), and the kappa coefficient was 0.63 (±0.19). Figure 8b presents the confusion matrix of four-class sleep stage classification in sub-study 1. The accuracy of BLSTM for four-class sleep stage classification was 82.80%, 78.47%, 66.27%, 74.85%, respectively. The classification of wake had the best performance (82.80%) due to its distinct patterns against other sleep stages. As shown in Fig. 8c, 8 out of 30 had an accuracy of more than 80%, and there were no cases with an accuracy below 70%. The best case by SensEcho was 87.73% and the worst case was 71.47%. Figure 9 presents the examples of the best case and the worst case, respectively. Determining sleep stages based on an EEG of patients with sleep apnea is believed to be challenging for specialists while following normal staging rules [3]. Our results were relatively satisfactory.

Results of Sleep Apnea/Hypopnea Event Detection. In the left figure of Fig. 10a, the middle horizontal dashed line indicated the average bias (mean of AHI = –2.94 events/h), the top and bottom dashed lines were the 1.96 standard deviation limits. The right figure of Fig. 10a depicts the reference AHI of PSG (x-axis) versus SensEcho AHI (y-axis). Two black dashed lines indicated the reference threshold (AHI = 5 events/h) and SensEcho's threshold (AHI = 5 events/h). A confusion matrix for the classification of all participants into two

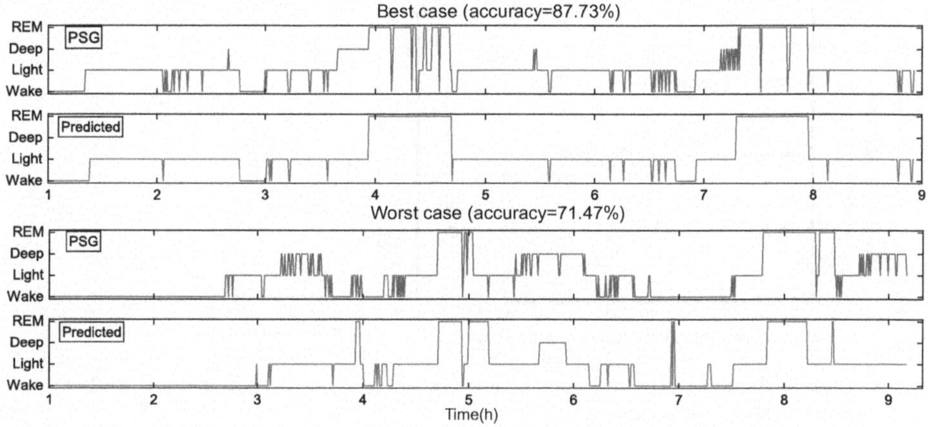

Fig. 9. Examples of the best and the worst cases of sleep stage classification in sub-study 1.

Table 2. Confusion matrix of sleep apnea detection using SensEcho in sub-study 1.

		PSG		
		AHI ≥ 5	AHI < 5	
SensEcho	AHI ≥ 5	25	1	PPV 96.15%
	AHI < 5	0	4	NPV 100%
		Sensitivity 100%	Specificity 80%	Accuracy 96.67%

categories is presented in Table 2. SensEcho had a sensitivity of 100% in detecting AHI of 5 and above. The specificity, positive predictive value (PPV), negative predictive value (NPV), and total accuracies were 80%, 96.15%, 100%, 96.67%, respectively.

3.2 Sub-study 2: SensEcho Compared with a CFDA-approved Device for Sleep Apnea/Hypopnea Event Detection

The dashed lines in the left figure of Fig. 10b referred to the average bias and the 1.96 standard deviation limits, and the dashed lines in the right figure of Fig. 10b denoted the reference threshold (AHI = 5 events/h) and SensEcho's threshold (AHI = 5 events/h). A confusion matrix for the classification of all participants into two categories is illustrated in Table 3. SensEcho had a sensitivity of 93.10% in detecting AHI of 5 and above. In addition, specificity, PPV, NPV, and the total accuracy was 83.33%, 96.43%, 71.43%, 91.43%, respectively.

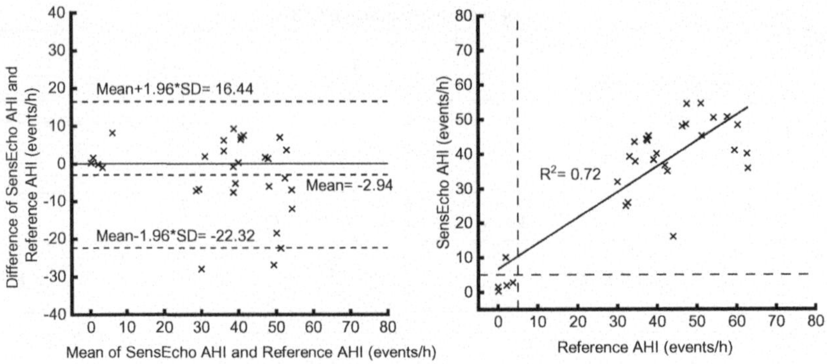

(a) Bland-Altman (left) and correlation (right) plots of SensEcho AHI and the reference AHI in sub-study 1

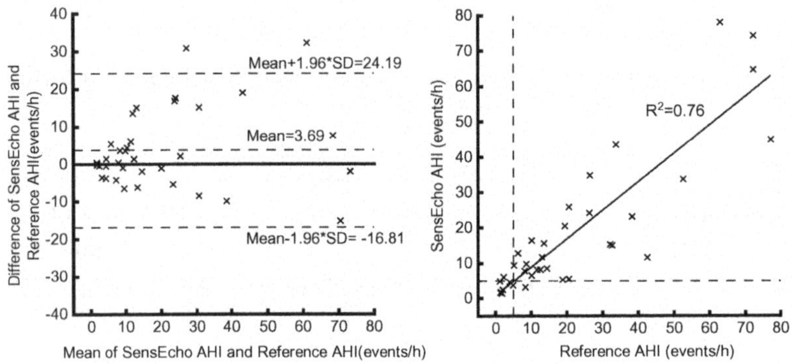

(b) Bland-Altman (left) and correlation (right) plots of SensEcho AHI and the reference AHI in sub-study 2

Fig. 10. Sleep apnea/hypopnea event detection in sub-study 1 and 2.

4 Discussion

In this study, we proposed two algorithms for sleep analysis with sleep stage classification and apnea/hypopnea event detection. We also validated our algorithms in different environmental settings via two independent sub-studies, enabling us to provide a comprehensive validation study on the two algorithms in both hospital and home scenarios. Compared with the gold standard, the results in both sub-studies indicate that the algorithms along with the wearable physiological monitoring system provide a reliable approach to sleep analysis. The satisfactory overall accuracy is attributed to the stability and robustness of the wearable physiological detection system. Based on a user survey of 30 subjects in sub-study 1, 85% of the subjects responded that they felt comfortable with SensEcho and

Table 3. Confusion matrix of sleep apnea detection using SensEcho in sub-study 2.

		PS		
		AHI $\geq$ 5	AHI $<$ 5	
SensEcho	AHI $\geq$ 5	27	1	PPV 96.43%
	AHI $<$ 5	2	5	NPV 71.43%
		Sensitivity 93.10%	Specificity 83.33%	Accuracy 91.43%

did not feel tight in their thoraxes. SensEcho is regarded as patient-friendly for long-term sleep monitoring.

In terms of sleep stage classification, numerous researches relied on PSG tests where EEG, EOG, and EMG were recorded for an accurate sleep stage classification [12,26]. However, those signal sources (EEG, EOG, EMG) were not available for typical wearable devices, making the sleep stage classification task more challenging. Some researchers utilized the public dataset (SIESTA, SHHS) and laboratory data to classify four sleep stages and reported an satisfactory accuracy [8,32]. However, most of them did not conduct further clinical validation studies. Asher Tal et al. validated a contact-free sleep monitoring device (EarlySense) in 2017 [31]. EarlySense achieved relatively high accuracy in two-class sleep stage classification (sleep and wake). However, the overall accuracy of four-class sleep stage classification was moderate (about 63.5%, calculated from the confusion matrix provided by the authors). Unlike the researches mentioned above, we performed validation studies in clinical settings. The average accuracy of our four-class sleep stage classification was satisfactory on the dataset collected from the enrolled patients.

Considering the performance of sleep apnea detection using wearable systems in existing studies, based on a threshold of AHI $\geq$ 5 events/h, Nox-T3 portable monitor had a sensitivity of 95%, a specificity of 69%, PPV of 94% and NPV of 75% when used to detect AHI compared to PSG [38], a photoplethysmography (PPG)-based device detected OSA with a sensitivity of 100%, specificity of 44%, PPV of 62%, and NPV of 100% compared to PSG on 48 patients [7]. Compared to those results, SensEcho had a satisfactory sensitivity, specificity, and accuracy in terms of sleep apnea/hypopnea event detection. The confident results could be attributed to the robust sleep apnea/hypopnea event detection algorithm presented in this study, as well as accurate measurement of respiratory signals from SensEcho. The sensitivity of the AHI detection in sub-study 2 was slightly lower than that in sub-study 1 possibly for the following reasons. Firstly, patients who wore PSG usually suffered from worse sleep problems than those who wore PS (shown in Fig. 10a and Fig. 10b). Secondly, PS was specifically designed for portable sleep apnea/hypopnea event detection. Its results might be influenced by factors such as wearing conditions of the patients and device performance so that the results might be not so reliable as those of PSG.

Admittedly, there are some limitations to our study. First, the participants enrolled in the two sub-studies were not identical. They were allowed to choose to sleep in clinical or home settings. However, since each sub-study was independent, there was no substantial impact on our validation results. Second, the number of patients and healthy individuals in sub-study 1 was not matched, which was why the sleep apnea/hypopnea event detection algorithm showed higher accuracy on the external test dataset than on the validation dataset. Third, since the experiments in sub-study 2 were performed in a home setting, there was some uncertainty about the device. For instance, some patches were displaced or not tightly connected by accident while the participants were not realizing such events, even though every participant was given instructions as to how to use the device by specialists before he/she conducted the experiment at home. Fourth, while our study significantly improved the accuracy of sleep stage classification, the accurate classification between N3 and N1/N2 remained challenging.

In our ongoing and future research, we will keep expanding the clinical sample size, recruiting patients who have sleep-related symptoms or diseases to continuously constitute our comprehensive sleep database. A large in-house database will also mitigate the possible bias introduced by ethnicity, age, and disease, etc. when a public database is used for model training. Second, we will optimize and fine-tune the sleep stage classification and sleep apnea/hypopnea event detection models based on large sample datasets to improve the accuracy and robustness. The current sleep event detection algorithm can effectively identify whether a patient has sleep apnea/hypopnea. In future studies, we will continue to explore sleep event detection algorithms based on the different severity levels of AHI to provide patients with a severity degree screening for sleep apnea/hypopnea events. Finally, despite the inability of SensEcho to fully achieve the accuracy of PSG's sleep analysis, it still provides sleep architecture and apnea/hypopnea event detection. We will apply the wearable system with algorithms to monitor patients' sleep conditions in both clinical and home scenarios to further validate the feasibility of the system and algorithms.

5 Conclusions

In this study, we developed algorithms for sleep stage classification and sleep event detection using cardiopulmonary signals based on a large sample dataset, and adopted a medical-grade wearable system to collect physiological data. To further validate the performance of the algorithms, we conducted validation studies in clinical and home settings, and the results showed high agreement with PSG for four-class sleep stage classification and sleep apnea/hypopnea detection in clinical settings, and good performance for sleep apnea/hypopnea screening in home settings. The results demonstrate that the sleep analysis algorithms proposed in this paper perform well in both sleep stage classification and sleep event detection, either in clinical scenarios and home settings, indicating that the wearable system of SensEcho can be used along with the two algorithms for sleep measurement and analysis.

Acknowledgment. This work is supported by The National Natural Science Foundation of China (62171471); Beijing Municipal Science and Technology (Z181100001918023); Big Data Research & Development Project of Chinese PLA General Hospital (2018MBD-09).

References

1. Berry, R.B., et al.: Aasm scoring manual updates for 2017 (version 2.4). J. Clin. Sleep Med. **13**(5), 665–666 (2017)
2. Berry, R.B., et al.: Aasm scoring manual version 2.2 updates: new chapters for scoring infant sleep staging and home sleep apnea testing. J. Clin. Sleep Med. **11**(11), 1253–1254 (2015)
3. Carskadon, M.A., Rechtschaffen, A.: Monitoring and staging human sleep. Principles Pract. Sleep Med. **5**, 16–26 (2011)
4. Chaiard, J., Weaver, T.E.: Update on research and practices in major sleep disorders: part ii-insomnia, willis-ekbom disease (restless leg syndrome), and narcolepsy. J. Nurs. Sch. **51**(6), 624–633 (2019)
5. Cheng, W., Rolls, E.T., Ruan, H., Feng, J.: Functional connectivities in the brain that mediate the association between depressive problems and sleep quality. JAMA Psychiatry **75**(10), 1052–1061 (2018)
6. Dean, D.A., et al.: Scaling up scientific discovery in sleep medicine: the national sleep research resource. Sleep **39**(5), 1151–1164 (2016)
7. Faßbender, P., Haddad, A., Bürgener, S., Peters, J.: Validation of a photoplethysmography device for detection of obstructive sleep apnea in the perioperative setting. J. Clin. Monit. Comput. **33**(2), 341–345 (2018). https://doi.org/10.1007/s10877-018-0151-2
8. Fonseca, P., Long, X., Radha, M., Haakma, R., Aarts, R.M., Rolink, J.: Sleep stage classification with ecg and respiratory effort. Physiol. Meas. **36**(10), 2027 (2015)
9. Irwin, M.R.: Sleep and inflammation: partners in sickness and in health. Nat. Rev. Immunol. **19**(11), 702–715 (2019)
10. Iwasaki, A., et al.: Screening of sleep apnea based on heart rate variability and long short-term memory. Sleep Breathing **25**(4), 1821–1829 (2021). https://doi.org/10.1007/s11325-020-02249-0
11. Klosh, G., et al.: The siesta project polygraphic and clinical database. IEEE Eng. Med. Biol. Mag. **20**(3), 51–57 (2001)
12. Lajnef, T., et al.: Learning machines and sleeping brains: automatic sleep stage classification using decision-tree multi-class support vector machines. J. Neurosci. Meth. **250**, 94–105 (2015)
13. Li, P., et al.: Mobicardio: a clinical-grade mobile health system for cardiovascular disease management. In: 2019 IEEE International Conference on Healthcare Informatics (ICHI), pp. 1–6. IEEE (2019)
14. Long, X., et al.: Measuring dissimilarity between respiratory effort signals based on uniform scaling for sleep staging. Physiol. Meas. **35**(12), 2529 (2014)
15. Magnusdottir, S., Hilmisson, H.: Ambulatory screening tool for sleep apnea: analyzing a single-lead electrocardiogram signal (ecg). Sleep Breathing **22**(2), 421–429 (2018). https://doi.org/10.1007/s11325-017-1566-6
16. Myllymaa, S., et al.: Assessment of the suitability of using a forehead eeg electrode set and chin emg electrodes for sleep staging in polysomnography. J. Sleep Res. **25**(6), 636–645 (2016)

17. Cho, J.H., Kim, H.J.: Validation of apnealink ox^{TM} plus for the diagnosis of sleep apnea. Sleep Breathing **21**(3), 799–807 (2017). https://doi.org/10.1007/s11325-017-1532-3
18. Peppard, P.E., Young, T., Barnet, J.H., Palta, M., Hagen, E.W., Hla, K.M.: Increased prevalence of sleep-disordered breathing in adults. Am. J. Epidemiol. **177**(9), 1006–1014 (2013)
19. Pigeon, W.R., Taylor, M., Bui, A., Oleynk, C., Walsh, P., Bishop, T.M.: Validation of the sleep-wake scoring of a new wrist-worn sleep monitoring device. J. Clin. Sleep Med. **14**(6), 1057–1062 (2018)
20. Pinheiro, G., Cruz, A., Genta, P., Lorenzi-Filho, G.: Validation of a wireless wearable oximeter using mobile technology and cloud computing for the diagnosis of obstructive sleep apnea. In: B68. Diagnosis and Treatment of Sleep Disordered Breathing, pp. A3976–A3976. American Thoracic Society (2018)
21. Pion-Massicotte, J., Godbout, R., Savard, P., Roy, J.F.: Development and validation of an algorithm for the study of sleep using a biometric shirt in young healthy adults. J. Sleep Res. **28**(2), e12667 (2019)
22. Iber, C., et al.: The sleep heart health study: design, rationale, and methods. Sleep **20**(12), 1077–1085 (1997)
23. Radha, M., et al.: Sleep stage classification from heart-rate variability using long short-term memory neural networks. Sci. Rep. **9**(1), 1–11 (2019)
24. Redmond, S.J., de Chazal, P., O'Brien, C., Ryan, S., McNicholas, W.T., Heneghan, C.: Sleep staging using cardiorespiratory signals. Somnologie-Schlafforschung und Schlafmedizin **11**(4), 245–256 (2007). https://doi.org/10.1007/s11818-007-0314-8
25. Ruehland, W.R., Rochford, P.D., O'Donoghue, F.J., Pierce, R.J., Singh, P., Thornton, A.T.: The new aasm criteria for scoring hypopneas: impact on the apnea hypopnea index. Sleep **32**(2), 150–157 (2009)
26. Shi, P., Zheng, X., Du, P., Yuan, F.: Automatic sleep stage classification based on LSTM. In: Sun, Y., Lu, T., Xie, X., Gao, L., Fan, H. (eds.) ChineseCSCW 2018. CCIS, vol. 917, pp. 478–486. Springer, Singapore (2019). https://doi.org/10.1007/978-981-13-3044-5_35
27. Silber, M.H., et al.: The visual scoring of sleep in adults. J. Clin. Sleep Med. **3**(02), 121–131 (2007)
28. Somers, V.K., et al.: Sleep apnea and cardiovascular disease: an American heart association/American college of cardiology foundation scientific statement from the american heart association council for high blood pressure research professional education committee, council on clinical cardiology, stroke council, and council on cardiovascular nursing in collaboration with the national heart, lung, and blood institute national center on sleep disorders research (national institutes of health). J. Am. Coll. Cardiol. **52**(8), 686–717 (2008)
29. Stephansen, J.B., et al.: Neural network analysis of sleep stages enables efficient diagnosis of narcolepsy. Nat. Commun. **9**(1), 1–15 (2018)
30. Strollo, P.J., Jr., Rogers, R.M.: Obstructive sleep apnea. N. Engl. J. Med. **334**(2), 99–104 (1996)
31. Tal, A., Shinar, Z., Shaki, D., Codish, S., Goldbart, A.: Validation of contact-free sleep monitoring device with comparison to polysomnography. J. Clini. Sleep Med. **13**(3), 517–522 (2017)
32. Tataraidze, A., Korostovtseva, L., Anishchenko, L., Bochkarev, M., Sviryaev, Y.: Sleep architecture measurement based on cardiorespiratory parameters. In: 2016 38th Annual International Conference of the IEEE Engineering in Medicine and Biology Society (EMBC), pp. 3478–3481. IEEE (2016)

33. Thomas, R.J., Mietus, J.E., Peng, C.K., Goldberger, A.L.: An electrocardiogram-based technique to assess cardiopulmonary coupling during sleep. Sleep **28**(9), 1151–1161 (2005)
34. Xiao, M., Yan, H., Song, J., Yang, Y., Yang, X.: Sleep stages classification based on heart rate variability and random forest. Biomed. Sign. Proces. Control **8**(6), 624–633 (2013)
35. Xu, H., et al.: Study on the accuracy of cardiopulmonary physiological measurements by a wearable physiological monitoring system under different activity conditions. Sheng wu yi xue gong cheng xue za zhi=J. Biomed. Eng.=Shengwu yixue gongchengxue zazhi **37**(1), 119–128 (2020)
36. Xu, H., et al.: Construction and application of a medical-grade wireless monitoring system for physiological signals at general wards. J. Med. Syst. **44**(10), 1–15 (2020). https://doi.org/10.1007/s10916-020-01653-z
37. Xu, H., et al.: Assessing electrocardiogram and respiratory signal quality of a wearable device (sensecho): semisupervised machine learning-based validation study. JMIR mHealth uHealth **9**(8), e25415 (2021)
38. Xu, L., et al.: Validation of the nox-t3 portable monitor for diagnosis of obstructive sleep apnea in chinese adults. J. Clin. Sleep Med. **13**(5), 675–683 (2017)
39. Yang, Z., Pathak, P.H., Zeng, Y., Liran, X., Mohapatra, P.: Vital sign and sleep monitoring using millimeter wave. ACM Trans. Sens. Netw. (TOSN) **13**(2), 1–32 (2017)
40. Zhang, Y., et al.: Breathing disorder detection using wearable electrocardiogram and oxygen saturation. In: Proceedings of the 16th ACM Conference on Embedded Networked Sensor Systems, pp. 313–314 (2018)
41. Zhang, Y., et al.: Automated sleep period estimation in wearable multi-sensor systems. In: Proceedings of the 16th ACM Conference on Embedded Networked Sensor Systems, pp. 305–306 (2018)
42. Zhao, M., Yue, S., Katabi, D., Jaakkola, T.S., Bianchi, M.T.: Learning sleep stages from radio signals: a conditional adversarial architecture. In: International Conference on Machine Learning, pp. 4100–4109. PMLR (2017)

Design Approaches for Executable Clinical Pathways at the Point of Care in Limited Resource Settings to Support the Clinical Decision Process: Review of the State of the Art

Geletaw Sahle Tegenaw[1,3](✉), Demisew Amenu[2], Girum Ketema[3], Frank Verbeke[1], Jan Cornelis[1], and Bart Jansen[1,4]

[1] Department of Electronics and Informatics ETRO, Vrije Universiteit Brussel (VUB), Pleinlaan 2, 1050 Brussel, Belgium
gtegenaw@vub.be, gelapril1985@gmail.com
[2] Department of Obstetrics and Gynecology, College of Health Science, Jimma University, Jimma, Ethiopia
[3] Faculty of Computing, JIT, Jimma University, Jimma, Ethiopia
[4] iMEC, Kapeldreef 75, 3001 Leuven, Belgium

Abstract. Decision support clinical pathways are used to improve the performance of the health-care management system. An effective clinical pathway (CP) helps to know the optimal treatment route that patients will follow. The extent of the CP goes from the first contact in the health-center (or hospital) to the completion of the treatment until the patient is dismissed. Up to now, far too little attention has been paid to a systematic review, the research and the development of CPs in a low resource setting (LRS). The main focus has been primarily on data-intensive environments where there is no shortage of resources. A systematic search in PubMed and Web of Science was conducted for bundling and categorizing the relevant approaches for LRS. Of 45 full reviewed articles, 25/45(55.6%) and 20/45(44.4%) of the studies were conducted using knowledge-based and data-driven approaches respectively. Among the knowledge-based studies, 9/25(36%) were reporting a stand-alone applications, 10/25(40%) attempting to deliver a paper-based CP, and the remaining focus was on web-based applications. In the data-driven approaches, 15/20(75%) tried to integrate with the electronic health record. The paper identifies the approaches for executing CPs and highlights key considerations for building LRS-compatible CPs. Data-driven CPs do not only resolve the challenges of improving the quality of existing knowledge-based CPs, but also enable evidence-based practice, improve outcomes, and reduce cost and delay.

Keywords: Limited resource setting · Clinical decision support system · Clinical workflow · Clinical pathway · Patient flow · Point of care service

X. Gao et al. (Eds.): MobiHealth 2021, LNICST 440, pp. 186–203, 2022.
https://doi.org/10.1007/978-3-031-06368-8_13

1 Introduction

Promoting healthy lives and the well-being of people is one of the main agenda points for Global Sustainable Development Goal 3 by 2030 [1]. Diverse tools have been implemented to improve the access and to assist the healthcare service in delivering patient-centered value. For instance, eHealth (telehealth) will play a leading role for universal health coverage [2] and is expected to bring *equity and extended access*, to *improve outcome* and fill the *gap in professional scarcity* at primary care level [3]. However, the success of eHealth depends on: (i) the policy environment, (ii) the flexibility of integration with the health-care delivery system, (iii) usability, (iv) public-private partnership, and (v) business models and protocols [4]. A case study on the Ethiopian Black Lion Hospital also noted that ensuring the compatibility with the medical practice and the physician's preferred work style facilitates the eHealth adoption [5].

The primary health-care management is seeking a point of care instrument to deliver appropriate, consistent, and integrated care. The Clinical pathway (CP) aims to deliver and outline an optimal logical path and plan of care from assessment to treatment at the primary and secondary health care level [6, 7, 10]. It is also known as "*care pathway, integrated care pathway, critical pathway, or care map*". CPs are utilized for various purposes, and studies demonstrated that adopting a decision support clinical pathway has a significant impact on: (I) managing the quality and standardization of health-care processes [6], (II) reducing delay [8–14], (III) improving outcomes [7, 8], (IV) increasing coherence between care units and professionals [7, 8, 10, 11, 14–22], (V) reducing the risk of errors and complications [7, 8, 15–17, 20], (VI) reducing cost [8, 10, 13–16, 18, 23], (VII) promoting evidence-based decision making [7, 8, 12, 15, 17, 18, 23–26], (VIII) improving communication and feedback e.g. within or between the health center and the hospital [12, 18–20, 25, 26], and (IX) increasing job satisfaction [6, 14]. However, previous studies on CP did not systematically consider contexts of low resource setting (LRS) but implicitly assumed a data and resource-intensive environment. For instance, Aspland et al. 2019 found, only 0.1% of the CP studies have been conducted outside America, Asia, and Europe [27]. The purpose of this review is to systematically confront existing CP publications with the low resource setting (LRS) context, explore the gaps and recommend approaches (important design considerations) for building and executing CPs. Furthermore, the motivation for this research arose from a desire to help frontline workers in low-resource settings who primarily make decisions based on hard-copy clinical guidelines (CGs), patient card-sheets, and point-of-care charts. Some of the challenges were a lack of health information infrastructure, as well as a lack of data management and decision support tools. We can also see that the patient card-sheets give insufficient information, lack referral feedback (which may result in unnecessary referrals and delays in seeking care), and many decision-support tools are out of reach for low-resource settings.

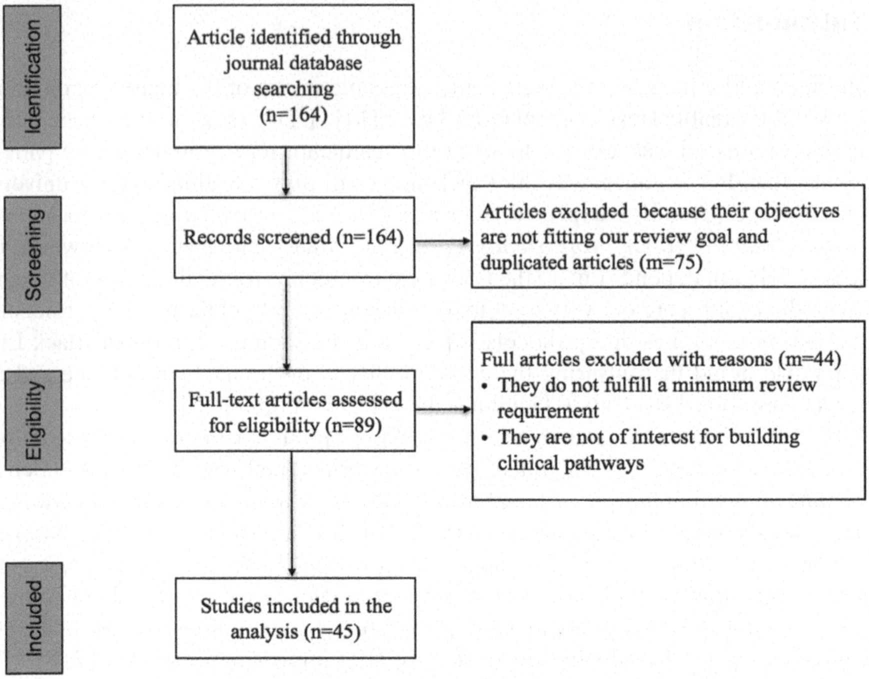

Fig. 1. Flowchart of study selection and inclusion (**n** is the number of papers at each step of inclusion and eligibility assessment, and **m** is the number of excluded papers)

2 Methods

The methodology of the review process was adopted from [28, 29] and customized to our needs. The review process was conducted based on the following steps: (I) defining the goal of the review, (II) identifying search strategies, (III) identifying databases for literature search, (IV) defining the inclusion and eligibility assessment criteria, and (V) extracting data and conducting data analysis. More information on the detailed flow of the review process is shown in Fig. 1.

2.1 Goal

The systematic review aims to explore the feasible approaches and strategies to develop an executable clinical pathway for low resource settings (LRS). To achieve this, the present review systematically confonted existing CP publications with the LRS context. Specifically, we explored: (I) which techniques and procedures are the most appropriate to design an executable clinical pathway at point of care services for better health outcomes in the context of low resource settings, and (II) what are the principles, challenges, and important considerations to build executable CPs? Furthermore, we also seek to map those techniques in the literature that have been identified with the point of care executable platforms.

2.2 Search Strategy and Literature Search

A literature search was performed using PubMed and Web of Science database. As shown in Table 1, search strategies were developed using various composite keywords. The summary of keywords and search strategies is presented in Table 1. The search criteria were intended to involve various decision support executable clinical pathway terms that have been labeled as 'clinical pathways' for promoting evidence-based management practice. We searched PubMed and Web of Science published in English without publication year restriction.

Table 1. Summary of the search strategy

Databases	Keywords and techniques
PubMed	Clinical Pathways
	((((((((clinical pathway) OR computerized clinical pathway) OR computerized clinical pathway system) OR decision support clinical pathway) OR interactive clinical pathway) OR data-driven clinical pathway) AND applicable clinical pathway) OR model-based clinical pathway) OR CDSS in low resource settings) OR patient flow analysis) OR low resource settings
	((((((((clinical pathway) OR computerized clinical pathway) OR computerized clinical pathway system) OR decision support clinical pathway) OR interactive clinical pathway) OR data-driven clinical pathway) AND applicable clinical pathway) OR model-based clinical pathway) OR CDSS in low resource settings) OR patient flow analysis) AND low resource settings
Web of Science	Ts = (clinical pathways) AND LANGUAGE: (English) Timespan: All years. Indexes: SCI-EXPANDED, SSCI, A&HCI, CPCI-S, CPCI-SSH, ESCI
	Ts = (clinical pathway OR computerized clinical pathway OR decision support clinical pathway OR interactive clinical pathway OR data-driven clinical pathway OR applicable clinical pathway OR model-based clinical pathway OR low resource settings) AND LANGUAGE: (English) Indexes = SCI-EXPANDED, SSCI, A&HCI, CPCI-S, CPCI-SSH, ESCI Timespan = All years
	Ts = (clinical pathway OR computerized clinical pathway OR decision support clinical pathway OR interactive clinical pathway OR data-driven clinical pathway OR applicable clinical pathway OR model-based clinical pathway AND low resource settings) AND LANGUAGE: (English) Indexes = SCI-EXPANDED, SSCI, A&HCI, CPCI-S, CPCI-SSH, ESCI Timespan = All years
	searched for: CITED WORK: (clinical pathways) Timespan: All years. Indexes: SCI-EXPANDED, SSCI, A&HCI, CPCI-S, CPCI-SSH, ESCI

(*continued*)

Table 1. (*continued*)

Databases	Keywords and techniques
Google Scholar	Clinical Pathways
	"clinical pathway" OR "clinical pathway management system" OR "computerized clinical pathway" OR "decision support clinical pathway " OR "interactive clinical pathway" OR "data-driven clinical pathway" OR "applicable clinical pathway" OR "model-based clinical pathway" AND "low resource settings"
	"clinical pathway" OR "clinical pathway management system" OR "computerized clinical pathway" OR "decision support clinical pathway " OR "interactive clinical pathway" OR "data-driven clinical pathway" OR "applicable clinical pathway" OR "model-based clinical pathway" OR "low resource settings"
Manual Search	Manual searching based on citation and related articles

Additionally, Google Scholar queries and manual searches of citations and related articles of the included studies were undertaken to identify any relevant articles that might have been missed. For example, on Google scholar, we searched using the keyword "computerized clinical pathway management" queries to extract publication year, number of citations and name of the publisher. The visual illustration is presented in Fig. 2.

2.3 Eligibility Assessment

A variety of steps were performed to examine the inclusion and eligibility assessments of a specific journal or conference article. The title, abstract and objectives of individual studies were reviewed to select eligible studies. In general, studies were included if they (I) demonstrated and reported the application of CPs, (II) examined the impact of CPs such as promoting evidence-based practice, improving outcomes, reducing cost and delay, improving communication and feedback, or a combination of these items, or (III) examined factors that impact the

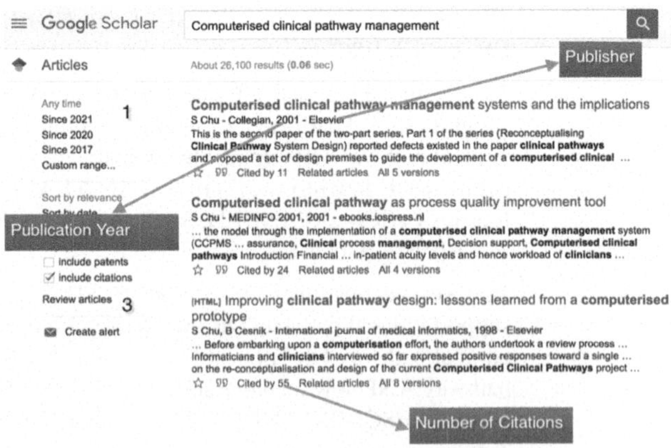

Fig. 2. Sample searching result

practice of CPs. In particular, studies that presented a situation in low resource settings were included for analysis. Then, we set the "number of citations" thresholds based on the publication year. We only considered articles with a minimum of five citations if they are published before 5 years (i.e. before 2014) and a minimum of one citation if they are published within 5 years. The search was conducted in 2019. Full articles were reviewed where it was not possible to decide about their inclusion based upon abstract-review alone. In the end, mixed-methods, cross sectional studies, survey, cohort studies, pilot studies, randomized control trails and case study reports were included and assessed based on their stated intent to bring and design effective decision support clinical pathways at the point of care service.

2.4 Data Extraction and Data Analysis

The data extraction template was adopted from [29] and customized for our needs based on the review objectives. Data from each article were extracted using a standardized excel database. the extracted information at the end of the review process are: the title, author, name of publisher, publication year, number of citations, context, mechanism and intervention strategies, characteristics (setting, platform, approaches, and techniques), the outcome of the study and the possibility to adapt (or reproduce) it in low resource settings. Data analysis and visualization were performed using our own python-based interactive tool. Then, we examined the CP design techniques, platforms, and approaches. We also summarised the included study using citations, publication year, intent, and outcomes.

3 Results

3.1 Search Results

A total of 164 articles were identified for inclusion and eligibility assessment. We excluded 75 articles after title and abstract screening and 89 articles were eligible for full article review. Of these, 45 articles were included for review and met the inclusion criteria. The included studies were published between 1992 and 2018. The review process for selecting articles with reasons is summarized in Fig. 1.

3.2 Summary Characteristics of Included Studies

Summary of the Studies Using Citations and Publication Years. Of the 45 included studies, 10/45 (22.2%), 7/45(15.6%), 5/45(11.1%), and 4/45(8.9%) were from Elsevier, BioMed Central (BMC), Springer, and IEEE respectively. The detailed summary of the studies using journal publications is presented in Fig. 3.

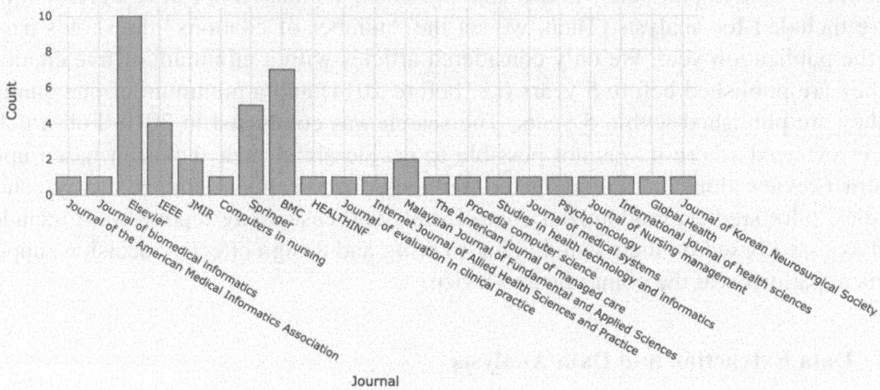

Fig. 3. Summary of journals

Of the 45 studies, 30/45(66.7%) of the articles have more than 10 citations and 33/45(73.3%) were published after 2012. Figures 4 and 5 are illustrating the detailed summary of citations and publication year respectively.

Summary of the Studies' Intent and Their Outcomes. Among the manuscripts, twenty-seven studies were demonstrating the use of CPs for the point of care decision support service and evidence based multidisciplinary care plans [9, 11–14, 20, 25, 26, 36–40, 44, 47–61]. These studies were describing that the introduction of automated and accessible CPs not only uncovered evidence and visualized specific care plans but they also compared and emphasized the contrasts between different CPs. Five studies demonstrated the advantage of computerized CPs, the functional requirements and the expected benefits [24, 31–34]. Three studies attempted to automate and generate computer interpretable CPs from CGs [23, 41, 42]. Two studies have focused on the challenge and practice of designing and implementing CPs [19, 22]. Three studies have explored

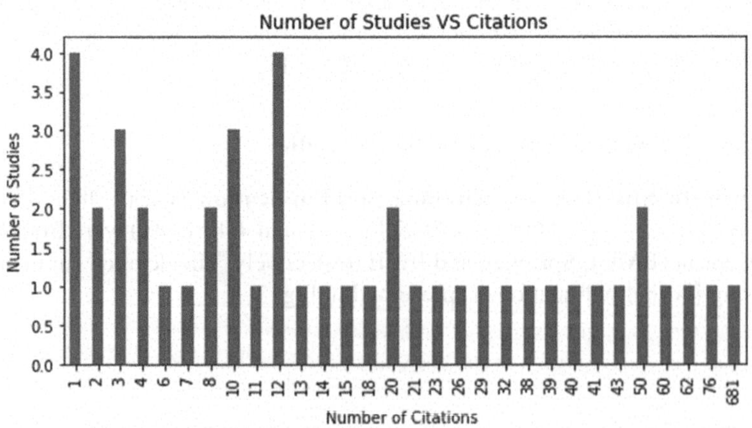

Fig. 4. Summary by citations

the patient current state, treatment intent, behavior, and outcomes [9, 52, 53]. These studies tried to characterize, cluster and visualize the visit sequence, patient condition, and progress to promote accessible and evidence-based CP. Four studies examined the use of CP for predicting and handling the variance or deviation from the specified care plan [21, 54, 62, 63]. Only one study examined the optimal mechanism for CGs and CPs representation and strategies for clinical-care improvement [45]. In this study, CGs and CPs were transformed into decision-tree for delivering quality service and coherent decision-making. However, very few studies were explicitly demonstrating CPs in low resource settings [20, 22, 26]. In low resource settings, the target of the studies was handling patient flow analysis, assisting critical care, and aiding resource management. Moreover, few studies also implement CPs for tracking performance and managing resources [49, 59, 61].

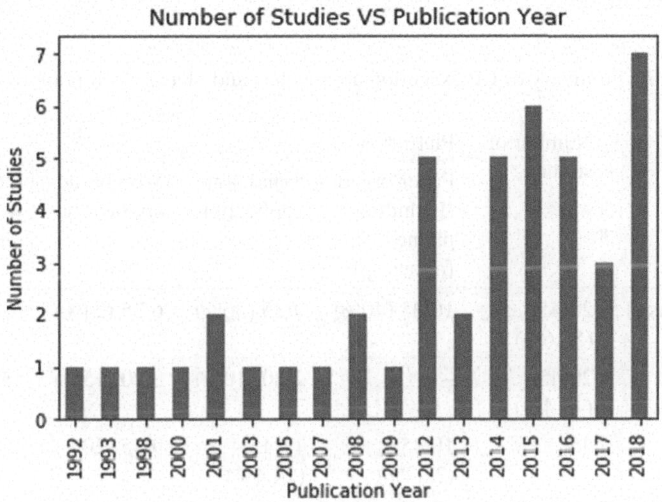

Fig. 5. Summary by publication year

In summary, among the reported outcomes, the included studies: (I) outlined the functional requirements for designing CPs, (II) disclosed the way to assist the process of intervention, and to reduce the treatment waiting times (visit sequence, condition, progress), outcome prediction, and quality of evidence, (III) brought easiness of data extraction for collaboration and monitoring, (IV) reported a significant impact on reducing errors, reducing cost and length of patient stay, and (V) described the variance (or deviation) from the specified care plan.

3.3 Clinical Pathway Design Approaches, Platforms, and Techniques

Of the 45 full reviewed articles, 25/45 (55.6%) and 20/45 (44.4%) of the studies were conducted using knowledge-based and data-driven approaches respectively. From the 25 knowledge-based studies, paper-based follow-up (10/25, 40%), stand-alone applications (9/25, 36%), and web-based applications (6/25, 24%) were the most commonly reported CP execution platforms. The paper-based follow-up mainly used face-to-face communication at the point of care services. Additionally, it also includes a telephone follow-up and conversation. In the data-driven approaches, 15/20(75%) of the studies tried to integrate with the electronic health record while the remaining focused on delivering web-based and standalone CP applications. Overall, paper-based follow-up (10/45, 22.2%), stand-alone applications (11/45, 24.4%), web-based applications (9/45, 20%), and integration with heath records (15/45, 33.3%) were the most commonly reported CP execution platforms. The results obtained from the analysis of platforms and approaches are summarized in Table 2.

Table 2. Summary of CP execution approaches and platforms at point of care

Approaches	Number of studies	Platforms			
		Paper-based (Including phone follow-up)	Standalone application	Web-based application	Integrated with health records (HR)
Knowledge-based approaches	25/45 (55.6%)	10/25 (40%)	9/25 (36%)	6/25 (24%)	–
Data-driven approaches	20/45 (44.4%)	–	2/20 (10%)	3/20 (15%)	15/20 (75%)
Total	45	10/45 (22.2%)	11/45 (24.4%)	9/45 (20%)	15/45 (33.3%)

As shown in Table 3, automation was demonstrated using stand-alone and web-based platforms. Additionally, rule-based logic and probabilistic techniques were used for the implementation of stand-alone and web-based CPs. Whereas learning algorithms, visualization, and recommendation techniques were employed on health records for delivering data-driven CPs. Results obtained from the mapping of CP platforms on implementation techniques are presented in Table 3. The mapping of CP platforms and implementation techniques includes CP execution platforms that have been integrated into health records (HR), stand-alone, and web-based applications. However, CP follow-ups, assessments, requirement analysis, and reviews were also conducted using paper-based platforms.

Table 3. Mapping of CP execution platforms with techniques

Platform	Techniques	Number of studies
Integrated into HR	Learning algorithm and clustering, Markov chain modeling	1
	Frequent sequence mining algorithm & visualization using Sankey diagram	1
	Hierarchical task networks or Hierarchical clustering and Markov chains	1
	Hybrid learning algorithm	1
	K-means with Levenshtein distance	1
	Neural network	2
	Probabilistic	1
	Rule Based or Fuzzy rule, extended fuzzy Petri net	3
	Statistical machine-learning algorithms	1
	Visualization techniques and/or, score system and graphical representation	2
	Rating based recommendation	1
Standalone APP	Automation	7
	Decision trees	1
	Hierarchical task networks or Hierarchical clustering and Markov chains	1
	Probabilistic	1
	Rule Based or Fuzzy rule, extended fuzzy Petri net	1
WEB APP	Automation	6
	Probabilistic	2
	Rule Based or Fuzzy rule, extended fuzzy Petri net	1

We also observed that the overall trend is moving towards integrating CPs with electronic health records for enabling the use of learning algorithms, improving data visualization and recommendation techniques. As can be seen from the Fig. 6, the trend of executing clinical pathways is shifting from knowledge-driven to data-driven approaches. In general, as illustrated on the y-axis in Fig. 7, a total of 14 techniques were extracted to design an executable CP. Information on the summary of CP studies based on their approaches, platforms, and implementation techniques between 1992 and 2018 are presented in Figs. 6 and 7.

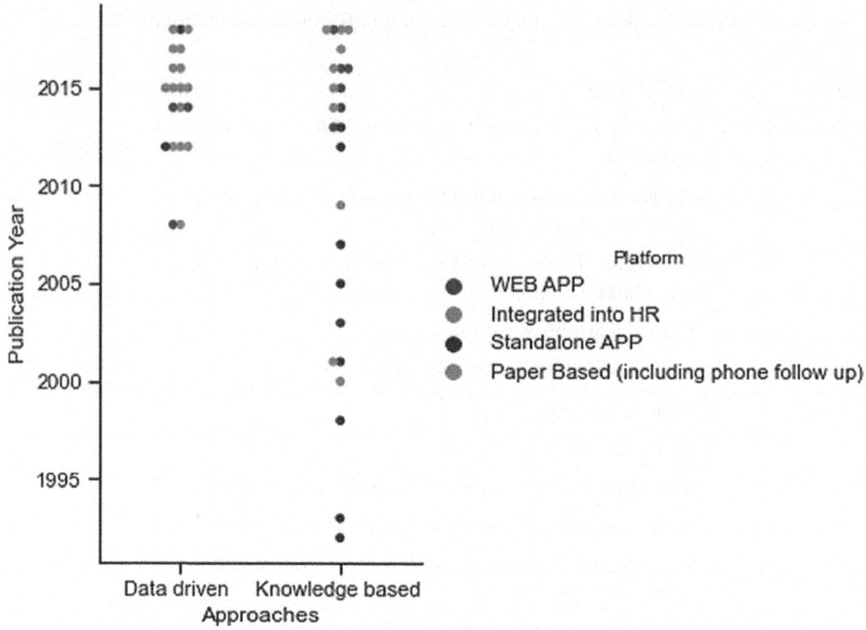

Fig. 6. Summary of CP studies publication year, approaches, and platforms

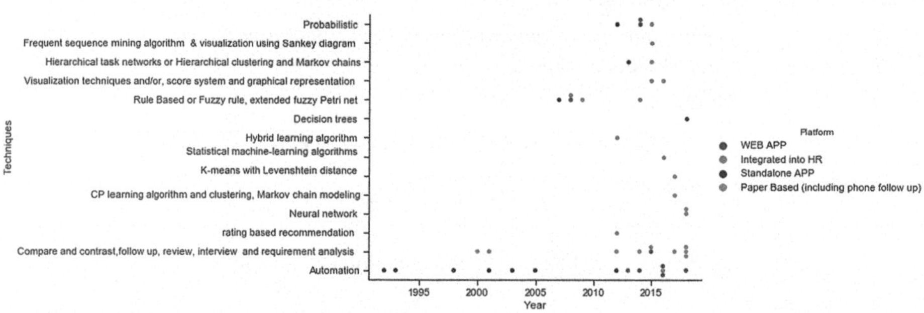

Fig. 7. Summary of CP studies based on platform and techniques over the years

4 Discussion

The clinical decision support system has improved over the years and is moving towards "*delivering ubiquitous accessibility and availability of data, any form of knowledge representation, shared decision making, continuous feedback and improvement*" [30]. Our systematic review was designed to explore the diversity and the relevance of the approaches used, and to identify the mechanisms and implementation strategies for designing CPs in LRS.

This review has shown that knowledge-based and data-driven approaches were found to be the major approaches for designing executable clinical pathways at the point of care to support the clinical decision process. Further analysis showed that the *knowledge-based* approaches can be categorized into paper-based, Information Technology (IT)-based, and model-based implementations for executing CPs at the point of care while the *data-driven* approaches can be subdivided into ontology, probabilistic, and artificial neural network (machine learning) techniques. The data-driven approach relies on the integration with the electronic health record, events, and logs. For instance, in the current review, among the data-driven approaches 75% of the studies demonstrated integration with the existing electronic health record. In all, based on our observations, we classify the CP approaches into two distinct categories (and three distinct sub-categories) depending on the design principles, strategies, and methodologies. A detailed summary of our observations is presented in Fig. 8.

The first group facilitates evidence-based decision-making using knowledge-based CPs. In this category, a group of experts and interdisciplinary teams will start designing knowledge-based CPs from the existing CGs, accepted standards, best practices or an extensive literature review. The knowledge-based CP can be executed in three ways:

- First, using a paper-based system. The main challenges of the paper-based approach are time-consumption, resource-intensiveness, lack of adaptiveness and flexibility to accommodate dynamic change [31, 32].
- The IT-based system is often based on the automation of the paper-based approach to facilitate the delivery and quality of healthcare service. The IT-based system [21, 24, 33–41] demonstrated the development of computerized management CPs through algorithms for recommendation or a management portal. However, there is still a need to differentiate clearly between the clinical pathway and automated clinical guidelines, and a need to put usable intelligent recommendation (or wizards) into the clinical routine [34, 36, 41]. IT is used for modeling tasks and activities, but it is challenging to model the whole life cycle management of clinical pathways. Moreover, communication between IT and the domain experts is often still an issue.
- Finally, using the model (CGs) based approach. The model-based approach attempted to bring the overall treatment of a specific disease in one concrete setting based on a clinical guideline [23, 42–44]. The paper- and IT-based systems focused on the development of CPs for one specific condition and setting. Commonly, guideline-based representation languages as rule-based languages and the ready-to-use (or executable) pathway models are generated to deliver assistance for the domain expert. However, as stated in [23, 42–44], it is important to consider the inter-sectoral pathway (multi-disease/case pathways) and cycle pathway during CGs based implementation.

Overall, the knowledge-based CP is concentrated on delivering static, stand-alone, disease-specific, and nonadaptive pathways. It is also practiced in a low resource setting, e.g. paper-based flow charts and integrated symptom-based guidelines used as a point of care instrument for assisting the frontline workers [46].

In the second group, the data-driven CPs, it was demonstrated that complex and heterogeneous scenarios can be captured. The goal is to learn CPs from actual practice data to enable shared decision-making, promote exploration for better understanding and management, and maximize clinical efficiency through evidence-based practice and optimal clinical outcomes. Many studies have explored the practice of data-driven approaches for different settings and disease conditions [9, 47–63]. However, the data driven CPs need to be integrated with ontology, probabilistic, or artificial neural network (machine learning) approaches for enabling an efficient and adaptive service. Ontology (semantics) based techniques [54–58] focused on the subjects and their relationships, not so much on the presentation of the data. However, a variety of factors have been described that limit the practicality of ontology-based CPs. For instance, the care plan [57]: (I) is too general and requires more detail, (II) lacks the required universally accepted standards, and (III) requires to consider the plan of care experience, hospital (health-center) characteristics, pathway summarization of different hospitals (health-centers) that need to be aggregated to deliver adaptively and universally accepted CPs. Probabilistic-based techniques [9, 59–61] employed probabilistic CPs to visualize, explore and discover a series of healthcare system challenges. However, when the number of attributes increases, the probabilistic techniques grow in size which results in an exponential increase of the number of lookups to perform the CP recommendations [59].Therefore, a trade-off is required to understand and manage CP complexity by probabilities of occurence. Though most of the existing clinical decision support systems appear to be aimed at assisting the clinical workflows, management of information, and decision-making, there is a need to

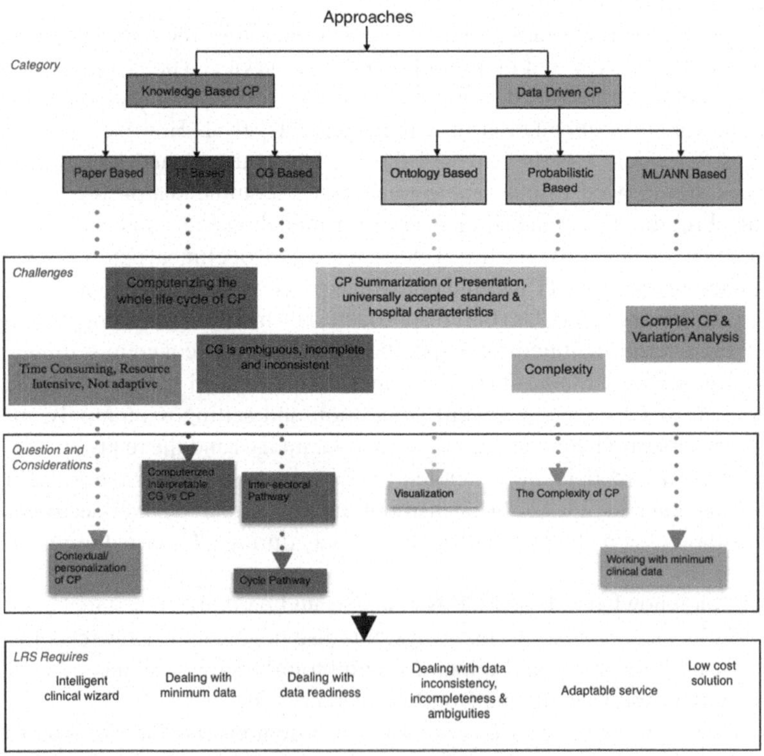

- **Color Clustering:** Follow the color and the broken line from top to bottom for getting the details of each approach, expected challenge, and design considerations. *e.g. The paper-based system is challenged to deliver flexible (adaptive) CPs. Need to consider; how a paper-based approach addresses the contextual (personalization) of CP?*

Fig. 8. Summary of approaches, challenges and considerations

deliver personalized care, evidence-based practice by keeping the latest practice guideline and react to the patient's condition. Artificial neural network (machine learning) techniques have been demonstrated to be successful for delivering personalized care, promoting evidence-based practice, slashing cost, and predicting variance [8, 62, 63].

Overall, we found that the trend of executing clinical pathways is shifting from knowledge-driven to data-driven approaches by integration with electronic medical records for assisting healthcare professionals and frontline workers. However, there is no "*one technology for all*" approach for designing applicable clinical pathways (or plans of care) to support and promote an evidence-based decision process. Both the knowledge-based and data-driven approaches have their own pros and cons. More information on the challenges, considerations, and LRS requirements is presented in Fig. 8. Even though data-driven clinical pathways are more advantageous than knowledge-driven approaches, enabling and putting evidence into practice is challenging in health systems with limited resources. Besides that, a complex healthcare decision must allow for many pathways, be updated in real time as new information is provided and encourage patient preference and participation.

Furthermore, a search of the literature revealed only few studies which attempt to examine the application of CPs in LRS. Hence, we considered it useful in this review to make a summary of previous observations [27] from a broader perspective than only the LRS one. In LRS, most of the primary and first-level care follows a paper-based system as a dominant practice. Designing a CP that is working with minimum clinical data is required while maintaining the CP's reliability and maneuverability. A need exists to design an executable clinical pathway solution that is accessible to low-resource health facilities that can tightly interface with the existing workflow. The LRS requires to deal with minimum clinical data, data readiness, data inconsistency, and incompleteness. Designing a low-cost solution, intelligent clinical wizards, and adaptable services is also crucial. It is also important to consider other available health information to explore the existing best practice and clinical guidelines. The lack of the expected resources and limited digitization will challenge the practice of data-driven CPs. Therefore, the implementation and selection of the CP approach depend on the strategies, resources (e.g. practical guidelines), principles, standards of care, best practices, and intended goals [10, 11, 15]. Besides these, as noted in [4, 7, 8], the effectiveness of CPs highly depends on (A) the recognized clinical guidelines and policy, (B) the key stakeholders and their drivers, (C) the quality of the evidence-based approach, (D) the integration of the existing workflow, (E) the complexity of the used techniques, logic, and ability to adopt contextual decision making - for example rule-based and decision tree logic are challenged to deliver meaningful contextual and non-linear workflow clinical pathways, (F) the accessibility and treatment options, and (G) patient preference and participation.

This review has limitations. In addition to PubMed and the Web of Science database, we have employed Google Scholar queries and manual searches. We were discarded articles from inclusion based on the citation threshold. However, potential studies from other sources not indexed to one of these databases might be missed. Moreover, studies published in languages other than English are often missed.

5 Conclusion

The purpose of this review was to explore feasible approaches and strategies to develop an executable clinical pathway for low resource settings. We have provided a review of the decision support clinical pathway by: (I) reviewing the applications and publications between 1992 and 2018, (II) summarizing the approaches, and (III) presenting the important considerations for designing executable CPs and it's expected benefits.

The included studies highlight the importance of CPs for promoting evidence-based healthcare, assisting the care process, and improving the quality of care. The CP can be designed based on the guidelines, the standard of care, and best practices. Findings from studies included in this review indicate that knowledge-based and data-driven approaches are the main approaches for designing CPs. Knowledge-driven CPs can be executed using a paper-based, IT-, or model-based system. Integrating with the existing electronic health record, web-based and standalone CP applications are the modalities of data-driven CP execution. Taken together, this review observed that the trend of executing clinical pathways is shifting from knowledge-driven to data-driven approaches. However, most of the primary and first-level care in low resource settings follows a paper-based system as a dominant practice in-comparison with the IT and model-based approaches. Therefore, it is required to design a mechanism for evidence-based practice to improve outcomes and feedback. Exploring a trade-off mechanism for promoting data-driven decision-making approaches may help to explore, visualize, and discover a series of health-care system challenges such as: (I) assisting low clinical competence, limited medical staff, and shortage of equipment, and (II) improving clinical outcomes, workflows and temporal relationships for clinical pathway workflow management. However, infrastructure, data readiness, data inconsistency, incompleteness, and ambiguities as well as adaptability (understanding the context) still are major challenges of clinical data.

Acknowledgments. The NASCERE (Network for Advancement of Sustainable Capacity in Education and Research in Ethiopia) program has assisted us in the work to date and will continue to assist us as we move forward with the planned activities.

References

1. Lee, B.X., et al.: Transforming our world: implementing the 2030 agenda through sustainable development goal indicators. J. Public Health Policy **37**, 13–31 (2016)
2. Marker, P., McNamara, K., Wallace, L.: The Significance of Information and Communication Technologies for Reducing Poverty. DFID, London (2002)
3. Wootton, R., Patil, N.G., Scott, R.E., Ho, K.: Telehealth in the Developing World. (IDRC) (2009)
4. Shiferaw, F., Zolfo, M.: The role of information communication technology (ICT) towards universal health coverage: the first steps of a telemedicine project in Ethiopia. Glob. Health Action **5**, 15638 (2012)
5. Mengesha, G.H., Garfield, M.J.: A contextualized it adoption and use model for telemedicine in Ethiopia. Inf. Technol. for Dev. **25**, 184–203 (2019)
6. Lawal, A.K., et al.: What is a clinical pathway? Refinement of an operational definition to identify clinical pathway studies for a Cochrane systematic review. BMC Med. **14**(1), 1–5 (2016)

7. Abrahams, E., et al.: Clinical pathways: recommendations for putting patients at the center of value-based care. Clin. Cancer Res. **23**, 4545–4549 (2017)
8. Siwicki, B.: Flagler Hospital uses AI to create clinical pathways that enhance care and slash costs (2018). https://www.healthcareitnews.com/news/flagler-hospital-uses-ai-create-clinical-pathways-enhance-care-and-slash-costs. Accessed June 2019
9. Huang, Z., et al.: Discovery of clinical pathway patterns from event logs using probabilistic topic models. J. Biomed. Inform. **47**, 39–57 (2014)
10. Schrijvers, G., van Hoorn, A., Huiskes, N.: The care pathway: concepts and theories: an introduction. Int. J. Integr. Care **12** (2012)
11. Huang, Z., Lu, X., Duan, H.: Using recommendation to support adaptive clinical pathways. J. Med. Syst. **36**(3), 1849–1860 (2012)
12. Butow, P., et al.: Clinical pathway for the screening, assessment and management of anxiety and depression in adult cancer patients: Australian guidelines. Psycho-Oncology **24**(9), 987–1001 (2015)
13. Chung, S.-B., et al.: Implementation and outcomes of a critical pathway for lumbar laminectomy or microdiscectomy. J. Korean Neurosurg. Soc. **51**(6), 338 (2012)
14. Sou, V., et al.: A clinical pathway for the management of difficult venous access. BMC Nurs. **16**(1), 64 (2017)
15. Gesme, D.H., Wiseman, M.: Strategic use of clinical pathways. J. Oncol. Pract. **7**, 54 (2011)
16. Rotter, T., et al.: The effects of clinical pathways on professional practice, patient outcomes, length of stay, and hospital costs: Cochrane systematic review and meta-analysis. Eval. Health Prof. **35**, 3–27 (2012)
17. Ellis, P.G., et al.: Clinical pathways: management of quality and cost in oncology networks in the metastatic colorectal cancer setting. J. Oncol. Pract. **13**, e522–e529 (2017)
18. Wylde, V., et al.: Clinical- and cost-effectiveness of the STAR care pathway compared to usual care for patients with chronic pain after total knee replacement: study protocol for a UK randomised controlled trial. Trials **19**(1), 132 (2018). https://doi.org/10.1186/s13063-018-2516-8
19. Jones, A.: Implementation of hospital care pathways for patients with schizophrenia. J. Nurs. Manag. **8**(4), 215–225 (2000)
20. Rickard, J., et al.: Critical care management of peritonitis in a low-resource setting. World J. Surg. **42**(10), 3075–3080 (2018). https://doi.org/10.1007/s00268-018-4598-6
21. Chen, K.S., et al.: Utilizing clinical pathways and web-based conferences to improve quality of care in a large integrated network using breast cancer radiation therapy as the model. Radiat. Oncol. **13**(1), 44 (2018). https://doi.org/10.1186/s13014-018-0995-0
22. Vukoja, M., et al.: A survey on critical care resources and practices in low- and middle-income countries. Glob. Heart **9**(3), 337–342 (2014). https://doi.org/10.1016/j.gheart.2014.08.002
23. Böckmann, B., Heiden, K.: Extracting and transforming clinical guidelines into pathway models for different hospital information systems. Heal. Inf. Sci. Syst. **1**, 13 (2013)
24. Hu, S.-C.: Computerized monitoring of emergency department patient flow. Am. J. Emerg. Med. **11**(1), 8–11 (1993)
25. Hilario, A.L., et al.: Utilization of clinical pathway on open appendectomy: a quality improvement initiative in a private hospital in the Philippines. Int. J. Health Sci. **12**(2), 43 (2018)
26. Dixon, C.A., et al.: Patient flow analysis in resource-limited settings: a practical tutorial and case study. Glob. Health: Sci. Pract. **3**(1), 126–134 (2015). https://doi.org/10.9745/GHSP-D-14-00121
27. Aspland, E., Gartner, D., Harper, P.: Clinical pathway modelling: a literature review. Health Syst. **10**, 1–23 (2019)

28. Liberati, A., et al.: The PRISMA statement for reporting systematic reviews and meta-analyses of studies that evaluate health care interventions: explanation and elaboration. J. Clin. Epidemiol. **62**(10), e1–e34 (2009)
29. Groot, G., et al.: Development of a program theory for shared decision-making: a realist review protocol. Syst. Rev. **6**(1), 114 (2017). https://doi.org/10.1186/s13643-017-0508-5
30. Middleton, B., Sittig, D., Wright, A.: Clinical decision support: a 25 year retrospective and a 25 year vision. Yearb. Med. Inform. **25**, S103–S116 (2016)
31. Chu, S.: Reconceptualising clinical pathway system design. Collegian **8**, 33–36 (2001)
32. Chu, S., Cesnik, B.: Improving clinical pathway design: lessons learned from a computerised prototype. Int. J. Med. Inform. **51**(1), 1–11 (1998)
33. Miller, T.W., Ryan, M., et al.: Utilizing algorithms and pathways of care in allied health practice. Internet J. Allied Heal. Sci. Pract. **3**, 7 (2005)
34. DiJerome, L.: The nursing case management computerized system: meeting the challenge of health care delivery through technology. Comput. Nurs. **10**, 250–258 (1992)
35. Khodambashi, S., Slaughter, L.A., Nytrø, Ø.: Computer-interpretable clinical guidelines: a review and analysis of evaluation criteria for authoring methods. In: MedInfo, p. 954 (2015)
36. Chu, S.: Computerised clinical pathway management systems and the implications. Collegian **8**, 19–24 (2001)
37. Donald, M., et al.: Development and implementation of an online clinical pathway for adult chronic kidney disease in primary care: a mixed methods study. BMC Med. Inform. Decis. Making **16**(1), 109 (2016). https://doi.org/10.1186/s12911-016-0350-z
38. Gibbs, J., et al.: The eclinical care pathway framework: a novel structure for creation of online complex clinical care pathways and its application in the management of sexually transmitted infections. BMC Med. Inform. Decis. Making **16**, 98 (2016)
39. Yang, H., Li, W., Liu, K., Zhang, J.: Knowledge-based clinical pathway for medical quality improvement. Inf. Syst. Front. **14**, 105–117 (2012)
40. Bouamrane, M.M., Mair, F.S.: Implementation of an integrated preoperative care pathway and regional electronic clinical portal for preoperative assessment. BMC Med. Inform. Decis. Making **14**, 93 (2014)
41. Peleg, M., et al.: Comparing computer-interpretable guideline models: a case-study approach. J. Am. Med. Informatics Assoc. **10**, 52–68 (2003)
42. GonzáLez-Ferrer, A., Ten Teije, A., Fdez-Olivares, J., Milian, K.: Automated generation of patient- tailored electronic care pathways by translating computer-interpretable guidelines into hierarchical task networks. Artif. Intell. Med. **57**, 91–109 (2013)
43. Heiden, K.: Model-based integration of clinical practice guidelines in clinical pathways. In: CAiSE (Doctoral Consortium). (Citeseer) (2012)
44. Rebbeck, T., et al.: Implementation of a guideline-based clinical pathway of care to improve health outcomes following whiplash injury (whiplash impact): protocol of a randomised, controlled trial. J. Physiotherapy **62**, 111 (2016)
45. Djulbegovic, B., Hozo, I., Dale, W.: Transforming clinical practice guidelines and clinical pathways into fast-and-frugal decision trees to improve clinical care strategies. J. Eval. Clin. Pract. **24**(5), 1247–1254 (2018). https://doi.org/10.1111/jep.12895
46. Ethiopian primary healthcare clinical guidelines: Care of children 5–12 years and Adults 15 years or older in Health Centers. Practical Approach to Care Kit (2017)
47. Bettencourt-Silva, J.H., Mannu, G.S., de la Iglesia, B.: Visualisation of integrated patient-centric data as pathways: enhancing electronic medical records in clinical practice. In: Holzinger, A. (ed.) Machine Learning for Health Informatics. LNCS (LNAI), vol. 9605, pp. 99–124. Springer, Cham (2016). https://doi.org/10.1007/978-3-319-50478-0_5
48. Zhang, Y., Padman, R.: An interactive platform to visualize data-driven clinical pathways for the management of multiple chronic conditions. Stud. Health Technol. Inform. 672–676 (2017)

49. Bettencourt-Silva, J.H., et al.: Building data-driven pathways from routinely collected hospital data: a case study on prostate cancer. JMIR Med. Inform. **3**, e26 (2015)
50. Zhang, Y., Padman, R.: Data-driven clinical and cost pathways for chronic care delivery. Am. J. Managed Care **22**, 816–820 (2016)
51. Funkner, A.A., Yakovlev, A.N., Kovalchuk, S.V.: Data-driven modeling of clinical pathways using electronic health records. Procedia Comput. Sci. **121**, 835–842 (2017)
52. Perer, A., Wang, F., Hu, J.: Mining and exploring care pathways from electronic medical records with visual analytics. J. Biomed. Inform. **56**, 369–378 (2015)
53. Zhang, Y., Padman, R., Patel, N.: Paving the cowpath: learning and visualizing clinical pathways from electronic health record data. J. Biomed. Inform. **58**, 186–197 (2015)
54. Ye, Y., Jiang, Z., Yang, D., Du, G.: A semantics-based clinical pathway workflow and variance management framework. In: 2008 IEEE International Conference on Service Operations and Logistics, and Informatics, vol. 1, pp. 758–763. IEEE (2008)
55. Hu, Z., et al.: Modeling of clinical pathways based on ontology. In: 2009 IEEE International Symposium on IT in Medicine & Education, vol. 1, pp. 1170–1174. IEEE (2009)
56. Alexandrou, D., Xenikoudakis, F., Mentzas, G.: Adaptive clinical pathways with semantic web rules. In: HEALTHINF (2), pp. 140–147 (2008)
57. Wang, H., Zhou, T., Tian, L., Qian, Y., Li, J.: Creating hospital-specific customized clinical pathways by applying semantic reasoning to clinical data. J. Biomed. Inform. **52**, 354–363 (2014). https://doi.org/10.1016/j.jbi.2014.07.017
58. Hurley, K.F., Abidi, S.S.R.: Ontology engineering to model clinical pathways: towards the computerization and execution of clinical pathways. In: Twentieth IEEE International Symposium on Computer-Based Medical Systems (CBMS 2007), pp. 536–541. IEEE (2007)
59. Liu, R., et al.: Pathway-finder: an interactive recommender system for supporting personalized care pathways. In: 2014 IEEE International Conference on Data Mining Workshop, pp. 1219–1222. IEEE (2014)
60. Tsoukalas, A., Albertson, T., Tagkopoulos, I.: From data to optimal decision making: a data-driven, probabilistic machine learning approach to decision support for patients with sepsis. JMIR Med. Inform. **3**, e11 (2015)
61. Yang, X., et al.: Modelling and performance analysis of clinical pathways using the stochastic process algebra pepa. BMC Bioinform. **13**, S4 (2012)
62. Du, G., Jiang, Z., Diao, X., Ye, Y., Yao, Y.: Variances handling method of clinical pathways based on TS fuzzy neural networks with novel hybrid learning algorithm. J. Med. Syst. **36**, 1283–1300 (2012)
63. Yazid, M.H.A., et al.: Clinical pathway variance prediction using artificial neural network for acute decompensated heart failure clinical pathway. Malays. J. Fundamental Appl. Sci. **14**, 116–124 (2018)
64. De-Arteaga, M., Herlands, W., Neill, D.B., Dubrawski, A.: Machine learning for the developing world. ACM Trans. Manag. Inf. Syst. **9**(2), 1–14 (2018). https://doi.org/10.1145/3210548
65. Ethiopian Federal Ministry of Health: Pathways to Improve Health Information Systems in Ethiopia. Analysis of report on the stage of continuous improvement - Defining the Current Status, Goal and Improvement roadmap of the HIS (2021)

Effectiveness of a mHealth Coaching Program on Predictors of Work Absenteeism

Bojan Simoski(✉) and Michel C. A. Klein

Department of Computer Science, VU Amsterdam, Amsterdam, The Netherlands
{b.simoski,michel.klein}@vu.nl

Abstract. Health-related work absenteeism has an extensive economic and societal impact. Digital health interventions at the workplace can play a beneficial role in reducing the risks of absenteeism. However, the effects of these health interventions are rarely explored in terms of predicting work absenteeism. This paper presents the outcomes of a six month coaching-based digital health intervention. In this intervention, employees receive health or lifestyle coaching by using a smartphone app. We define eight predictors of absenteeism based on an extensive validated health check that the participants have filled throughout the program participation. The predictors are related to mental health, work ability, work stress, physical activity, perceived health and need to recovery after work. We show statistically significant effects of change in multiple predictors of absenteeism as a result of being part of the intervention. Additionally, we define multiple app usage scores founded on the coaching-based smartphone app. They are related to frequency of coach-coachee communication or doing healthy activities. We correlate these app scores with the predictors of absenteeism scores, and detect moderately-strong and significant correlations.

Keywords: Mobile health · Workplace digital health intervention · Coaching program

1 Introduction

The estimated economic and societal impact of health related absenteeism is enormous. For example, estimates of the costs of absence in the UK range from £270 to £659 per employee per year [8]. In an estimation of the costs in the US, the economic burden of illness was assessed up to $392 per employee per year [10]. The costs of just back pain to society in the Netherlands in 1991 were assessed to be 1.7% of the GNP [25]. Interventions focusing on improving health and lifestyle via employers are therefore attractive. A meta-analysis of workplace disease prevention and wellness programs shows that such interventions have both economic and health benefits [1]. In their critical meta-analysis of the

X. Gao et al. (Eds.): MobiHealth 2021, LNICST 440, pp. 204–220, 2022.
https://doi.org/10.1007/978-3-031-06368-8_14

literature on costs and savings associated with disease prevention and wellness programs to improve health, it was found that absenteeism costs fall by about $2.73 for every dollar spent on these programs. Programs focusing on physical activity (PA) have also reported positive results. For example, [12] found that an individually tailored intelligent physical exercise training with recommendations of leisure-time PA significantly decreased absenteeism when following the protocol. Participation in an employee fitness program resulted in a significant decline in sick days (4.8 days) for people in the high participation group [14]. However, a systematic review on the effectiveness of physical activity programs at worksites reported limited evidence of an effect on absenteeism [19].

In this paper, we investigated the effect of a mhealth coaching program in which employees receive health coaching from lifestyle coaches by using an smartphone app. VitalityPlatform (anonymous industry partner) is a platform that combines software with human coaching, where a lifestyle coach professional - a coach, communicates with an employee participating in the program - a coachee, via a smartphone app. This paper analyses the changes on different predictors of absenteeism (measured via questionnaires) through the participation in the program. We investigate the effects of the health intervention on these absenteeism predictors. In addition, we define a set of VitalityPlatform app usage measurements related to the frequency of coach-coachee communication, and the activities performed by the coachee. We investigate the relationship between these app measurements and the predictors of absenteeism scores.

This paper is structured as follows. In Sect. 2 we present the related work on predictors of sick leave and absenteeism, followed by an overview of coaching-based digital health interventions in the workplace. The methodology (Sect. 3) gives more details on the health intervention program, the predictors of absenteeism scores and VitalityPlatform app scores, and the data analysis methods. Section 4 shows the results of the study related to the effect of the intervention on the predictor scores, and the relationship between the app measurements and these scores. These outcomes are discussed in the final Sect. 5.

2 Related Work

2.1 Predictors of Sick Leave and Absenteeism

A literature study has been performed to investigate predictors of sick leave and absenteeism. In [18], the effect of PA on sick leave is investigated. No differences was found in mean sick leave duration between those who met the moderate intensity recommendation and those who did not. However, a significant reduction in amount of sick leave in workers meeting the vigorous intensity activity recommendation was found, as well as a dose-response relation between frequency of vigorous intensity activity up to a frequency of 3 times a week and sick leave duration. Workers not carrying out vigorous activity at all had the most days of sick leave, whereas those who were vigorously active three times a week had the least sick leave. PA was measured using the SQUASH questionnaire [26].

In [2], it is investigated which factors can improve work participation for people with a chronic illness. The effects of perceived health and limitations at work were investigated. The conclusion is that the association between health and sick leave can be explained by limitations at work, work characteristics, and work adjustments. Perceived health was assessed with a single question: 'how do you evaluate your health in general?'.

In [7], the effectiveness of a worksite social and physical environment intervention on need for recovery (i.e., early symptoms of work-related mental and physical fatigue), PA and relaxation was investigated. The "need for recovery after work" is mentioned as an early indicator for mentally and physically work-induced fatigue. Also, PA helps unwinding from work and reduces levels of stress. Measurements that are used are the SQUASH [26] for physical activity, the Oldenburg Burnout Inventory [20], the Need for recovery questionnaire [9], and a generic question about the perceived health. In [21], depression and low self-rated health are identified as risk factors for longer sick-leave periods. Measurements that are used are the ability to work [11] and the PHQ-9 [13].

2.2 Health Coaching Programs in the Workplace

Workplace interventions to improve health are popular for several reasons. People spend much time at work, there are existing social structures that can be used in the interventions, and it is possible to combine them with incentives from the employer [38]. Health interventions at the workplace may have different aims. Many of them focus on increasing PA. A meta-review by [27] has identified more than 138 reports describing studies on workplace PA interventions, showing that the interventions are very diverse and some can improve health. Another review [28] also shows a growing evidence base that workplace PA-based interventions can positively influence PA behaviour. Another, more recent focus for workplace interventions is breaking prolonged sedentary behavior. A systematic review of 26 studies aiming at reducing sitting among white-collar working adults concludes that there is significant overall effect on workplace sitting reduction [34]. A review of 25 interventions using mobile technology concludes that there is reasonable evidence for mHealth in a workplace context as a feasible, acceptable and effective tool to promote PA and reduce sitting time [35].

Mental health is another target of workplace interventions. Many interventions use mindfulness [29] to reduce stress at the workplace [30], others apply psycho-education [31] or psycho-social approaches [32]. A recent review has found evidence for the effectiveness of workplace interventions on the prevention of mental health problems [33].

Several workplace interventions focus on multiple health goals, e.g. a combination of dietary behaviour and PA [36,37]. Overall, health coaching to improve lifestyle behaviors seems to be a promising way to prevent diseases. In a 2010 literature review, significant improvements in one or more of the behaviors of nutrition, physical activity, weight management, or medication adherence were found in six (40%) of the fifteenth studies [17]. A more recent review of 18 interventions found small positive effect sizes, which were partly determined by intervention characteristics and experimental setup [38].

A few studies focus specifically on coaching as the means of the intervention. Coaching is about enhancing well-being and performance in personal life and work domains with normal, non-clinical populations, underpinned by models of coaching grounded in established adult learning or psychological approaches [39]. A recent meta-analysis has shown a positive effect of coaching in organizations. Interestingly, no difference in effect was found for different coaching formats (comparing face-to-face, with blended face-to-face and e-coaching) or duration of coaching (number of sessions or longevity of intervention). A study about the effect of coaching on the reduction of workplace stress has shown mixed outcomes: anxiety and stress had decreased more in the coaching group compared to the control group, but levels of depression had decreased more in the control group compared to the coaching group. However, participants reported high levels of perceived coaching effectiveness [40].

Overall we can conclude that there is some evidence that health coaching, also in a blended from, could have positive effects on the factors related to physical and mental health. In the remainder of this paper, we describe the methods and results of our study on the effectiveness of a specific online health coaching program on predictors of absenteeism.

3 Methodology

3.1 Recruitment and Timeline

Employees from 10 different companies were recruited to potentially participate in the program. Companies were offered a fixed number of places for their employees in the program. Potential participants received an email with an invitation to perform a "vitality scan", an online pre-scan on motivation and potential for improvement. This scan assessed their motivation for increasing physical activity using the SRQ-E [4]. In addition, their current health behavior was assessed by measuring physical activity (using the SQUASH questionnaire [26]), sleep quality (using the PSQ [5]), eating habits (using the RIVM VCP questionnaire [3]) and a work-related burnout [6,23]. All subscales for health behavior have been normalized to a scale between −2,5 and +2,5, where a score of −2,5 represent extremely unhealthy behaviors and a score of +2,5 represent the most healthy behaviors. The total score for health behavior was calculated by summing up all subscores. The exact questions and the normalization used are available per request.

Based on the outcome of the vitality check, a subset of employees were invited to join the health coaching program. The aim was to include people that were motivated to increase their health behavior and for whom there was some room for improvement. This has been operationalized by inviting people that scored above 0 on the motivation scale and below 1 on the health behavior scale, as shown in Fig. 1.

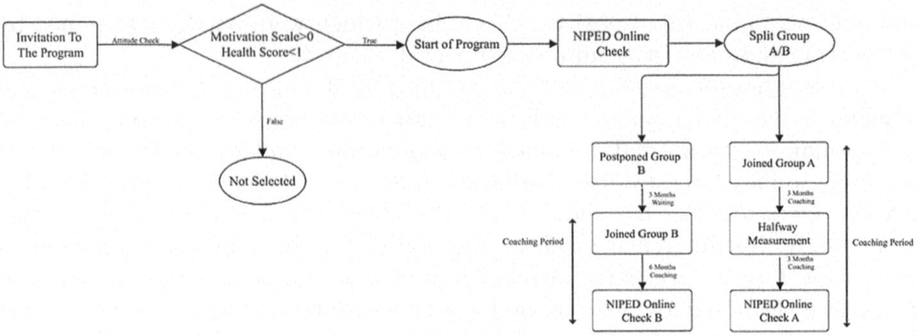

Fig. 1. VitalityPlatform Recruitment flowchart

The selected participants were then randomly assigned and divided in two groups. Group A participants have started the coaching program directly, while group B participants had to wait for three months (control group).

Both groups were invited to fill in a baseline questionnaire, the NIPED personal health check (time0). When the number of places in the program was not filled up by people in group A after two weeks, people were randomly selected from group B to switch to group A. Three months after the baseline measurements, group A participants were invited for a halfway-program NIPED check, while group B started their coaching program (time1). From this time point, group A participants took three more months to finish the program (time2), while group B participants, having started later, finished the program and filled their final NIPED survey after six months (time3).

3.2 NIPED

The NIPED health check [15,16,24] is a modular health check consisting of questionnaires and physical tests, which has been used by more than 325.000 people. The check is often offered by employers or insurance companies. The version used in this research contains 92 questions of items related to mental health, work ability, work stress, nutrition, physical activity, perceived health and the need for recovery, mostly based on existing scales. These questions were used to calculate scores for predictors of sick leave. Table 1 shows the 8 predictors of sick leave (absenteeism), most of them being based on validated questionnaires. The workability predictor is sourced from WAI [11], burnout is based on the UBOS [23], depressive symptoms are derived from the PHQ-2 questionnaire [41], perceived health as used in WHO survey [22], and the need for recovery based on NFR [9]. The last three predictors are based on a single questions about PA. PA/w refers to number of PA minutes per week, VPA/w refers to the number of minutes per week in which participants performed moderate/vigorous PA activities. The dPA30 question asked participants about the number of days in a week in which they move more than 30 min (referring to moderate and vigorous exercises).

Table 1. Predictors of sick leave.

Predictor	Composite score	Final score
Workability	Nine questions, combination of choice-questions and 5-points likert scale	0 (very bad) - 50 (very good)
Burnout	Five questions, 7-points likert scale	0 (very good) - 6 (very bad)
Depression	Two questions, 4-points scale (not at all - several days - more than half the days - nearly every day)	0 (never depressive symptoms) - 6 (nearly every day depressive feelings and no pleasure in doing things)
Perceived Health	One question, 5-points likert scale	1 (very bad) - 5 (very good)
Need for recovery	Eleven questions, yes/no	0 (very good) - 100 (very bad)
PA/w	One question	Number of minutes
VPA/w	One question	Number of minutes
dPA30	One question	Number of days, 0 to 7

3.3 VitalityPlatform Health Coaching Platform

The participants have installed the app that is part of the VitalityPlatform health coaching platform on their smartphones. The app offers mobile coaching experience, where an employee (coachee) can pick their own professional coach. The platform first gives a recommendation for a set of coaches, based on the requirements of coachees for certain lifestyle improvement. If needed, the coachee can anytime change the coach. One coach can have multiple coachees under their guidance. The communication is done via the app, by using chat messages or doing face-to-face video calls. The coachee can inform their coach when a certain exercise has been completed and connect the app to a fitness tracker. In this way, the coach is able to track the daily progress. The coach will continuously update the coachee' activity schedule based on their mutual communication. The coachee can undertake activities divided in several categories: mental, workout, lifestyle, physical and nutrition.

Only the meta-data of the VitalityPlatform usage is available for analysis. Data items are related to the frequency of coach-coachee (dyad) communication: number_messages, number_conversations, number_calls, duration_calls; and the coachee activities: ratio_done, number_done, number_liked. Table 2 gives a more detailed description of these variables.

3.4 Data Analysis

A Wilcoxon signed-rank was applied to the predictors of absenteeism scores at different time points for both groups. We test the effect of change in the predictors of absenteeism as a result of using the app (6 months period, for both groups). Wilcoxon signed-rank test was used as a non-parametric univariate test, applicable when the data violates the assumption of normality, which is the case for the predictors of absenteeism data as we will show in the next chapter.

Table 2. Variables derived from the VitalityPlatform app.

Variable name	Variable description	Possible values
number_messages	Total number of dyad text messages	[0, inf+]
number_conversations	Total number of dyad conversations	[0, inf+]
number_calls	Total number of dyad video/audio calls	[0, inf+]
avg_duration_calls	Average minutes of dyad video/audio calls	[0, inf+]
ratio_done	Ratio of planned versus done activities	[0, 1]
number_done	Total number of done activities	[0, inf+]
number_liked	Total number of liked activities	[0, inf+]

Spearman's rank-order correlation method was used in order to report the relationship between the app measurements and the predictors of absenteeism. For this analysis, the difference in the predictors of absenteeism scores before and after using the VitalityPlatform app, was used as a measure of change.

4 Results

4.1 Descriptive Statistics

Program Participation. In total 560 participants met the selection criteria (for motivation and health check scores) and were thus invited to participate in the coaching program. Figure 2 gives an overview of the number of participants per group, at different time points of the program, based on completing the NIPED questionnaires.

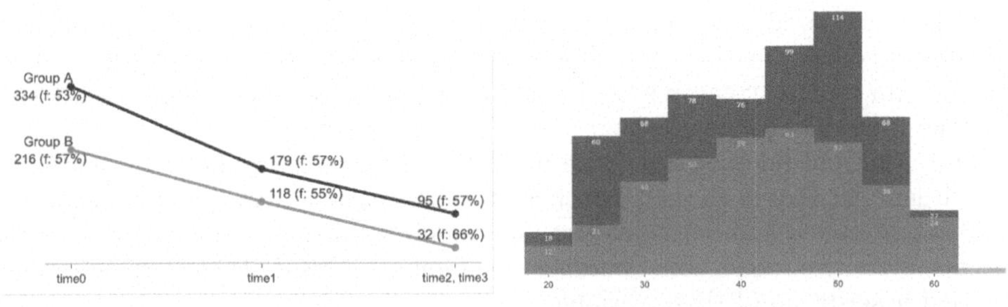

Fig. 2. Completed Niped measurements - program participation. Age distribution.

A group of 334 participants was invited to start directly after taking the baseline survey - group A, another group of 216 participants was offered to start the coaching in 3 months after filling in the baseline survey - group B. As can be seen in Fig. 2, there is a significant dropout in the number of participants who filled the second NIPED questionnaire (time1). At the final point, after completion of group A and group B participation programs (at time points time2 and time3, respectively), we observe another wave of dropout. In total, 95 participants of group A and 31 participants of group B filled the final round of the survey. For the upcoming analysis we consider 93 participants (group A) and 31 participants (group B), as they have completed the three NIPED questionnaires.

Predictors of Absenteeism Scores. Eight predictors of absenteeism were derived based on the NIPED questionnaire, as shown in Table 1. These scores were obtained at all multiple time points of the program for both group A and group B. Below we present an exploratory analysis obtained at the baseline questionnaire (time0), summarized for group A and group B participants (total n = 550, average age = 43.2, 60% female). This analysis was conducted for reporting purposes, and the outcomes were used in order to decide on the relevant statistical tests for answering our research questions.

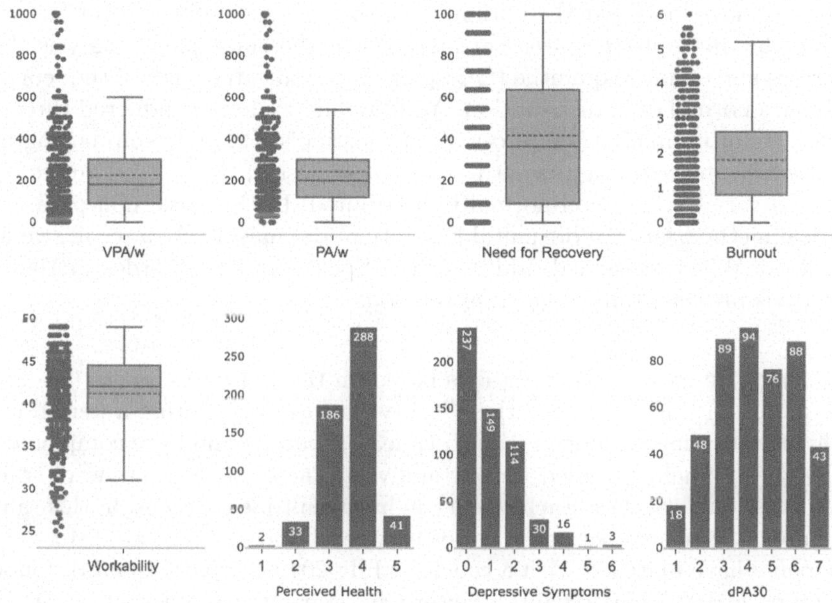

Fig. 3. Data distribution - Predictors of absenteeism scores

Figure 3 visualizes the data distribution of the predictors of absenteeism scores. Five scores are considered as continuous ratio variables, namely: VPA/w, PA/w, need for recovery, burnout and workability scores. The remaining three scores are classified as categorical nominal variables: perceived health, depressive symptoms and dPA30. The participants have self-reported an average of 243.7 min (s = 181.1) of physical activity per week, and an average of 224.9 (s = 194.7) moderate to vigorous minutes activity per week. The average need for recovery after work score was 41.7 (s = 30.78) where a score of 100 is the least favorable score (i.e. a very high need for recovery). The participants have reported a mean score of 1.79 (s = 1.37) for the risk of burnout, where 6 indicates the highest risk of burnout and 0 is the lowest risk. The average workability (or work capacity) score was 41.16 (s = 4.83), with 50 indicating the highest work capacity. Looking at the perceived health score, we can observe that most commonly participants have answered 4-good (n = 288) and 3- not bad, not good (n = 186) with an average response of 3.6 (s = 0.72). Regarding the depression score, participants have dominantly reported 0 - never depressive symptoms (n = 237), followed by 1 - several days either depressive feelings or no pleasure in doing things (n = 149), followed by 2 (n = 114) and 3 (n = 30), 4 (n = 16), 5 (n = 1) and three participants with a score of 6 (almost every day depressive feelings and no pleasure in doing things). The average is 1.00 (s = 1.13). Finally, participants were asked how many days in a week they do at least 30 min of physical activity (score dPA30). The bottom right plot of Fig. 3 shows a relatively uniform distribution with 3-, 4-, 5- and 6- days of more than 30 min activities.

Next we have looked at the normality of the data, as an important factor for selecting the appropriate statistical methods in the subsequent analysis. Both histograms and quantile-quantile (QQ) plots have indicated that all the scores do not follow a normal data distribution. Additionally we have conducted three statistical tests of normality (shapiro-wilk, d'agostino's K2, anderson-darling test) none of which showed a significant p-value regardless of the score. Therefore the considered variables are non-normally distributed. In this case, non-parametric statistical methods are a more suitable solution for analysis. As a result, we have selected the Wilcoxon signed-rank test and Spearman's rank-order method for the analysis presented in the next subsections.

App Usage Scores. This analysis is based on the 124 participants (93- group A, 31- group B) that have used the VitalityPlatform app during a period of six months (time0, time2- group A, time1, time3 - group B) and have completed the NIPED questionnaires needed for our analysis. These participants were trained by 25 professional coaches. Each coach can have multiple coachees, in this sample the number of coachees per coach varies between 1 and 12 (avg = 5). Most of the participants have matched with a coach in July 2019 (65 participants), followed by October 2019 (37 participants). Fewer have started in August and September (10 and 3 participants), or November and December 2019 (3, 4 participants). Five participants got their coach in January 2020.

Figure 4 shows the data distribution of the seven app usage scores. These scores belong to two categories: dyad communication and activity trends. The communication scores are related to number of exchanged messages, number of conversations, number of calls (audio/video) and the duration of the calls (audio/video). The activity scores are related to the coachee performance during the app usage. We look into the number of done activities, the number of liked activities and the ratio of done versus planned activities. All the scores are considered as continuous ratio variables. The dyads have exchanged on average

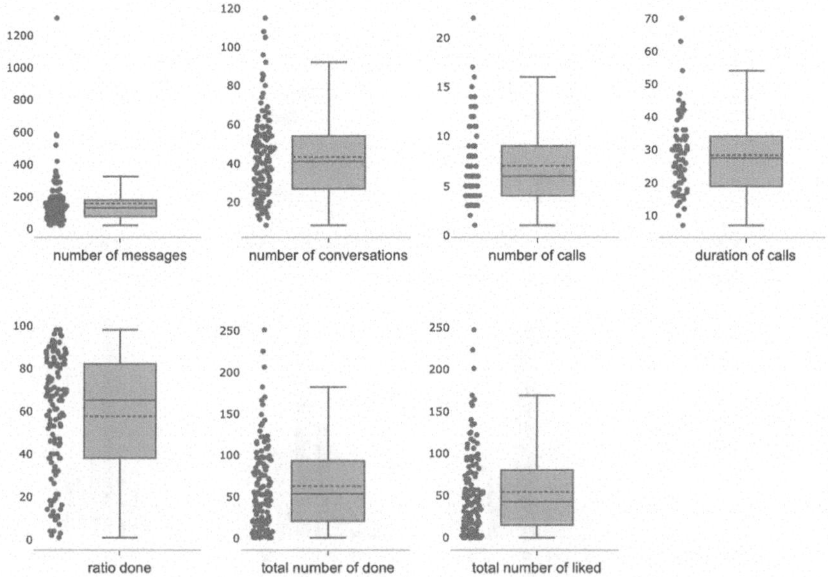

Fig. 4. App measurements data distribution

155 messages (s = 146.50) while using the app. A conversation is defined as any day in which there was a message exchanged between the dyad. On average there were 43 conversations between dyads (s = 21.41). The dyads have communicated via video/audio calls on average 7 times during the app usage (s = 4.2), with an average call time of 28 min (s = 12). Only 70 coachees have used the app for video/audio calls. Moving to the activities, we observe that the coachees did on average 58% (s = 27) of the planned activities. Looking at the total number of finished exercises, the participants did 62 activities on average while using the app (s = 51), and have liked 54 activities (s = 50) out of the ones done on average. In total there were 7728 activities performed via the app. Among them, the most common categories were lifestyle (n = 2128), mental health (n = 2184) and nutrition (n = 2012), followed by physical (n = 1365) and workout (n = 39). The activities were 94% initiated by the coach.

4.2 Effects of the Intervention

Intervention Effect on Predictors of Sick Leave. For analyzing the effects of the intervention on the predictors of sick leave, the absenteeism scores at the end of the program (time2 - group A, time3 - group B) were subtracted from the ones at the beginning of using the app (time 0 - group A, time 1 - group B). These scores are referred to as 'absenteeism difference scores' in the remainder of the paper. They give an indication of potential improvement or deterioration in absenteeism as a result of intervention participation and using the VitalityPlatform app.

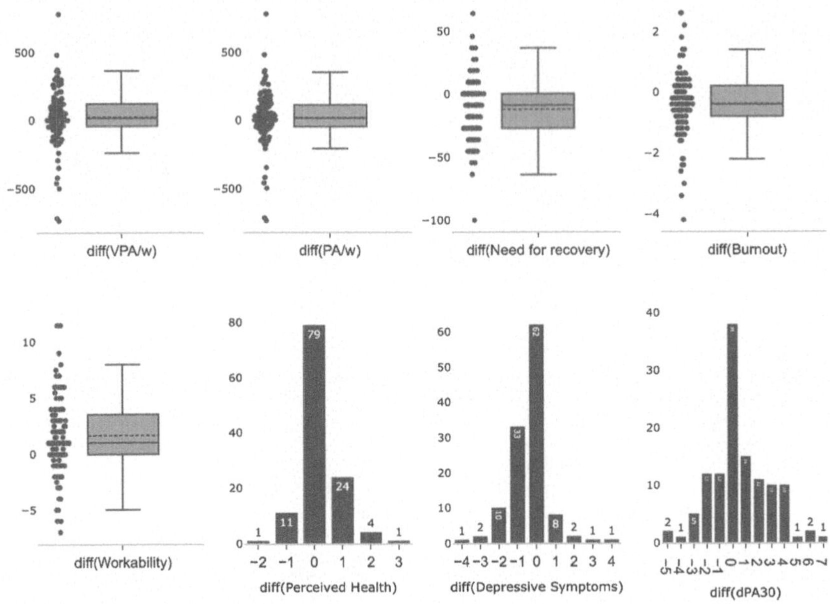

Fig. 5. Data Distribution - absenteeism difference scores

Figure 5 gives a visual overview of the absenteeism difference scores. The depicted results are summarized for group A (n = 93) and group B (n = 31). The participants have reported on average 22.7 min (s = 200.7) more vigorous activities per week - diff(VPA/w), at the end of the program participation. In a related manner, they have reported on average 16.5 more minutes (s = 190) of weekly activities. The reported need for recovery (measured on a scale 0–100, 100 - very bad) was lowered by an average of 12.4 points (s = 24.03). The participants have assessed on average 0.38 (s = 1.03) lower risk of burnout, and reported increased workability of 1.64 (s = 3.43). The five reported absenteeism difference scores are considered as interval continuous variables. The next three scores are categorical variables. First, looking at the diff(Perceived Health) we observe that most of the participants have reported no change (64%), followed by 19% that improved their score by 1, and 3% improved by two. On the other hand, 8% of participants have reduced their score by 1. The depressive symptoms score also sees improvement. While 50% of the participants have no change, 27% have improved their score by 1 (in this case the lower the better), followed by 8% improving the score by 2. One score of deterioration was reported by 6% of the participants. Finally, the diff(dPA30) score shows that 30% of participants have been doing activities in the same number of days of the week. One more day a week of activity reported 12% of participants, followed by 9% reporting doing activities in two more days. Another 8% have seen an improvement of doing three and four more days of activity after finishing the program. Looking at the opposite side, 10% of the participants reported reducing the number of days of activity by one and two days, while 4% did three less days per week.

Table 3. Wilcoxon tests results

	Workability	Burnout	Depressive symptoms	Perceived health	Need for recovery	PA/w	VPA/w	dPA30
Group A	881.5*	899.5*	300.5*	369.0	451.0*	1420.5	1361.5	679.0*
Group B	75.5*	166.5	20.0	8.0*	72.5*	167.0	143.5	95.0

Next we report the effects of change in the predictors of absenteeism as a result of the 6 month intervention for both groups. Table 3 presents the outcomes of running the Wilcoxon tests, with a T statistics and a star mark (*) for statistical significance results. The T statistics is a float value representing the sum of the ranks of the differences above or below zero, whichever is smaller. In Table 3, each T score is associated with a * mark in case of a statistically significant difference between the two means, indicated when p-value < 0.05. We note statistically significant mean differences among five scores for group A participants, namely: workability, burnout, depressive symptoms, need for recovery and dPA30. For group B, we found a statistically significant effect at three scores: workability, perceived health and need for recovery. These results indicate statistically significant changes in the corresponding predictor scores comparing before and after the intervention.

Effects of App Usage Patterns on Predictors of Sick Leave. This analysis is conducted to answer our research question if changes in NIPED scores can be associated with certain app usage patterns, regarding coach-coachee communication or the frequency of activities. We assess the relationship between the app measurements scores and the absenteeism difference scores. The relationships are examined by performing Spearman rank correlation coefficient tests for two reasons: the data is not normally distributed (to use Pearson test) and the reported type of variables. All the app scores are ratio variables, while the absenteeism difference scores are interval (n = 5) and categorical (n = 3). The results are presented separately for group A and group B, as reported in Table 4 and Table 5. The statistically significant correlation coefficients (with $p < 0.05$) are marked with a star sign (*). Among group A participants we observe four statistically significant relationships between the app usage measurements and the absenteeism difference scores. The number of dyad audio/video calls is linked with higher PA/w ($r = 0.30$) and need for recovery ($r = 0.49$), the number of exchanged messages has a moderate relation with the increase of perceived health ($r = 0.24$), and the number of liked activities with the workability score ($r = 0.24$). As observed in Table 5, among group B participants, the exchanged number of messages could be related to reducing the risk of burnout ($r = -0.40$), while the ratio of done activities lead to increase of the depressive symptoms ($r = -0.39$).

Table 4. Correlation outcomes - groupA

	avg_dur	num_calls	num_conv	ratio_done	num_mes	total_done	total_liked
diff(Workability)	0.14	0.04	0.10	−0.04	0.07	0.19	0.24*
diff(Burnout)	0.01	−0.02	−0.08	0.04	−0.05	0.05	0.04
diff(Depressive symptoms)	−0.04	−0.14	−0.03	−0.05	−0.05	−0.01	0.05
diff(Perceived Health)	−0.24	0.15	0.12	−0.01	0.24*	0.10	0.08
diff(Need recovery)	−0.04	0.49*	0.07	0.14	0.09	0.02	0.02
diff(PA/w)	−0.11	0.30*	0.06	−0.04	−0.01	−0.02	0.01
diff(VPA/w)	−0.14	0.24	0.08	−0.03	0.03	−0.03	−0.01
diff(dPA30)	−0.14	0.10	0.03	0.07	0.02	−0.04	0.03

Table 5. Correlation outcomes - groupB

	avg_dur	num_calls	num_conv	ratio_done	num_mes	total_done	total_liked
diff(Workability)	−0.32	0.35	0.02	−0.15	0.22	0.10	0.08
diff(Burnout)	0.24	−0.20	−0.36	0.11	−0.40*	−0.13	−0.10
diff(Depressive symptoms)	−0.17	0.05	0.34	0.39*	0.20	0.30	0.23
diff(Perceived Health)	−0.29	0.25	0.12	0.02	0.18	0.14	0.14
diff(Need recovery)	0.35	−0.10	−0.32	−0.03	−0.36	−0.32	−0.28
diff(PA/w)	0.07	−0.34	−0.20	0.17	−0.17	0.01	0.01
diff(VPA/w)	0.15	−0.41	−0.20	0.12	−0.19	−0.05	−0.04
diff(dPA30)	−0.20	0.37	0.26	0.07	0.15	0.04	0.06

5 Discussion and Conclusions

This paper presents the outcomes of a coaching-based digital health intervention and its effects on predictors of absenteeism. This makes our work distinguishable from previous research, as most commonly the intervention effects are measured (linked to) health outcomes such as increasing PA or weight loss. The predictors of absenteeism scores were analyzed after 6 months of coach-based intervention via smartphone app. The summarized results show improvement in all the absenteeism difference scores. The participants have reported lower risk of burnout (0.38 points), showing less depressive symptoms and need for recovery (12.4 points). On the other hand, they have performed more PA activities per week (any activities 16.5 min, vigorous 22.7 min), increased their workability (1.64), improved their perceived health and had slightly more days of PA per week. These results indicate that the mhealth intervention had a positive effect on the participants, if one is to observe the difference in the reported scores before and after the intervention. Furthermore, the outcome of the Wilcoxon tests shows statistically significant effects of change in the predictors of absenteeism as a result of using the app. This has been observed separately in both group A and group B participants. The effects are detected in the following absenteeism scores: workability, burnout, depressive symptoms, need for recovery and dPA30 (group A); perceived health, workability and need for recovery (group B).

Additionally, we have investigated the relationship between the VitalityPlatform app usage (in terms of frequency of dyad communication and performing activities) and the observed changes in the absenteeism predictor scores. The spearman correlation coefficients did not find any strong and significant correlation between the two. However, we are able to detect moderately-strong and significant correlations. Regarding the frequency of dyad communication we found significant relationships between the number of audio/video calls with need for recovery and PA/w (group A), and the number of exchanged messages correlates with the perceived health (group A), and burnout (group B). Looking at the performed activities, the total number of liked activities was linked to the workability score (group A), and surprisingly the depressive symptoms increase with the ratio of done exercises (group B).

This work comes with certain limitations. Only a limited number of people filled in the NIPED questionnaire after three months. Engagement data shows that 90% of the participants were active after 3 months. Therefore, the reason behind the relatively low number of participants who completed the second test was not that they dropped out of the health coaching program. We suspect that that the relative cumbersome health check (it takes 30 to 45 min to complete the entire test) is the primary reason for people not completing the second questionnaire. For a more thorough analysis of the effect of the coaching program on itself, we ideally need a control group data that is not invited to participate in a health coaching program. With the current experimental setup, we cannot explicitly investigate this, as group B participants were put on a waiting list. One possible additional analysis could be whether the participation in the programme or already filling in the first health questionnaire (for group B) is causing a potential positive effect among participants.

The investigated coaching aspect also comes with certain constraints. For example, we cannot rule out that there have been other interactions between the dyad then via the app. We have focused on quantifying the dyad relationship through frequency of communication. However, textual analysis of the chat interactions can offer additional valuable information on their relationship. The defined app usage measurements are of course a simplification. Many other (non) latent factors might potentially influence the effects of the coaching program, for example seasonal effects. Therefore a larger and more complete study would be prefered to investigate the relation between the app usage and change in predictors of absenteeism.

References

1. Baicker, K., Cutler, D., Song, Z.: Workplace wellness programs can generate savings. Health Aff. (2010). https://doi.org/10.1377/hlthaff.2009.0626
2. Boot, C.R.L., Koppes, L.L.J., van den Bossche, S.N.J., Anema, J.R., van der Beek, A.J.: Relation between perceived health and sick leave in employees with a chronic illness. J. Occup. Rehabil. **21**(2), 211–219 (2011). https://doi.org/10.1007/s10926-010-9273-1
3. van den Brink, C., Ocké, M., Houben, A., van Nierop, P., Droomers, M.: Validering van Standaardvraagstelling voeding voor Lokale en Nationale Monitor Volksgezondheid. RIVM Rapport 260854008 (2005)
4. Brown, J.M., Miller, W.R., Lawendowski, L.A.: The Self-Regulation Questionnaire (SRQ). Innovations in Clinical Practice: A Source Book, vol. 17 (1999)

5. Buysse, D.J., Reynolds, C.F., Monk, T.H., Berman, S.R., Kupfer, D.J.: The Pittsburgh sleep quality index: a new instrument for psychiatric practice and research. Psychiatry Res. (1989). https://doi.org/10.1016/0165-1781(89)90047-4
6. Champion, D.F., Westbrook, B.W.: Maslach burnout inventory. Meas. Eval. Couns. Dev. (1984). https://doi.org/10.1080/07481756.1984.12022754
7. Coffeng, J.K., Boot, C.R.L., Duijts, S.F.A., Twisk, J.W.R., Van Mechelen, W., Hendriksen, I.J.M.: Effectiveness of a worksite social & physical environment intervention on need for recovery, physical activity and relaxation; results of a randomized controlled trial. PLoS ONE (2014). https://doi.org/10.1371/journal.pone.0114860
8. Cooper, C., Dewe, P.: Well-being-absenteeism, presenteeism, costs and challenges. Occup. Med. **58**(8), 522–524 (2008). https://doi.org/10.1093/occmed/kqn124
9. de Croon, E.M.: Psychometric properties of the Need for Recovery after work scale: test-retest reliability and sensitivity to detect change. Occup. Environ. Med. **63**(3), 202–206 (2006). https://doi.org/10.1136/oem.2004.018275
10. Goetzel, R.Z., Long, S.R., Ozminkowski, R.J., Hawkins, K., Wang, S., Lynch, W.: Health, absence, disability, and presenteeism cost estimates of certain physical and mental health conditions affecting U.S. employers. J. Occup. Environ. Med. (2004). https://doi.org/10.1097/01.jom.0000121151.40413.bd
11. Ilmarinen, J.: The work ability index (WAI). Occup. Med. **57**(2), 160–160 (2006). https://doi.org/10.1093/occmed/kqm008
12. Justesen, J.B., Søgaard, K., Dalager, T., Christensen, J.R., Sjøgaard, G.: The effect of intelligent physical exercise training on sickness presenteeism and absenteeism among office workers. J. Occup. Environ. Med. (2017). https://doi.org/10.1097/JOM.0000000000001101
13. Kroenke, K., Spitzer, R.L., Williams, J.B.W.: The PHQ-9: validity of a brief depression severity measure. J. Gen. Intern. Med. (2001). https://doi.org/10.1046/j.1525-1497.2001.016009606.x
14. Lechner, L., De Vries, H., Adriaansen, S., Drabbels, L.: Effects of an employee fitness program on reduced absenteeism. J. Occup. Environ. Med. (1997). https://doi.org/10.1097/00043764-199709000-00005
15. Niessen, M.A.J., et al.: Short term reduction in absenteeism after implementation of a personalized prevention program. Eur. J. Cardiovasc. Prev. Rehabil. (2010)
16. Niessen, M.A.J., Kraaijenhagen, R.A., Dijkgraaf, M.G.W., Van Pelt, D., Van Kalken, C.K., Peek, N.: Impact of a web-based worksite health promotion program on absenteeism. J. Occup. Environ. Med. (2012). https://doi.org/10.1097/JOM.0b013e31824d2e43
17. Olsen, J.M., Nesbitt, B.J.: Health coaching to improve healthy lifestyle behaviors: an integrative review. Am. J. Health Promot. **25**(1), e1–e12 (2010)
18. Proper, K.I.: Dose-response relation between physical activity and sick leave. Br. J. Sports Med. **40**(2), 173–178 (2006). https://doi.org/10.1136/bjsm.2005.022327
19. Proper, K.I., Staal, B.J., Hildebrandt, V.H., van der Beek, A.J., van Mechelen, W.: Effectiveness of physical activity programs at worksites with respect to work-related outcomes. Scand. J. Work Environ. Health **28**(2), 75–84 (2002). https://doi.org/10.5271/sjweh.651
20. Reis, D., Xanthopoulou, D., Tsaousis, I.: Measuring job and academic burnout with the Oldenburg Burnout Inventory (OLBI): factorial invariance across samples and countries. Burn. Res. (2015). https://doi.org/10.1016/j.burn.2014.11.001
21. Salomonsson, S., Hedman-Lagerlöf, E., Öst, L.G.: Sickness absence: a systematic review and meta-analysis of psychological treatments for individuals on sick leave

due to common mental disorders. Psychol. Med. (2018). https://doi.org/10.1017/S0033291718000065
22. Subramanian, S.V., Huijts, T., Avendano, M.: Self-reported health assessments in the 2002 World Health Survey: how do they correlate with education? Bull. World Health Organ. **88**(2), 131–138 (2010). https://doi.org/10.2471/BLT.09.067058
23. Schaufeli, W., Van Dierendonck, D.: Utrechtse Burnout Schaal (UBOS). De Psycholoog (2001)
24. Van Den Brekel-Dijkstra, K., Rengers, A.H., Niessen, M.A.J., De Wit, N.J., Kraaijenhagen, R.A.: Personalized prevention approach with use of a web-based cardiovascular risk assessment with tailored lifestyle follow-up in primary care practice - a pilot study. Eur. J. Prev. Cardiol. (2016). https://doi.org/10.1177/2047487315591441
25. van Tulder, M.W., Koes, B.W., Bouter, L.M.: A cost-of-illness study of back pain in The Netherlands. Pain (1995). https://doi.org/10.1016/0304-3959(94)00272-G
26. Wendel-Vos, G.C.W., Schuit, A.J., Saris, W.H.M., Kromhout, D.: Reproducibility and relative validity of the short questionnaire to assess health-enhancing physical activity. J. Clin. Epidemiol. (2003). https://doi.org/10.1016/S0895-4356(03)00220-8
27. Conn, V.S., Hafdahl, A.R., Cooper, P.S., Brown, L.M., Lusk, S.L.: Meta-analysis of workplace physical activity interventions. Am. J. Prev. Med. **37**(4), 330–339 (2009)
28. Dugdill, L., Brettle, A., Hulme, C., McCluskey, S., Long, A.F.: Workplace physical activity interventions: a systematic review. Int. J. Workplace Health Manag. (2008)
29. Chiesa, A., Serretti, A.: Mindfulness-based stress reduction for stress management in healthy people: a review and meta-analysis. J. Alternative Complement. Med. **15**(5), 593–600 (2009)
30. Wolever, R.Q., et al.: Effective and viable mind-body stress reduction in the workplace: a randomized controlled trial. J. Occup. Health Psychol. **17**(2), 246 (2012)
31. Kagan, N.I., Watson, M.G.: Stress reduction in the workplace: the effectiveness of psychoeducational programs. J. Couns. Psychol. **42**(1), 71 (1995)
32. Czabała, C., Charzyńska, K., Mroziak, B.: Psychosocial interventions in workplace mental health promotion: an overview. Health Promotion Int. **26**(Suppl. 1), i70–i84 (2011)
33. Proper, K.I., van Oostrom, S.H.: The effectiveness of workplace health promotion interventions on physical and mental health outcomes-a systematic review of reviews. Scand. J. Work Environ. Health **45**(6), 546–559 (2019)
34. Chu, A.H., Ng, S.H., Tan, C.S., Win, A.M., Koh, D., Müller-Riemenschneider, F.: A systematic review and meta-analysis of workplace intervention strategies to reduce sedentary time in white-collar workers. Obes. Rev. **17**(5), 467–481 (2016)
35. Buckingham, S.A., Williams, A.J., Morrissey, K., Price, L., Harrison, J.: Mobile health interventions to promote physical activity and reduce sedentary behaviour in the workplace: a systematic review. Digit. Health **5**, 2055207619839883 (2019)
36. Hutchinson, A.D., Wilson, C.: Improving nutrition and physical activity in the workplace: a meta-analysis of intervention studies. Health Promot. Int. **27**(2), 238–249 (2012)
37. Verweij, L.M., Coffeng, J., van Mechelen, W., Proper, K.I.: Meta-analyses of workplace physical activity and dietary behaviour interventions on weight outcomes. Obes. Rev. **12**(6), 406–429 (2011)
38. Rongen, A., Robroek, S.J., van Lenthe, F.J., Burdorf, A.: Workplace health promotion: a meta-analysis of effectiveness. Am. J. Prev. Med. **44**(4), 406–415 (2013)

39. Palmer, S., Tubbs, I., Whybrow, A.: Health coaching to facilitate the promotion of healthy behaviour and achievement of health-related goals. Int. J. Health Promot. Educ. **41**(3), 91–93 (2003)
40. Gyllensten, K., Palmer, S.: Can coaching reduce workplace stress? A quasi-experimental study. Int. J. Evidence Based Coaching Mentoring **3**(2), 75–85 (2005)
41. Arroll, B., et al.: Validation of PHQ-2 and PHQ-9 to screen for major depression in the primary care population. Ann. Family Med. **8**(4), 348–353 (2010)

eHealthCare - A Medication Monitoring Approach for the Elderly People

António Pinto, Ana Correia, Rui Alves(✉), Paulo Matos, João Ascensão, and Diogo Camelo

Polytechnic Institute of Bragança, Bragança, Portugal
{a36727,a39944,a34505,a36739}@alunos.ipb.pt, {rui.alves,pmatos}@ipb.pt

Abstract. For the regularly medicated population, the management of the posology is of utmost importance. With increasing average life expectancy, people tend to become older and more likely to have chronic medical disorders, consequently taking more medicines. This is predominant in the older population, but it's not exclusive to this generation. It's a common problem for all those suffering from chronic diseases, regardless of age group. Performing a correct management of the medicines stock, as well as, taking them at the ideal time, is not always easy and, in some cases, the diversity of medicines needed to treat a particular medical disorder is a proof of that. Knowing what to take, how much to take, and ensuring compliance with the medication intervals, for each medication in use, becomes a serious problem for those who experience this reality. The situation is aggravated when the posology admits variable amounts, intervals, and combinations depending on the patient's health condition. This paper presents a solution that optimizes the management of medication of users who use the services of institutions that provide health care to the elderly (e.g., day care centers or nursing homes). Making use of the NB-IoT network, artificial intelligence algorithms, a set of sensors and an Arduino MKR NB 1500, this solution, in addition to the functionalities already described, eHealthCare also has mechanisms that allow identifying the non-adherence to medication by the elderly.

Keywords: Medication · Elderly · Non-adherence · Sensors network

1 Introduction

Forgetting to take a dose or two of a certain medication may not seem critical. Sometimes ignored doses do not cause obvious problems, but many medications will not work properly if they are not ingested at the right time and in the right way. Non-adherence to medication is unfortunately quite common, especially among patients with chronic diseases and the elderly [1–3]. This non-adherence [4,5] is usually associated with factors such as [6]: fear of possible related effects; mistrust, making many patients believe that prescriptions passed by doctors are

X. Gao et al. (Eds.): MobiHealth 2021, LNICST 440, pp. 221–234, 2022.
https://doi.org/10.1007/978-3-031-06368-8_15

for pharmaceutical benefits; the absence of symptoms leading many patients to believe that they do not require medication.

Regardless of the causes that lead to medication non-adherence, depending on the chronic disease in question, the incorrect medicines ingestion quickly becomes a problem for the patients health. However, identifying whether the medication was taken correctly, in many cases and especially in the elderly, is an extremely complicated task since many of them do not have permanent caregivers to assist in the management of medicines. A good example of this difficulty, is the case of schizophrenia [7], where there are patients who can survive treatment failures for considerable periods without adverse consequences. However, in the case of schizophrenia, recidivism rates are very high after treatment interruption, and in many cases they occur within weeks of interruption. In these cases, to aggravate the situation, there are no reliable signs of early warning for caregivers or doctors in identifying individuals with an imminent risk of relapse whose symptoms, instead of gradually appearing, usually return quickly. Thus, a careful observation approach to patients suspected of non-adherence, with a view to introducing rescue medication at the first sign of recurrence, is unlikely to be effective in real-world contexts.

In this way, it's important to prepare institutions that provide support services for medication with solutions that make possible not only to identify non-adherence to medication, as well as allowing better medication management, for both final users and their staff. Additionally, the COVID-19 pandemic [8], which exposed inequalities in social assistance different social groups, especially in the older one [9–11], makes medication monitoring an even more difficult task to perform, since the measures adopted worldwide to contain the pandemic do not promote direct contact with the population.

Through a small set of sensors, chips and artificial intelligence processes, the solution illustrated in this paper presents as its main scientific contribution, a tool that allows to identify possible users who do not adhere to medication. In addition, the restrictions implemented to contain the COVID-19 pandemic, which, as already mentioned, encourage the reduction of physical and social contacts, further reinforce the importance of building tools such as the one presented.

The remainder of the paper is organized as follows: Sect. 2 offers a brief analysis of the others possible solutions to the problems presented; Sect. 3 describes the architecture constructed as a response to the problems identified; Sect. 4 illustrates the conclusions of the paper and the goals for future work.

2 State of the Art

The development of solutions to help identify non-adherence to medication is not something new in the market [12]. During this section it will be detailed a set of solutions similar to the tool presented in this paper. Despite eHealthCare has similar functionalities to the following solutions, it's important to clarify that its target audience is different.

Thus, while the solutions presented in the following section are targeting of any user who needs medication, the eHealthCare solution, as already illustrated, is aimed at institutions (e.g., day care centers, nursing homes) and was conceived as a monitoring and control solution for the detection of medication non-adherence. So, this solution has as main purpose, assist institutions that provide medication control services and will not be available to the end-users.

As shown in Table 1 there is already a set of solutions that are intended to assist the taking of medication, which may reinforce the importance of the theme addressed in this article.

Table 1. Comparisons between solutions

	Config	Alarm	Management	Stock	Tool
eHealthCare	Simple	Yes	Non adherence alerts; Mobile and Web control	Auto pharmacy contact; Automatic meds refill	Web; Mob; Organizer
TabTime Timer [13]	Nonex	Yes	No	No	Organizer
e-pill TimeCap [14]	Nonex	Yes	"Last Opened" display; Same meds in a row prevention	No	Online pharmacy
PillPack [15]	Nonex	Yes	Doctor is contacted	Auto purchase and recharge	Mob
MedMinder [16]	Hard	Yes	Missed dose alerts; Weekly reports; Wrong meds prevention	No	Pill Dispenser
MediSafe [17]	Nonex	Yes	App synchronization with someone	Specific company contact	Mob
CareZone [18]	Nonex	Yes	Doctor is contacted	Automatic meds refill	Mob

Despite the great diversity of solutions, the great advantage of eHealthCare, in addition to the technical functionalities that its architecture presents, is in the simplicity of use and target of the population for which it is intended - the elderly who live in more remote regions.

Thus, although most of the solutions illustrated in Table 1 present a set of quite interesting functionalities, some even surpass the functionalities presented in eHealthCare.

A general overview, shows that all presented solutions have some sort of alarm/reminder to help the user remember to take the medicines, and almost all of them provide one or more features to medication management.

However, unlike eHealthCare where only the medication organizer is delivered to the patient, in the solutions presented in this section it is always necessary to integrate them with other technologies/mechanisms (internet/smartphones), where often older people and especially the ones living in more remote regions do not have.

Due to this reason, the authors considered that a comparison between eHealthCare and the other solutions isn't that feasible, since, as mentioned above, the remaining solutions are not optimized for older people to use them.

3 Implementation

In Fig. 1, it's possible to analyze the overview of the built architecture, consisting of 4 elements:

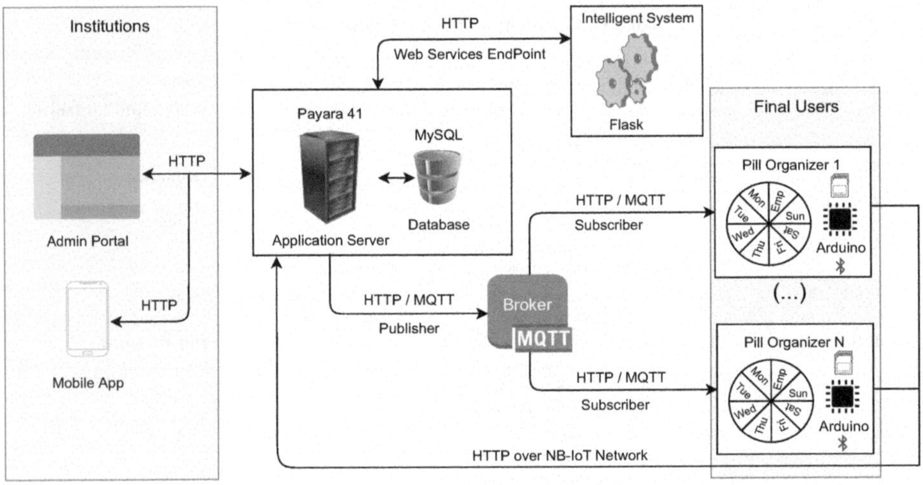

Fig. 1. Overview of eHealthCare architecture.

- a web server that provides a set of endpoints (see Sect. 3.4), used by the mobile application and the administration portal. It can control distributed organizers, registered users and interact with the intelligent part of the architecture.
- the medication organizers described in the Sect. 3.1, adapted to the users which have a strong rejection of the use of technologies [19,20];
- a broker who will be responsible for managing the exchange of messages between the web server and the Arduino MKR 1500 board (the first and only Arduino to be compatible with LTE Cat M1 and NB-IoT [21,22]) inserted in the organizers of medication;
- a set of intelligent processes, available through the Flask framework, described in the Sect. 3.2 that will be responsible for identifying users who are not non-adherent to medication. Additionally, these processes will be responsible for trying to predict the likelihood of new users not adhering to medication based on their characteristics and data already entered in the system.

The operation of eHealthCare can be defined in 3 phases. The first phase corresponds to the preparation of the pill organizer (described in Sect. 3.1) which will be delivered to each user. This preparation corresponds to the filling of the medication for the corresponding user, as well as the transfer of the timetables of each dose to the memory of the Arduino Board. The second phase corresponds to the normal detection by the system of the intakes medication, that is, as the user withdraws/ignores medication from the organizer. For each occurrence, the Arduino Board sends a message, to a server, that will be processed later by the intelligent part of the architecture. The last phase, is the presentation of the results, that is, where the institutions can monitor almost in real time the state of the medication of each one of its users, being clearly identified the users who are suspected of not adhering to the medication.

Finally, all components of the solution intended for majority use by the elderly, were designed to make them as simple as possible and according to the capabilities of this target audience as will be illustrated in the next sections.

3.1 Pill Organizer

In the Fig. 2 it is illustrated the organizer created and introduced in the architecture of the eHealthCare solution. This organizer contains 29 slots[1] that correspond, for the 7 days of the week, to the morning, lunch, snack and dinner periods, very similar to what already happens in common pill organizers. The last slot (Empty slot) corresponds to the medication collection slot.

All the remaining 28 slots are blocked, that is, their upper limit is covered with a plastic layer preventing the users to take the medication out of their intake time. However, the collection slot (represented in Fig. 2 by an Empty slot) is the only one that does not contain such protection. This allows, when it is reaching the given time to intake the medication, the Arduino to activate the stepper motor so that it positions the division corresponding to this intake in the collection slot, making possible for the user to withdraw the medication.

When the institution prepares an organizer, it already contains all the timetables by which the medication should be available for the user to ingest. Added to this information, a timeout value that corresponds to the time that the Arduino must wait until it blocks the slot of the corresponding portion is also defined. Thus, when the Arduino detects a timeout related to the actual time of ingestion of the medication, it activates the stepper motor in order to position in the collection slot, the division that corresponds to the time of the taking. In parallel, a LED is activated, and a horn is issued to alert the user that medication is available and should be taken.

Each slot contains a [23] force sensor that makes it possible to identify when the user changes the content of the medication. Thus, in the tests performed, it was identified that four situations may occur when the medication becomes available: total removal of the contents of the slot; partial removal of the contents of the slot; removal of the content with addition in the near instance; not removal

[1] In the Fig. 2 only 8 are represented to facilitate the understanding of the architecture.

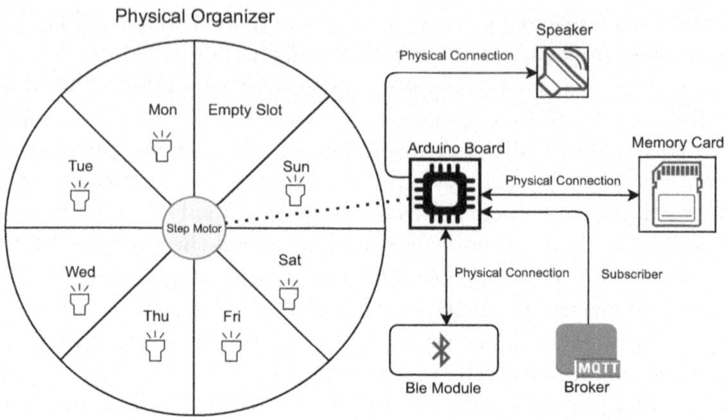

Fig. 2. Detailed architecture of the pill organizer.

of the content inside the slot. Thus, only in the first situation is that the system considers that non-adherence to medication did not occur and the remaining are considered situations of non-adherence to medication.

Listing 1.1. Example of JSON string sent by Arduino board to webserver


```
{
    "id_pill_organizer":150,
    "state":0,
}
```


When Arduino identifies one of the four situations described above, it sends a message to the web server, using NB-IoT, with information similar to that represented in Listing 1.1. The information sent contains only two fields: id_pill_organizer that identifies the organizer in question and the state field that identifies which of the four previously identified situations occurred, where the medication in question is identified by the time the message is sent to the server through the current timestamp. For cases where NB-IoT support does not exist, Arduino stores all records generated on a memory card added for this purpose. In this context, the data will then be collected by the collaborators of the institutions using the mobile application (see in the Sect. 3.4).

Finally, it should also be noted that Arduino performs Subscriber in the Broker illustrated in Fig. 3. This action allows the Arduino to perform any unlocking of the slots triggered in the administration portal (see Sect. 3.4). It also makes it possible to receive the information necessary to monitor and make available the medication of the user concerned.

3.2 Intelligent System

Nowadays, artificial intelligent systems/processes are becoming helpful tools in countless tasks, since forecasting academic dropout [24] to plant classification

[25]. In this paper, the authors explored artificial intelligent processes to classify the level of non-adherence to medication of a new patient with the collected data. In addiction, an intelligent algorithm was implemented to monitor the medication non-adherence rate of the eHealthCare system patients.

For better understanding, in Fig. 3 can be observed the architecture of the intelligent system proposed by the authors.

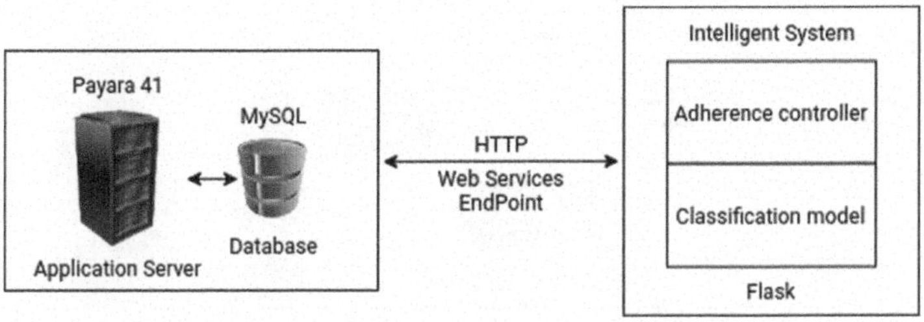

Fig. 3. Overview of the intelligent system of the eHealthCare system.

The eHealthCare intelligent system is composed by two components, the adherence controller and the classification model. The adherence controller is responsible for controlling the rate of non-adherence to medication of the patients of the eHealthCare system by receiving the messages send by the Arduino when a patient does not consume the pills that he has to consume. The classification model is responsible to classify the level of non-adherence to medication of a new patient.

For the usage of the intelligent system, two metrics were associated/added to the patients, the level of non-adherence to medication and the rate of non-adherence to medication. Both this metrics were stored in the database of the system. The levels of non-adherence to medication and their description can be seen in the Table 2.

Table 2. Levels of non-adherence to medication.

Level	Range of rates	Description
Green	[0%, 5%[	The patient is rarely non-adherent to medication
Yellow	]5%, 40%[	The patient is sometimes non-adherent to medication
Orange	]40%, 80%[	The patient is non-adherent to medication with some frequency
Red	]80%, 100%]	The patient is totally non-adherent to medication

The level of non-adherence to medication is used in the classification and to monitor the rate of non-adherence to medication. Another value added for the usage of the intelligent system, was the effect in the rate of non-adherence to medication of every medication. This value was added because the effect of not consuming some medications is greater than other medications. Thus, if a medication A has more importance than a medication B, the medication A will have a higher effect value than medication B. All values mention before are key elements to the operation of the adherence controller.

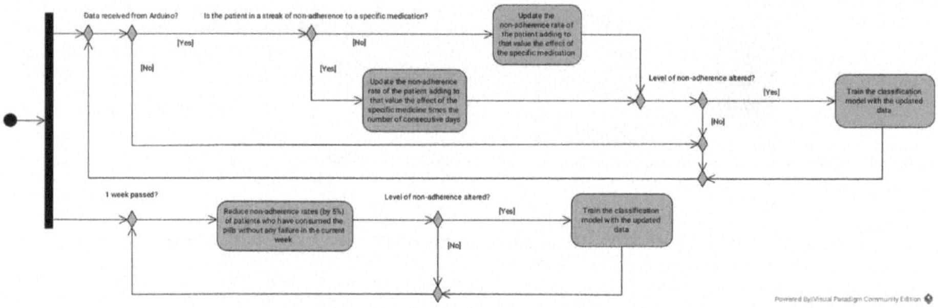

Fig. 4. Overview of the operation of the adherence controller.

In Fig. 4 can be observed an activity diagram that represents a detailed overview of the operation of the adherence controller of the intelligent system. The adherence controller has two processes that are always running, where the first is waiting for the data sent by the Arduino but forwarded by the HTTP Server (Payara 41) when a patient does not consume the medication; the second runs periodically, once per week. When triggered, the first process is going to update the non-adherence rate of the patient in question, adding to that value the effect of the specific medication, if the patient is in a streak of adherence to a specific medication, or adding to that value the effect of the specific medication times the number of consecutive days if the patient is in a streak of non-adherence. If that update changes the level of non-adherence of the patient, the classification model that will be discussed further ahead, will be trained with the updated data. The training process occurs every time the conditions described above are met, to ensure that the classification model is based on up-to-date data. Relatively to the second process, it will update the non-adherence rates of patients who have consumed the medication without any failure in the current week, reducing that value by 5%. This update is done to "reward" the patients that are becoming more adherent to medication. So, the system will always have up-to-date data about the patients. As in the first process, if that update changes the level of non-adherence of the patient, the classification model will be trained with the updated data. The main objective of this component and its processes, is to always monitor and adjust the rates of non-adherence of the patients, increasing their rates when they don't consume their medication and reducing their rates when they consume their medication without any failure in a week. Like that, the institutions that use the eHealthCare system will always have updated data of their patients.

Since the adherence controller is training the model every time the level of non-adherence of the patients changes, there was a need for a machine learning algorithm that could be fast and computationally light. In addition, that machine learning algorithm needed to be a supervised machine learning algorithm, since the authors had labelled data to train, and solve a classification problem, since the objective of the model is to classify patients into four classes (green, yellow, orange, red) [26]. The supervised machine learning algorithm chosen was the K-Nearest Neighbors, since it fulfills the intended requirements and because the authors relied on simplicity and functionality to implement this solution, however for future work, testing of new machine learning algorithms will be done to perceive the effect of other machine learning algorithms in the intelligent system of the eHealthCare system [27–31].

Before the training of adherence controller classification model, the data needs to be prepared to be feed to the model. The first step in the preparation of data is the pre-processing of the data related to the patients. In this step, several data related to the patients are extracted from the database of the system, like age, education and gender. One of the most important data that is extracted is the target variable of the classification that is the level of non-adherence to medication. The queries responsible for the extracting of all variables were manually pre-coded by the authors and are just invoked by the adherence controller. After the pre-processing of the data, the next step is the identification of the type (nominal, ordinal, discrete, continuous and logical) of each variable. For example, the age will be a discrete variable since it's a number. However, the gender will be a nominal variable since it's a categorical value where there is no ordination between categories. With every variable identified, the next step is to normalize every value of every variable, e.g. between 0 and 1 [32,33]. This process is necessary to ensure that the different variables have the same range of values, so that no variable has more influence on the result than another, making the classification model more accurate.

After that, the classification model will be trained with the resulted variables. After the training, the classification model will be available through a REST endpoint that will be consumed by the applications. With that, every time a new patient is registered in the eHealthCare system, the classification model will classify the level of non-adherence to medication of the patient, and if the level is high, the staff of the institutions can observe that information and closely monitor that patient.

3.3 NB-IoT Comunication

Designing solutions that identify non-adherence to medication is not an easy task as explained in previous sections. Although the target institutions often have physical support and human resources for the use of this type of tools, on the end user side, this is often not the case. Thus, in contexts where users, who use the services of these institutions, and live in isolated locations, the use of tools such as eHealthCare is compromised due to the weak support for the Internet [34].

It was, therefore, necessary to add mechanisms to the presented solution in this paper that make it possible to overcome the difficulties identified. To overcome the lack of Internet support in some regions, communication between medication organizers and institutional servers is carried out using NB-IoT.

This technology is currently part of the LTE network and any place on the planet with network coverage, is fertile ground for NB-IoT that significantly improve IoT devices energy consumption. Currently expanding, NB-IoT already present in 69 countries by 2019 [35,36]. Since NB-IoT is a mobile IoT network, security is not a problem as mobile operators ensure the encryption of customer/user data, or in some cases, VPNs with encrypted connections and APNs. Other security features are included, like Data over NAS (DoNAS), Non-IP Data Delivery (NIDD), or white-lists [37]. Resuming, NB-IoT uses licensed spectrum and secure communication channels, being this an vantage that releases programmers and end-users of concerns related with security.

3.4 Admin Portal and Mobile Application

The portal of administration and the mobile application has as main function assist the institutions in the preparation and monitoring of the medication. In Fig. 5 it is possible to see the layout built for the administration portal.

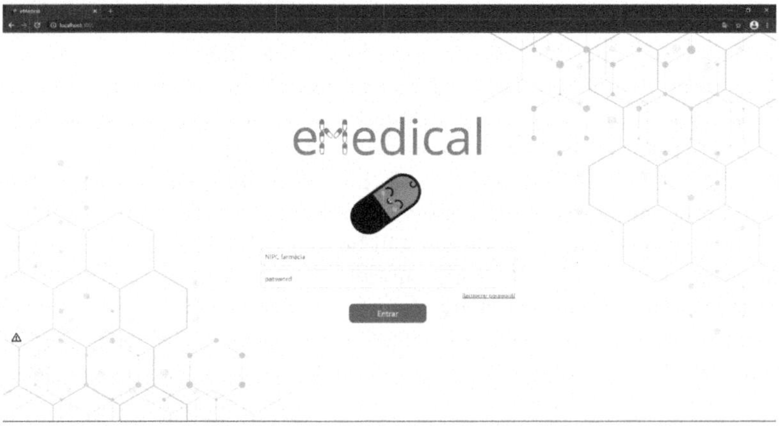

Fig. 5. Layout web portal eHealthCare

This portal has as main functions: the registration of new users; the real-time consultation of the medication taken that each user should take/made every instant; the unblocking of divisions in the drug organizers; the recording of medication-related information to be passed on to the organizers.

For the patient's registration, it's presented, based on the parameters already described in the previous section, the probability that a new user have to not adhere to the medication. For the divisions unblocking, it is guaranteed by the Broker, that is, when it is necessary to unlock a division, the web portal publishes in Broker a message that is later passed to Arduino. To record the medication information passed to the organizers, this is accomplished through a combination of touches on the button placed on the organizer, which obliges the organizer in question to establish an HTTP request over the NB-IoT network.

The layout of the mobile application can be analyzed in Fig. 6. This application allows the management of the parameters related to users and their medications. The great utility of this application is to enable the collection of data stored on the memory card added to each organizer. However, the collection of this data, performed using BLE, is only necessary in contexts where NB-IoT network is very weak or inaccessible. After collecting the data, the application sends it to the server to be processed as with the data sent by Arduino.

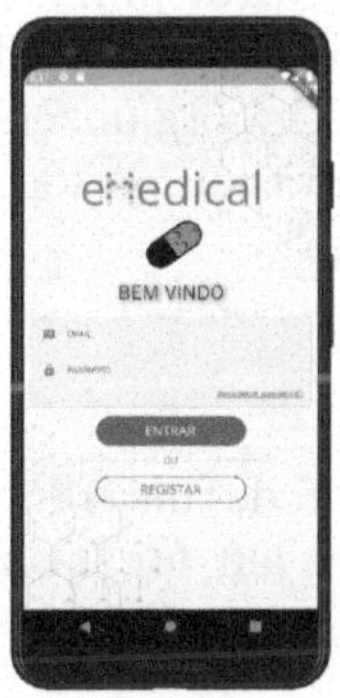

Fig. 6. Layout mobile application eHealthCare

4 Conclusion

This paper introduces a new tool that will allow institutions that provide assistance in medication to perform a better monitoring of their users as well as user's medication and to optimize some processes related to the preparation of medication. Through rigorous control, this tool allows caregivers/institutions a more agile mechanism to identify possible errors (non-adherence) in the consumption of medicines, contributing to increase the quality of life of its users. In the context of a pandemic, such as the current COVID-19 pandemic, the importance of such tools is even greater, because despite all measures of social estrangement, this solution may be something viable, since it allows support to users by greatly reducing social contacts.

However, the fact that the NB-IoT network is not yet supported in all regions, despite the existing mechanisms presented in the Sect. 3 to mitigate this issue, it may constitute a major disadvantage for the solution, since, although the data are collected and processed in it, this treatment presents a small delay (collection time) which in certain diseases can be a critical problem.

Although it is possible to clearly control the presence/absence of medication of the organizer, this solution, and unfortunately none of the reported in the Sect. 2, ensures that the medication is effectively ingested. The medicine may be removed from the correct division, but the user may not ingest it, a situation that it's very frequently in patients with medical disorders such as Alzheimer, dementia, schizophrenia, etc.

Finally, it should also be noted that, although the entire implementation cycle has already been tested and validated, that is to say, the sending of data from the organizers to the web platform, it has not yet been possible to carry out studies with the population, since the existing specimen is only for testing (it contains all wires and sensors completely disorganized). The production costs of this tool in the current state of the project, it is not yet possible to advance with an exact value, however, given the simplified architecture, it is estimated that the value is relatively low compared to similar approaches illustrated in Sect. 2.

Thus, at this moment, the current state of the work is dependent on the elaboration of 2/3 prototypes of the organizers presented to distribute among the small group of population, and then perform tests to understand the degree of success of the solution presented.

4.1 Future Work

Despite the great potential presented, this solution still has a long way to go. In this way, the following points were left for future work:

- Devise a solution to identify errors in the medication intake in the percentage of users who do not use the medication organizer.
- Conduct a study to quantify the impact of the detection of errors in medication intake with the use of eHealthCare.
- Append the medication stock replenishment detection process.
- Optimize methods to detect user's non-adherence.
- Consider/Use other machine learning algorithms and check their effect on the intelligent system of the eHealthCare solution.

References

1. Midão, L., Giardini, A., Menditto, E., Kardas, P., Costa, E.: Adherence to Medication in Older Adults as a Way to Improve Health Outcomes and Reduce Healthcare System Spending (2020). https://www.intechopen.com/books/gerontology/adherence-to-medication-in-older-adults-as-a-way-to-improve-health-outcomes-and-reduce-healthcare-sy. Accessed 27 Dec 2020
2. Yap, A.F., Thirumoorthy, T., Kwan, Y.H.: Medication adherence in the elderly. J. Clin. Gerontol. Geriatr. **7**(2), 64–67 (2016)
3. Jaul, E., Barron, J.: Age-related diseases and clinical and public health implications for the 85 years old and over population. Front. Public Health **5**(335) (2017)

4. Jin, H., Kim, Y., Rhie, S.J.: Factors affecting medication adherence in elderly people. Patient Preference Adherence **10**, 2117–2125 (2016)
5. Wick, J.Y.: RPh, MBA, and FASCP. Adherence Issues in Elderly Patients (2021). https://www.pharmacytimes.com/publications/issue/2011/January2011/RxFocus-0111. Accessed 27 July 2021
6. 8 reasons patients don't take their medications (2021). https://www.ama-assn.org/delivering-care/patient-support-advocacy/8-reasons-patients-dont-take-their-medications. Accessed 27 July 2021
7. Emsley, R.: Non-adherence and its consequences: understanding the nature of relapse. World Psychiatry Official J. World Psychiatric Assoc. (WPA) **12**, 234 (2013)
8. EClinicalMedicine. COVID-19 and older adults: more support is needed (2020). www.thelancet.com/journals/eclinm/article/PIIS2589-5370(20)30276--5/fulltext. Accessed 27 Dec 2020
9. Cugmas, M., Ferligoj, A., Kogovšek, T., Batagelj, Z.: The social support networks of elderly people in Slovenia during the Covid-19 pandemic. PLOS ONE **16**(3), 1–16 (2021)
10. Falvo, I., Zufferey, M.C., Albanese, E., Fadda, M.: Lived experiences of older adults during the first Covid-19 lockdown: a qualitative study. PLOS ONE **16**(6), 1–18 (2021)
11. Townsend, L., Wallace, C., Fairhurst, G.: Stuck out here': the critical role of broadband for remote rural places. Scott. Geogr. J. **131**(3–4), 171–180 (2015)
12. 6 of the Best Reminders for Your Medications. Brian Krans (2020). https://www.healthline.com/health/best-medication-reminders. Accessed 29 Dec 2020
13. TabTime. TabTime Super 8 - Pill Box (2020). https://tabtime.com/collections/all/products/tabtime-super-8-vat-free. Accessed 29 Dec 2020
14. epill. TimeCap Bottle Last Opened Time Stamp with Reminder (2020). https://www.epill.com/timecap.html. Accessed 29 Dec 2020
15. pillpack. Your medication, sorted and delivered (2020). https://www.pillpack.com/. Accessed 29 Dec 2020
16. medminder. The MedMinder Medication Dispenser (2020). https://www.medminder.com/. Accessed 29 Dec 2020
17. medisafe. Digitally-integrated ecosystem provides complete support (2020). https://www.medisafe.com/. Accessed 29 Dec 2020
18. carezone. Manage your health, without the headache (2020). https://carezone.com/. Accessed 29 Dec 2020
19. Pirhonen, J., Lolich, L., Tuominen, K., Jolanki, O., Timonen, V.: "These devices have not been made for older people's needs" - older adults' perceptions of digital technologies in Finland and Ireland. Technol. Soc. **62**, 101287 (2020)
20. Renstrom, J.: Why Older People Really Eschew Technology (2020). https://slate.com/technology/2020/07/seniors-technology-illiteracy-misconception-pandemic.html. Accessed 29 Dec 2020
21. Arduino MKR NB 1500. https://dev.telstra.com/iot-marketplace/arduino-mkr-nb-1500. Accessed 05 June 2021
22. MKR family. https://store.arduino.cc/arduino/mkr-family. Accessed 05 June 2021
23. Force Sensing Resistor (FSR) with Arduino Tutorial. Makerguides.com (2020). https://www.makerguides.com/fsr-arduino-tutorial/. Accessed 29 Dec 2020
24. Camelo, D.M.A., Santos, J.C.C., Martins, M.P.G., Gouveia, P.D.F.: Modelling academic dropout in computer engineering using artificial neural networks. In: Rocha, Á., Adeli, H., Dzemyda, G., Moreira, F., Ramalho Correia, A.M. (eds.)

WorldCIST 2021. AISC, vol. 1366, pp. 141–150. Springer, Cham (2021). https://doi.org/10.1007/978-3-030-72651-5_14
25. Pacifico, L., Macario, V., Oliveira, J.: Plant classification using artificial neural networks, pp. 1–6 (2018)
26. Géron, A.: Hands-On Machine Learning with Scikit-Learn, Keras, and TensorFlow: Concepts, Tools, and Techniques to Build Intelligent Systems. O'Reilly Media (2019)
27. K-nearest neighbors algorithm in python and scikit-learn. https://stackabuse.com/k-nearest-neighbors-algorithm-in-python-and-scikit-learn. Accessed 24 July 2021
28. K nearest neighbor algorithm in python. https://towardsdatascience.com/k-nearest-neighbor-python-2fccc47d2a55. Accessed 24 July 2021
29. Tutorial: K nearest neighbors in python. https://www.dataquest.io/blog/k-nearest-neighbors-in-python/. Accessed 24 July 2021
30. A quick introduction to KNN algorithm. https://www.mygreatlearning.com/blog/knn-algorithm-introduction/. Accessed 24 July 2021
31. Nearest neighbors. https://scikit-learn.org/stable/modules/neighbors.html. Accessed 24 July 2021
32. Why data normalization is necessary for machine learning models. https://medium.com/@urvashilluniya/why-data-normalization-is-necessary-for-machine-learning-models-681b65a05029. Accessed 24 July 2021
33. Understand data normalization in machine learning. https://towardsdatascience.com/understand-data-normalization-in-machine-learning-8ff3062101f0. Accessed 24 July 2021
34. Ruiz-Martínez, I., Esparcia, J.: Internet access in rural areas: brake or stimulus as post-covid-19 opportunity? Sustainability **12**(22) (2020)
35. GSA. Narrow band IoT & M2M - global narrowband IoT - LTE-M networks, March 2019. https://gsacom.com/paper/global-narrowband-iot-lte-m-networks-march-2019/. Accessed 01 Mar 2021
36. GSMA. Mobile IoT deployment map. https://www.gsma.com/iot/deployment-map/. Accessed 01 Mar 2021
37. GSMA. Security Features of LTE-M and NB-IoT Networks (2019). https://www.gsma.com/iot/wp-content/uploads/2019/09/Security-Features-of-LTE-M-and-NB-IoT-Networks.pdf. Accessed 07 Mar 2021

The Case for Symptom-Specific Neurological Digital Biomarkers

John Michael Templeton[1](✉), Christian Poellabauer[2], and Sandra Schneider[1]

[1] University of Notre Dame, Notre Dame, IN 46556, USA
{jtemplet,sschnei8}@nd.edu
[2] Florida International University, Miami, FL 33199, USA
cpoellab@fiu.edu

Abstract. Digital biomarkers provide novel and objective assessment of neurodegenerative diseases, such as Parkinson's Disease (PD). This paper demonstrates that objective digital biomarkers, obtained from mobile-based functional assessments, can be used for symptom-specific insights on neurological deficiencies. These digital biomarkers were found to be sensitive to change in relation to structured physical interventions. In this pilot study, 54 participants (n = 36 PD; n = 18 control) completed 13 neurocognitive functional tasks with 115 digital biomarkers being identified and compared between groups for objective assessment, evaluation, and monitoring of disease progression. 36 (31.30%) of these biomarkers were significant ($p < 0.10$) between groups. Of the 36 significant biomarkers, 10 were motor, 6 were memory, 1 was speech, 6 were executive function, and 13 were multi-functional. 8 biomarkers were significant ($p < 0.10$) between groups regardless of intervention, which may indicate strong biomarkers to assess PD. Further, 15 (13.04%) digital biomarkers showed significance ($p < 0.10$) in relation to structured physical intervention. Overall, mobile-based digital biomarkers provide promising measures and sensitivity to functional change that can be used in assessment and monitoring of Parkinson's Disease. Further integration of mobile device capabilities can enhance the understanding of how neurodegenerative diseases present and aid clinicians in the diagnosis and monitoring of conditions.

Keywords: Digital biomarkers · Neurocognitive assessment · Mobile app · Parkinson's disease

1 Introduction

Mobile devices are becoming increasingly prevalent in the area of neurocognitive assessments as their capabilities allow for the collection of more objective information than is currently achievable using pen-and-paper style tests (e.g., the Montreal Cognitive Assessment (MoCA) [1] or Mini Mental State Examination

X. Gao et al. (Eds.): MobiHealth 2021, LNICST 440, pp. 235–255, 2022.
https://doi.org/10.1007/978-3-031-06368-8_16

(MMSE) [2]) [3,4]. These pen-and-paper assessment instruments are administered by clinicians to 'score' neurological and cognitive functional tasks (e.g., motor, speech, memory, and executive function). These tasks are often difficult for individuals with neurodegenerative conditions including Parkinson's Disease (PD) [5–9]. This paper focuses on individuals with Parkinson's Disease as they demonstrate impaired functionality in both motor and cognitive areas [10].

The transition to mobile-based versions of neurocognitive assessments has become increasingly popular within the healthcare sector for the administration of functional tasks, objective scoring, and the interpretation of symptoms relating to neurological health or illness [11]. This transition also allows for the collection of additional unique digital biomarkers for specific functional tasks of interest (e.g., a Trail Making Task), and allows for the creation of multi-functional assessments with more expansive digital biomarker sets [12,13]. As Parkinson's Disease is often described as a "designer disease", meaning no two diagnosed individuals manifest the exact same symptoms, personalized medicine should be the goal and is required to optimize care and individuals' quality of life [14,15]. However, to reach personalized medicine for individuals with PD (e.g., the formation of individualized intervention protocols in an evidence-based manner), clinicians need further knowledge on specific patient characteristics to develop personalized rehabilitation programs [16].

The objective of this pilot study was to demonstrate that objective digital biomarkers, collected from mobile-based functional assessments, can be used to provide symptom-specific insights on neurological deficiencies of individuals with PD. Further, this work was to demonstrate that these digital biomarkers are sensitive to functional change in relation to structured physical interventions. This was completed by comparing subjects with Parkinson's Disease to age-matched controls across 13 mobile-based neurocognitive functional tasks, in addition to monitoring digital biomarkers for the PD group in relation to structured physical interventions.

2 Related Work

Neurodegenerative diseases, such as PD, present with progressive degeneration which can involve both movement disorders and neurological and/or cognitive deficits [17]. Neurocognitive assessments that evaluate this degeneration consist of functional tasks involving motor, speech, memory, and executive functions [7–9]. Previous works have identified sensor-based digital assessments (e.g., accelerometry based gait assessments or speech recognition systems for healthcare) which provide promising applications and user-device interactions for the collection of objective digital biomarkers across functional areas of neurocognition [5,13,18–22]. This pilot study further assesses mobile device capabilities by implementing mobile-based neurocognitive tasks that use device sensors to objectively collect information (e.g., digital biomarkers) that will provide clinicians with symptom-specific information that can assist with diagnosis, monitoring, and rehabilitation of individuals with PD [5,13].

2.1 Functional Assessments

Currently the assessment and monitoring of individuals with PD is primarily based on a set of clinical criteria from functional assessments, as physical biomarkers alone (e.g., blood based) are not able to reliably confirm the presence of the disease [23]. Mobile-based neurocognitive assessments have the capability and promise to expand functional assessments to allow for objective scoring, the interpretation of results relating to the initial diagnosis, and monitoring of disease progression [6,24]. Inherent device sensors (e.g., accelerometers, gyroscopes, cameras, microphones, and timers), along with human device interactions, can enhance the monitoring of neurocognitive functions (e.g., motor, memory, speech, and executive function) for individuals with neurodegenerative conditions such as PD [13,18,20,21,25]. The transition of these assessments to mobile devices also allows for standardized administration which is unaffected by examiner bias [26].

2.2 Physical Interventions

Currently there are both pharmacological and physical therapeutic interventions available for individuals diagnosed with PD. Previous work suggests that physical activity during the critical window of early- and mid-stage of the disease is vital to the management of PD symptoms and disease progression [27,28]. These activities encompass both routine activities of daily living (ADLs) (e.g., household activity, walking) and dedicated exercise (e.g., aerobics, strength training) [29]. Further, supervised and structured exercise is noted to be effective at improving functional performance outcomes (e.g., balance and functional ambulation) in individuals with PD [30,31]. However, many studies evaluate physical interventions as a one-size-fits-all concept as current evidence is not sufficient to develop personalized rehabilitation programs [16]. To gain further insights for intended personalized rehabilitation programs, it is imperative to administer precise and objective assessments providing symptom-specific information on physical rehabilitative efforts and for the understanding of various intervention approaches [32].

3 Methodology

Fifty four adults between the ages of 52 and 84 were divided into two groups-those with a confirmed diagnosis of Parkinson's Disease and age-matched healthy controls participated in this pilot study. Of those, the PD population included 36 individuals; with slightly less than half of the population being female (n = 17 or 47.22%). The age-matched control population included 18 individuals; more than half (n = 10 or 55.56%) being female. Participants were recruited through advertisements, physician and clinician referrals, spouses or caretakers of the diagnosed population, and prior studies from our laboratory. The inclusion criteria for this study consisted of being age 50 years or older. As the mean onset age for PD in the Western world is early-to-mid 60s [33], recruitment efforts for this pilot study were limited to diagnosed individuals age 50 years or older and appropriate age-matched controls. Participants were excluded from the current study if they were unable to provide informed consent or if their native language was not English (as all tasks were formatted in English).

3.1 Mobile Application Testing

All participants were administered a tablet-based neurocognitive assessment designed for individuals with Parkinson's Disease that focused on user-device interactions for the collection of objective measures [34]. Each participant completed mobile versions of 13 neurocognitive functional tasks across the areas of motor, memory, speech, and executive function. Functional tasks included single functional tasks (e.g., having focus on only one area of neurocognition; motor or memory) and multi-functional tasks (e.g., combining two or more single functional tasks into a functional task). The 13 administered neurocognitive tasks collected 74 objective mobile-based digital biomarkers for all participants. All task descriptions are listed below. For a fine-motor tracing task the individual was instructed to use their index finger to trace a depicted shape. For a gross-motor task the user was instructed to manipulate the mobile device to "air"-trace a depicted shape. For reflex tasks, the user was to tap on the screen to interact with a set of targets. For a memory task the user was to tap on depicted cards, in pairs, until all cards have been matched. For a trail making task the user was instructed to draw a line using their index finger connecting all shapes in increasing numerical order. For a set of speech based tasks, the user was prompted to read a sentence out loud or name prompted objects. Examples of multi-functional tasks include both fine (e.g., tracing an object) and gross (e.g., manipulating the mobile device) motor tasks paired with either an automatic (e.g., listing the months of the year in order from January to December) or non-automatic speech task (e.g., listing the months of the year, aloud, in reverse order; December to January). For an executive function/multi-functional task a digital version of the Stroop Word Color Test (SWCT) [35] was utilized where the user was required to discern the difference between prompted colors and words and then speak the correct response. For an expanded multi-functional task approach (e.g., Narration Writer), the user was instructed to narrate a sentence while also writing the sentence word by word (e.g., writing the same word being said aloud) in the space provided.

A subset of both PD and age-matched control populations ($n = 12$ and $n = 8$ respectively) were given an updated version of this neurocognitive assessment containing an expanded set of objective digital biomarkers ($n = 115$). All digital biomarkers collected in this expanded set made use of additional inherent device capabilities (e.g., device timers between instances of screen interactions, speech recognizers/dictionaries, and user interactions with relative positions on the device screen). This expanded digital biomarker set was implemented to give further monitoring of neurological and cognitive deficits.

3.2 Physical Interventions

All individuals with PD participated regularly (e.g., at least twice a week) in structured rehabilitation/intervention programs designed for PD. The supervised physical intervention activities included, but were not limited to, non-contact boxing, functional strength, yoga, dancing, and cycling. Each intervention training session lasted between 45 and 60 min and consisted of guided warm-up, main, and cool-down activities. All sessions were led by certified personal trainers. Individuals were given a mobile device assessment, consisting of the functional tasks discussed above, both prior to and directly after these supervised physical intervention programs. This testing protocol was included to see if the collected mobile-based digital biomarkers showed sensitivity to functional changes seen as a direct response to the intervention programs. In addition, the participants were required to take the functional assessment twice within a period of 2 h. Therefore, the tasks included in this assessment were internally randomized to avoid the test-retest phenomena (e.g., for a memory task, the location of matching card pairs; or in the Stroop Word Color Test, the order of colors and word combinations).

3.3 Statistical Analysis

All collected digital biomarker scores were compared for individuals with PD prior to a structured physical intervention (e.g., 'Before'), following a structured physical intervention (e.g., 'After'), and healthy age-matched controls (e.g., 'Control') using statistical methods (e.g., ANOVA and post hoc t-tests).

4 Results

4.1 Mobile Application Testing

The results from this work are discussed in two parts- Symptom-Specific Digital Biomarkers (i.e., to demonstrate that objective digital biomarkers can be used to provide symptom-specific insights on neurological deficiencies of individuals with PD), and Digital Biomarker Sensitivity (i.e., to demonstrate that these digital biomarkers are sensitive to functional change in relation to structured physical interventions).

The average scores for each digital biomarker for individuals with PD prior to a structured physical intervention (e.g., 'Before'), following a structured physical intervention (e.g., 'After'), and healthy age-matched controls (e.g., 'Control') are shown in supplemental Tables 5, 6, 7, 8 and 9 (Sect. A). The significance between groups for all digital biomarker scores ($p < 0.05$) is denoted by the following symbols: diagnosed PD populations prior to a physical intervention versus age-matched controls ($*$), diagnosed PD populations following a physical intervention versus age-matched controls (†), and diagnosed PD populations prior to a structured physical intervention versus directly following physical intervention (‡).

4.2 Symptom-Specific Digital Biomarkers

74 device-calculated, objective digital biomarkers were collected from all individuals (36 PD and 18 Control). Of the 74 digital biomarkers, 28 were collected from single functional tasks and the remaining 46 were collected from multi-functional tasks. Assessment results are seen in Table 1, Fig. 1, and supplemental Tables 5, 6 (Sect. A).

Table 1. Significant digital biomarker summary ($n = 74$ digital biomarkers).

Digital Biomarkers	Before/Control(∗)	After/Control(†)	Before/After(‡)
Significant Digital Biomarkers ($p < 0.05$)	17 (22.97%)	7 (9.46%)	7 (9.46%)
Single Functional Task	8 (10.81%)	4 (5.41%)	2 (2.70%)
Motor	*7 (9.46%)*	*4 (5.41%)*	*2 (2.70%)*
Memory	*1 (1.35%)*	*0 (-)*	*0 (-)*
Speech	*0 (-)*	*0 (-)*	*0 (-)*
Multi-Functional Task	9 (12.16%)	3 (4.05%)	5 (6.76%)
Executive Funciton	*5 (5.41%)*	*2 (2.70%)*	*3 (4.05%)*

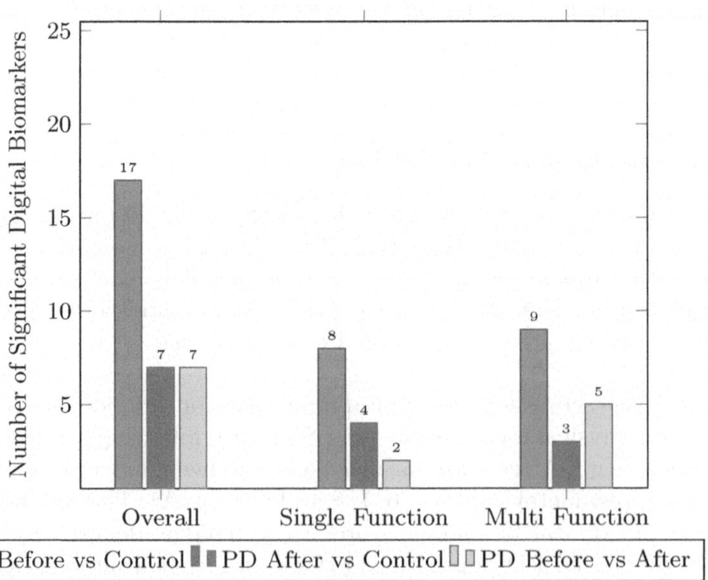

Fig. 1. Preliminary Assessment's Significant Digital Biomarkers. ($n = 74$) for the Total Number of Collected Biomarkers in the Preliminary Assessment.

Table 1 and Fig. 1 give a summary of the number of significant digital biomarkers between groups ($p < 0.05$) across task type (e.g., single or multi-functional tasks) and symptoms (e.g., motor or memory). Of the 74 collected digital biomarkers, 17 or 22.97% were significant ($p < 0.05$) when comparing individuals with PD prior to physical interventions, and age-matched controls.

A representative subset of the overall population (e.g., $n = 20$ individuals; $n = 12$ PD and $n = 8$ Control) interacted with an expanded version of the digital biomarker assessment. Of the 115 device-calculated, objective digital biomarkers, 41 were collected from single functional tasks and the remaining 74 were collected from multi-functional tasks. The expanded digital biomarker set results are seen in Table 2, Fig. 2, and supplemental Tables 7, 8 and 9 (Sect. A).

Table 2 and Fig. 2 give a summary of the number of significant digital biomarkers between groups ($p < 0.05$), across task types (e.g., single or multi-functional tasks) and symptoms (e.g., motor or memory) for the expanded digital biomarker assessment. Of the 115 digital biomarkers from the expanded set assessment, 20 were significant ($p < 0.05$) when comparing individuals with PD prior to physical interventions, and age-matched controls.

Table 2. Significant digital biomarker summary ($p < 0.05$) ($n = 115$ digital biomarkers).

Digital Biomarkers	Before/Control∗)	After/Control(†)	Before/After(‡)
Significant Digital Biomarkers ($p < 0.05$)	20 (17.39%)	15 (13.04%)	8 (6.96%)
Single Functional Task	10 (8.70%)	9 (7.83%)	2 (1.73%)
Motor	*7 (6.09%)*	*4 (3.48%)*	*2 (1.74%)*
Memory	*3 (2.61%)*	*4 (3.48%)*	*0 (-)*
Speech	*0 (-)*	*1 (0.87%)*	*0 (-)*
Multi-Functional Task	10 (8.70%)	6 (5.22%)	6 (5.22%)
Executive Function	*5 (4.35%)*	*2 (1.74%)*	*4 (3.48%)*

Given the sample size of this pilot study, the definition of significant digital biomarkers was expanded to $p < 0.10$. Increasing the p-value to $p < 0.10$ allows for a better understanding of PD given the nature of the condition; as individuals with PD do not always manifest the same symptoms [14]. Digital biomarkers with a p-value of less than $p < 0.10$ indicate functional biometrics that should be included in future functional assessments with a larger sample size as they have a higher likelihood of being significant within a p-value of $p < 0.05$. Table 3 and Fig. 3 depicts the number of significant digital biomarkers ($p < 0.10$) needed for inclusion in mobile-based neurocognitive assessments containing the aforementioned tasks. Out of 115 collected digital biomarkers in the expanded test set, 36 digital biomarkers (31.30%) were significant ($p < 0.10$). A breakdown of single and multi-functional tasks is also seen in Table 3 and Fig. 3. Of the 41 collected single functional task digital biomarkers, 17 (41.46%) were significant ($p < 0.10$) between individuals with PD and control groups. However, only 19

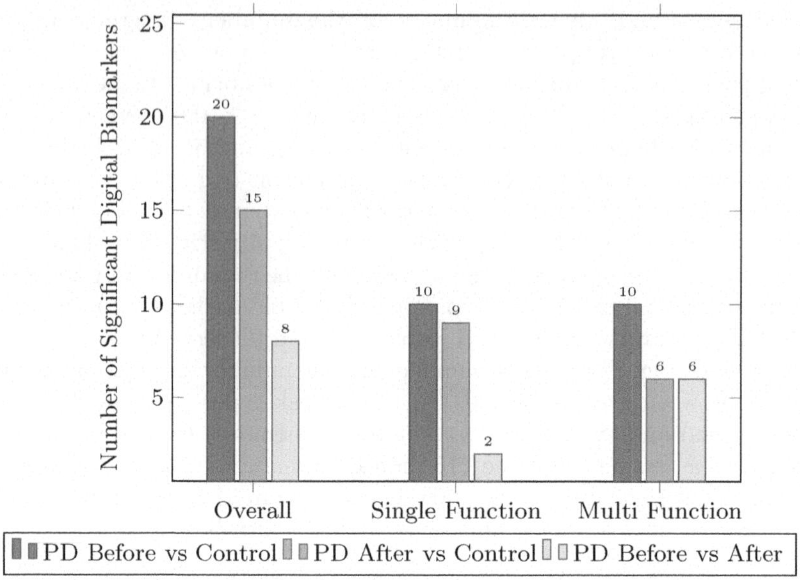

Fig. 2. Expanded Assessment's Significant Digital Biomarkers. ($n = 115$) for the Total Number of Collected Biomarkers in the Expanded Assessment.

of 74 (25.68%) digital biomarkers from multi-functional tasks were significant ($p < 0.10$) between groups.

For a more in depth understanding of how individuals with PD exhibit different neurocognitive functions of interest in a symptom-specific manner, a breakdown of the digital biomarkers by functional area was included in Fig. 4. A total of 36 (31.30%) mobile-based digital biomarkers were significant ($p < 0.10$) when comparing individuals with PD (e.g., before or after physical intervention) to age-matched controls. Further, Fig. 4 shows the number of collected digital biomarkers and the number of significant digital biomarkers ($p < 0.10$) for the categories of motor, memory, speech, executive function, and multi-functional tasks. The multi-functional task category includes all tasks that involve two or more areas of neurocognition in a single task. It should be noted that all executive function tasks are inherently multi-functional in nature (e.g., an individual needs to move or speak to carry out the executive function) and therefore are a subset of the multi-functional task digital biomarker set (e.g., denoted by an * in Fig. 4). Of the single functional tasks, 10 of 26 (38.46%) motor digital biomarkers, 6 of 10 (60.00%) memory digital biomarkers, and 1 of 5 speech digital biomarkers (20.00%) were significant ($p < 0.10$). 19 multi-functional digital biomarkers were also significant ($p < 0.10$); with 6 executive function digital biomarkers being included in this group. Lastly, all remaining significant multi-functional digital biomarkers (13; 17.57%) relate to both speech and motor function as the main components of the configured tasks (e.g., completing a motor task paired with an automatic or non-automatic speech task).

Table 3. Significant digital biomarker summary ($p < 0.10$) ($n = 115$ digital biomarkers).

Digital Biomarkers	Before/Control(∗)	After/Control(†)	Before/After(‡)
Significant Digital Biomarkers ($p < 0.10$)	30 (26.09%)	21 (18.26%)	15 (13.04%)
Single Functional Task	16 (13.91%)	12 (10.43%)	4 (3.48%)
Motor	*10 (8.70%)*	*7 (6.10%)*	*4 (3.48%)*
Memory	*6 (5.22%)*	*4 (3.48%)*	*0 (-)*
Speech	*0 (-)*	*1 (0.87%)*	*0 (-)*
Multi-Functional Task	14 (12.17%)	9 (7.83%)	11 (9.57%)
Executive Function	*5 (4.35%)*	*4 (3.48%)*	*6 (5.22%)*

4.3 Digital Biomarker Sensitivity

Of the 74 device-calculated, objective digital biomarkers collected from all individuals ($n = 36$ PD; $n = 18$ Control) 7 digital biomarkers were significant ($p < 0.05$) between individuals with PD following a physical intervention compared to controls (Table 1 and Fig. 1). 7 digital biomarkers were also significant ($p < 0.05$) when comparing those individuals with PD before and after physical intervention.

Of the 115 device-calculated digital biomarkers in the expanded set for a representative subset of the overall population (e.g., $n = 20$ individuals; $n = 12$ PD and $n = 8$ Control), 15 digital biomarkers were significant ($p < 0.05$) between individuals with PD following a physical intervention compared to controls (Table 2 and Fig. 2). Further, 8 digital biomarkers were significant ($p < 0.05$) when comparing individuals with PD before and after physical intervention in the expanded set. Given the expanded definition of significant digital biomarkers ($p < 0.10$), 21 digital biomarkers were significant between individuals with PD following a physical intervention compared to controls (Table 3 and Fig. 3). Finally, 15 digital biomarkers were significant ($p < 0.10$) when comparing those with PD before and after physical intervention in the expanded set.

5 Discussion

This pilot study implemented an assessment tool specifically designed for individuals with Parkinson's Disease that focused on tablet-based user-device interactions for the collection of function-specific digital biomarkers [34]. Mobile-based neurocognitive assessments allow for objective scoring of novel and relevant digital biomarkers with the use of device sensors and human device interactions to provide insights on neurological deficiencies specific to individuals with PD [13,24]. Following acquisition and analysis, objective digital biomarkers were found to provide symptom-specific insights on neurological deficiencies of individuals with PD. Further, these digital biomarkers were found to be sensitive to functional change in relation to structured physical interventions for individuals with PD. A task-specific list of these metrics is depicted in Table 4 which gives rise to symptom-specific digital biomarkers. Of the 36 digital biomarkers that were significant ($p < 0.10$), 10 were motor, 6 were memory, 1 was speech, 6 were executive function, and 13 involved multi-functional tasks. Additionally, 8 of the 36 digital biomarkers were found to be significant regardless of intervention which may indicate strong biomarkers for PD. These 8 digital biomarkers are denoted by (∗) in Table 4. The 36 significant digital biomarkers ($p < 0.10$) are listed in Table 4. Each of these biomarkers were found to be important in the configuration of mobile-based neurocognitive assessments as they provide insights regardless of physical intervention when comparing outcomes of PD populations to age-matched controls.

Future work should involve analyzing digital biomarkers across larger populations (e.g., PD populations in different stages of disease progression and other populations with other neurodegenerative diseases) and across the different stages of diagnoses. The analysis of different neurodegenerative diseases (e.g., Alzheimer's Disease, dementia) and their stages would help in extracting significant disease-specific digital biomarkers and aid in the prediction and monitoring of these various conditions over time. Additionally, a larger sample size would allow for adjusted statistical analyses and confidence intervals. Next, further exploration and expansion of all digital biomarkers, but particularly single functional digital biomarkers (e.g., memory and speech) should occur. Although individuals with PD exhibit difficulty in performing multi-functional tasks [36], single functional task digital biomarkers are still highly necessary in the understanding of how PD symptoms manifest. Similarly, while Parkinson's Disease is a progressive neurodegenerative disease primarily characterized by the hallmarks of motor symptoms (e.g., akinesia, rigidity, and tremor) [9,37] memory task digital biomarkers were shown to be important in the understanding of Parkinson's Disease with 60% of collected memory metrics being significant. The number of single functional memory and speech based digital biomarkers should also be increased for a more even distribution across all neurocognitive functions of interest. This expansion should include digital biomarkers collected using different device sensors (e.g., speech frequency, amplitude, timing using audio samples; or gait, using accelerometers, gyroscopes, and/or device cameras) or comprehensive systems (e.g., IoT or wearable devices).

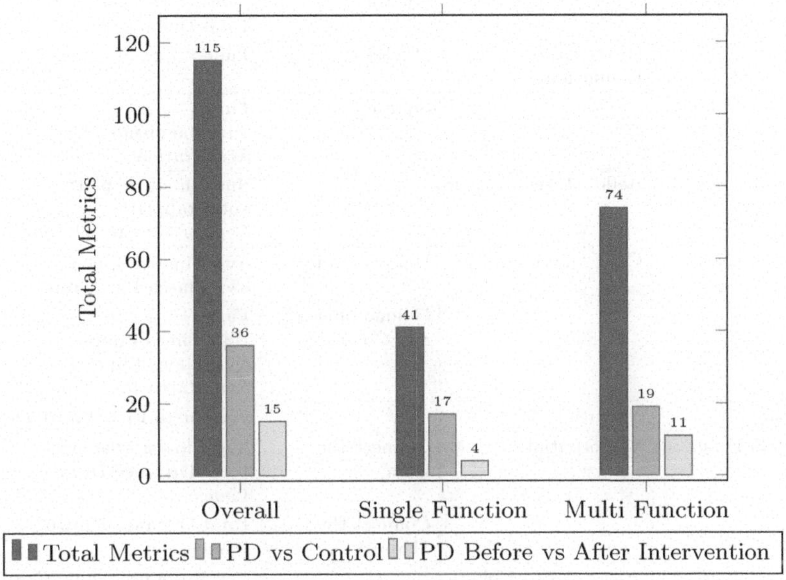

Fig. 3. Metrics Needed in Mobile-based Neurocognitive Assessments for Individuals with PD.

This study found that the number of significant digital biomarkers of the PD group following structured physical interventions decreased compared to the age-matched control group. Future work should include an investigation on how different activities (e.g., non-contact boxing, functional strength, yoga, dancing, and cycling) affect neurocognitive functions of interest through the collection of objective digital biomarker sets with relation to each activity [16,29]. Future work should also explore the extent to which these digital biomarkers are affected by different intervention types, across different stages, and populations. The knowledge gained through the use of objective and comprehensive digital assessments would aid clinicians and healthcare workers in the formation of specific recommendations for personalized therapeutic programs based on the

Table 4. Significant Digital Biomarkers ($p < 0.10$) by Task and Category

Category	Task		Digital Biomarker
Motor	Fine Motor Tracing	Circle	Average Distance Total Distance*
		Square	Average Distance Total Distance
	Gross Motor Emulation	Circle	Time
		Square	Time Min Magnitude of Acceleration
	Reflex Target Tapping		Num small tapped* Total tapped* Avg. prompt to hit time
Memory	Card Matching	Unique Shapes	Avg Times Flipped Avg Match Pair Time*
		Unique Shapes and Colors	Time Max Times Flipped Avg Times Flipped Avg Match Pair Time
Speech	Narration		Prompt to First Word Time
Executive Function	Visuospatial	Connect the Dots	Avg Closest Distance* Total Distance Drawn Time
		Connect the Shapes	Total Distance Drawn* Time
	Stroop Word Color		Avg Response Time (Correct)
Multi-Functional	Fine Motor Tracing (speech)	Circle	Writing Time Avg Distance Total Distance *Outline Crossings* Num of Additional Words Max Time Between Words Speaking Time
		Square	Writing Time Outline Crossings
	Gross Motor Emulation (Speech)	Circle	Num of Additional Words
		Square	Max Mag of Acceleration* Min Mag of Acceleration Num of Additional Words

functional deficits of each diagnosed individual [32]. Additionally, the inclusion of individuals with PD who do not interact with physical interventions should be completed to gain further insights on PD in addition to demonstrating quantifiable benefits of structured physical interventions. Finally, the expansion of these functional assessments for other neurodegenerative diseases (e.g., Alzheimer's disease, ALS, or dementia) should be completed.

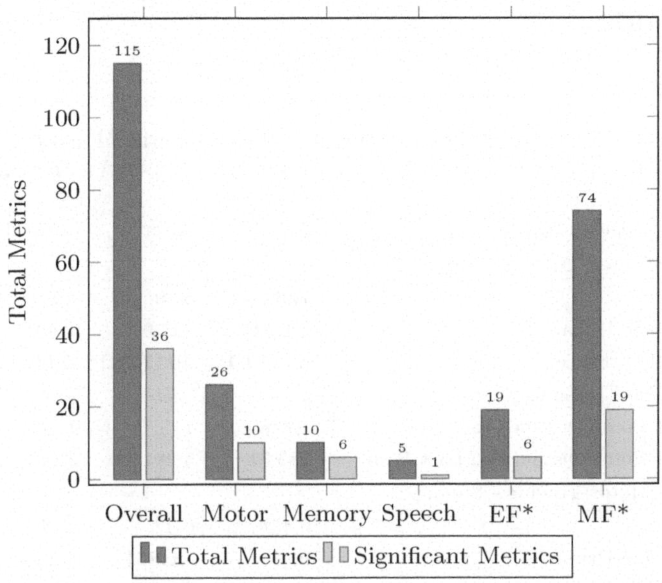

Fig. 4. Number of Significant Metrics ($p < 0.10$) by Neurocognitive Function Category.

6 Conclusions

Mobile-based digital biomarkers provide promising measures that can be useful in the diagnostic and monitoring processes that currently rely on subjective clinical judgements and self-reported information. Further integration of these mobile capabilities for the collection of objective measures can enhance the understanding of how neurodegenerative diseases present, and provide necessary personalized diagnostic and monitoring information.

This pilot study gives both an understanding of digital biomarkers specific to Parkinson's Disease that should be included in mobile-based neurocognitive assessment systems while also yielding further updates to be considered when expanding data collection efforts. Collected digital biomarkers in this work were used to (1) demonstrate that objective digital biomarkers, collected from mobile-based functional assessments, can be used to provide symptom-specific insights on neurological deficiencies of individuals with PD and (2) demonstrate that these digital biomarkers are sensitive to functional change in relation to structured physical interventions for individuals with PD.

A Appendix

Table 5. List of collected digital biomarkers from single functional tasks ($n = 54; PD = 36; Control = 18$). (* = Sig. BvC) († = Sig. AvC) (‡ = Sig. BvA); ($p < 0.05$)

Digital Biomarker	Before	After	Control
Fine Motor Tracing - Circle			
Time	7.95	6.59	7.29
Average Distance	**14.21***	14.39	**9.45***
Total Distance	**5687.01***	**4957.74†**	**2867.15*†**
Outline Crossings	5.89	5.71	5.17
First Point Distance to Shape	109.89	118.71	96.11
First Point Distance to Last Point	285.31	309.14	240.27
Fine Motor Tracing - Square			
Time	6.45	6.42	5.84
Average Distance	9.98	**11.85†**	**7.24†**
Total Distance	5086.28	5186.20	3012.72
Outline Crossings	6.87	6.56	4.56
First Point Distance to Shape	19.98	22.48	7.47
First Point Distance to Last Point	121.52	169.83	66.06
Gross Motor Emulation - Circle			
Time	**7.02*‡**	**5.266‡**	**4.70***
Average Magnitude of Acceleration	1.01	1.01	1.00
Maximum Magnitude of Acceleration	1.22	1.24	1.20
Minimum Magnitude of Acceleration	0.82	0.81	0.79
Gross Motor Emulation - Square			
Time	**7.82*‡**	**5.92‡**	**4.97***
Average Magnitude of Acceleration	1.00	1.01	1.01
Maximum Magnitude of Acceleration	1.26	1.30	1.34
Minimum Magnitude of Acceleration	**0.79***	0.75	**0.68***
Reflex - Target Tapping			
Number of Small Tapped	**21.24***	**21.74†**	**34.83*†**
Number of Large Tapped	15.02	16.67	16.58
Number of Total Tapped	**36.26***	**38.41†**	**51.42*†**
Memory - Card Matching - Unique Colors & Shapes			
Time	**52.21***	45.75	**36.91***
Memory - Card Matching - Unique Shapes			
Time	53.34	45.97	36.95
Speech - Narration			
Time	4.48	4.30	4.81
Missed Words	2.00	0.50	0.50
Additional Words	0.50	0.167	0.00

Table 6. List of collected digital biomarkers from multi-functional tasks ($n = 54; PD = 36; Control = 18$). (* = Sig. BvC) († = Sig. AvC) (‡ = Sig. BvA); ($p < 0.05$)

Digital Biomarker	Before	After	Control
Fine Motor Tracing with Speech - Circle			
Writing Time	**13.42‡**	**9.71‡**	9.51
Average Distance	**11.97***	10.73	**6.56***
Total Distance	12939.79	8758.14	4857.14
Outline Crossings	9.12	8.79	11.00
First Point Distance to Shape	89.40	97.94	92.43
First Point Distance to Last Point	226.24	247.87	407.05
Number of Missing Months	1.50	0.00	0.25
Number of Additional Words	2.62	0.375	0.25
Speaking Time	14.643	10.87	9.19
Fine Motor Tracing with Speech - Square			
Writing Time	**10.08*‡**	**8.54‡**	**7.92***
Average Distance	10.87	10.54	7.13
Total Distance	9842.72	8272.29	5073.25
Outline Crossings	8.02	7.88	10.17
First Point Distance to Shape	8.41	23.60	5.90
First Point Distance to Last Point	208.91	174.42	297.80
Number of Missing Months	1.50	0.00	0.25
Number of Additional Words	2.62	0.375	0.25
Speaking Time	14.875	10.88	9.25
Gross Motor Emulation with Speech - Circle			
Movement Time	8.72	7.97	6.85
Average Magnitude of Acceleration	1.00	1.01	1.01
Maximum Magnitude of Acceleration	1.17	1.20	1.18
Minimum Magnitude of Acceleration	0.87	0.84	0.82
Number of Missing Months	0.50	0.25	0.00
Number of Additional Words	1.50	0.00	0.50
Speaking Time	14.82	11.56	11.73
Gross Motor Emulation with Speech - Square			
Movement Time	10.15	8.24	7.98
Average Magnitude of Acceleration	1.00	1.00	1.00
Maximum Magnitude of Acceleration	**1.17***	**1.20†**	**1.31*†**
Minimum Magnitude of Acceleration	**0.83***	0.81	**0.731***
Number of Missing Months	0.25	0.00	0.50
Number of Additional Words	0.75	0.00	0.75
Speaking Time	13.97	11.41	11.58
Visuospatial Task - Connect the Dots			
Average Closest Distance	**12.56***	**13.20†**	**9.66*†**
Total Distance Drawn	**394.52*‡**	**333.09‡**	**293.67***
Time	**15.43*‡**	**12.39‡**	**11.32***

(*continued*)

Table 6. (*continued*)

Digital Biomarker	Before	After	Control
Visuospatial Task - Connect the Shapes			
Average Closest Distance	12.26	12.02	11.90
Total Distance Drawn	**368.28***	**336.11†**	**252.58*†**
Time	**15.53*‡**	**13.07‡**	**10.84***
Stroop Word Color Task			
Total Generated	8.50	9.83	7.5
Total Correct	6.00	8.83	6.00
Object Naming			
Total Generated	14.5	14.83	14.33
Total Correct	12.83	13.16	14.00
Narration Writer			
Writing Time	31.872	29.66	26.81
Speaking Time	22.96	24.30	21.54
Missed Words	1.667	1.667	1
Additional Words	3.167	0.833	0.00

Table 7. Expanded list of collected digital biomarkers from single functional tasks ($n = 20; PD = 12; Control = 8$). (* = Sig. BvC) († = Sig. AvC) (‡ = Sig. BvA); ($p < 0.05$)

Digital Biomarker	Before	After	Control
Reflex - Target Tapping			
Number of Missed Targets	2.0	2.25	1.67
Average Miss Distance	140.55	65.72	99.12
Average Time between Prompt and Hit	0.74	**0.77†**	**0.58†**
Memory - Card Matching - Unique Colors & Shapes			
Maximum Flipped	4.00	**4.82†**	**3.25†**
Average Times Flipped	2.23	**2.53†**	**1.90†**
Average Time for Match Pair	1.29	**1.39†**	**1.07†**
Average Time of Non-Match Pair	1.49	1.43	1.49
Memory - Card Matching - Unique Shapes			
Maximum Flipped	4.55	4.91	3.63
Average Times Flipped	**2.46***	2.59	**1.98***
Average Time for Match Pair	**1.38***	**1.30†**	**1.06*†**
Average Time of Non-Match Pair	1.51	1.43	1.28
Speech - Narration			
Time Between Prompt and First Word Spoken	2.58	**2.15†**	**3.14†**
Average Time Between Words	0.32	0.31	0.25

Table 8. Expanded list of collected digital biomarkers from multi-functional tasks ($n = 20; PD = 12; Control = 8$). (* = Sig. BvC) († = Sig. AvC) (‡ = Sig. BvA); ($p < 0.05$)

Digital Biomarker	Before	After	Control
Fine Motor Tracing with Speech - Circle			
Writing Time	**21.84‡**	**16.06‡**	16.08
Average Distance	**12.90***	10.98	**9.12***
Total Distance	**24402.72***	16995.06	**12778.22***
Outline Crossings	**20.00***	**14.46†**	**8.29*†**
First Point Distance to Shape	106.36	97.58	103.31
First Point Distance to Last Point	308.60	284.58	334.38
Number of Missing Months	3.73	3.27	4.43
Number of Additional Words	**2.82***	1.73	**0.43***
Start Time to First Word	5.41	4.64	3.53
Average Time Between Words	1.31	1.12	1.32
Maximum Time Between Words	4.24	**2.87†**	**7.55†**
Speaking Time	**21.30‡**	**14.83‡**	18.95
Fine Motor Tracing with Speech - Square			
Writing Time	22.58	18.60	15.17
Average Distance	13.62	9.30	9.09
Total Distance	22669.22	16074.48	12681.91
Outline Crossings	8.024	**15.27†**	**8.86†**
First Point Distance to Shape	20.25	38.67	7
First Point Distance to Last Point	312.38	235.26	209.48
Number of Missing Months	4.55	3.46	5.27
Number of Additional Words	2.55	1.82	0.57
Start Time to First Word	3.66	2.72	1.50
Average Time Between Words	1.91	2.76	1.79
Maximum Time Between Words	5.56	5.64	6.02
Speaking Time	21.13	19.23	18.90
Gross Motor Emulation with Speech - Circle			
Movement Time	14.87	13.62	15.65
Average Magnitude of Acceleration	1.01	1.01	1.00
Maximum Magnitude of Acceleration	1.14	1.20	1.15
Minimum Magnitude of Acceleration	0.88	0.83	0.85
Speaking Time	14.78	13.86	14.98
Number of Missing Months	1.75	0.75	0.00
Number of Additional Words	**2.25***	1.75	**0.67***
Average Time Between Words	1.20	0.96	1.02
Maximum Time Between Words	2.69	1.60	1.92

(continued)

Table 8. (*continued*)

Digital Biomarker	Before	After	Control
Gross Motor Emulation with Speech - Square			
Movement Time	21.26	16.60	15.63
Average Magnitude of Acceleration	1.01	1.01	1.01
Maximum Magnitude of Acceleration	1.24	1.26	1.36
Minimum Magnitude of Acceleration	0.79	0.78	0.75
Speaking Time	23.69	16.03	15.36
Number of Missing Months	1.00	0.75	0.33
Number of Additional Words	2.25	**2.75**†	**0.33**†
Average Time Between Words	1.62	1.08	1.10
Maximum Time Between Words	4.47	2.59	2.04

Table 9. Expanded list of collected digital biomarkers from multi-functional tasks continued ($n = 20; PD = 12; Control = 8$). (* = Sig. BvC)(† = Sig. AvC) (‡ = Sig. BvA); ($p < 0.05$)

Digital Biomarker	Before	After	Control
Visuospatial Task - Connect the Dots			
Number of Hits	9.83	9.00	9.00
Number of Misses	0.167	1.00	1.00
Average Time Between Correct Dots	0.96	0.51	0.43
Max Time Between Correct Dots	2.46	0.89	0.91
Visuospatial Task - Connect the Shapes			
Number of Hits	9.83	9.33	10.00
Number of Misses	0.17	0.67	0.00
Average Time Between Correct Shapes	0.88	0.71	0.50
Max Time Between Correct Shapes	2.73	1.27	1.58
Stroop Word Color Task			
Average Response Time - Correct	**2.57**‡	**2.20**‡	2.78
Average Response Time - Incorrect	3.23	3.29	1.29
Max Response Time	5.67	2.76	4.39
Object Naming			
Average Response Time - Correct	2.34	2.23	2.35
Narration Writer			
Total Number of Points	836.33	8.13.67	717.00
Total Number of Strokes	28.50	26.33	33.00
Average Stroke Time	0.66	0.70	0.40
Average Time Between Strokes	0.27	0.27	0.21
Time from Start to First Word	3.91	4.23	4.61
Average Time Between Words	3.59	2.96	3.05

References

1. Nasreddine, Z.S., et al.: The Montreal cognitive assessment, MoCA: a brief screening tool for mild cognitive impairment. J. Am. Geriatr. Soc. **53**, 695–699 (2005)
2. Tombaugh, T.N., McIntyre, N.J.: The mini-mental state examination: a comprehensive review. J. Am. Geriatr. Soc. **40**, 922–935 (1992)
3. Chen, K.B., Savage, A.B., Chourasia, A.O., Wiegmann, D.A., Sesto, M.E.: Touch screen performance by individuals with and without motor control disabilities. Appl. Ergon. **44**, 297–302 (2013)
4. Byrom, B., Wenzel, K., Pierce, J., Wenzel, K., Pierce, J.: Computerised clinical assessments: derived complex clinical endpoints from patient self-report data, pp. 179–202, May 2016
5. Goñi, M., Eickhoff, S., Sahandi Far, M., Patil, K., Dukart, J.: Limited diagnostic accuracy of smartphone-based digital biomarkers for Parkinson's disease in a remotely-administered setting
6. Vianello, A., Chittaro, L., Burigat, S., Budai, R.: MotorBrain: a mobile app for the assessment of users' motor performance in neurology. Comput. Methods Programs Biomed. **143**, 35–47 (2017)
7. Pettersson, A.F., Olsson, E., Wahlund, L.-O.: Motor function in subjects with mild cognitive impairment and early Alzheimer's disease. Dement. Geriatr. Cogn. Disord. **19**, 299–304 (2005)
8. Barbosa, A.F., et al.: Cognitive or cognitive-motor executive function tasks? Evaluating verbal fluency measures in people with Parkinson's disease. BioMed. Res. Int. **2017**, 7893975 (2017)
9. Yang, Y., Tang, B.S., Guo, J.F.: Parkinson's disease and cognitive impairment (2016)
10. Löfgren, N., Conradsson, D., Rennie, L., Moe-Nilssen, R., Franzén, E.: The effects of integrated single- and dual-task training on automaticity and attention allocation in Parkinson's disease: a secondary analysis from a randomized trial. Neuropsychology **33**, 147–156 (2019)
11. Bauer, R.M., Iverson, G.L., Cernich, A.N., Binder, L.M., Ruff, R.M., Naugle, R.I.: Computerized neuropsychological assessment devices: joint position paper of the American academy of clinical neuropsychology and the national academy of neuropsychology †
12. Fellows, R.P., Dahmen, J., Cook, D., Schmitter-Edgecombe, M.: Multicomponent analysis of a digital trail making test. Clin. Neuropsychol. **31**, 154–167 (2017)
13. Templeton, J.M., Poellabauer, C., Schneider, S.: Enhancement of neurocognitive assessments using smartphone capabilities: systematic review. JMIR mHealth uHealth **8**, e15517 (2020)
14. Blake-Krebs, B.: When Parkinson's Strikes Early: Voices, Choices, Resources and Treatment, 1st edn. HunterHouse (2001)
15. Ryu, J., Vero, J., Dobkin, R.D., Torres, E.B.: Dynamic digital biomarkers of motor and cognitive function in Parkinson's disease. J. Vis. Exp. **2019**, e59827 (2019)
16. Nonnekes, J., Nieuwboer, A.: Towards personalized rehabilitation for gait impairments in Parkinson's disease, January 2018
17. Zlokovic, B.V.: Neurovascular pathways to neurodegeneration in Alzheimer's disease and other disorders, December 2011
18. Yang, C.-C., Hsu, Y.-L., Yang, C.-C., Hsu, Y.-L.: A review of accelerometry-based wearable motion detectors for physical activity monitoring. Sensors **10**, 7772–7788 (2010)

19. Mathie, M.J., Coster, A.C.F., Lovell, N.H., Celler, B.G.: Accelerometry: providing an integrated, practical method for long-term, ambulatory monitoring of human movement. Physiol. Meas. **25**, 1–20 (2004)
20. Bhatia, M., Sood, S.K.: Temporal informative analysis in smart-ICU monitoring: M-healthcare perspective. J. Med. Syst. **40**, 1–15 (2016)
21. Vacher, M., Fleury, A., Portet, F., Serignat, J.-F., Noury, N.: Complete sound and speech recognition system for health smart homes: application to the recognition of activities of daily living. Technical report (2010)
22. Rosenblum, L.D.: Speech perception as a multimodal phenomenon. Curr. Dir. Psychol. Sci. **17**, 405–409 (2008)
23. Linares-del Rey, M., Vela-Desojo, L., Cano-de la Cuerda, R.: Mobile phone applications in Parkinson's disease: a systematic review. Neurología (English Edition) **34**, 38–54 (2019)
24. Maguire, Á., Martin, J., Jarke, H., Ruggeri, K.: Psychological services getting closer? Differences remain in neuropsychological assessments converted to mobile devices (2018)
25. Kobayashi, M., Hiyama, A., Miura, T., Asakawa, C., Hirose, M., Ifukube, T.: Elderly user evaluation of mobile touchscreen interactions. In: Campos, P., Graham, N., Jorge, J., Nunes, N., Palanque, P., Winckler, M. (eds.) INTERACT 2011. LNCS, vol. 6946, pp. 83–99. Springer, Heidelberg (2011). https://doi.org/10.1007/978-3-642-23774-4_9
26. Zygouris, S., Tsolaki, M.: Computerized cognitive testing for older adults: a review. Am. J. Alzheimer's Dis. Dementias **30**(1), 13–28 (2015)
27. Borrione, P.: Effects of physical activity in Parkinson's disease: a new tool for rehabilitation. World J. Methodol. **4**(3), 133 (2014)
28. Lauzé, M., Daneault, J.F., Duval, C.: The effects of physical activity in Parkinson's disease: a review, January 2016
29. Mantri, S., Wood, S., Duda, J.E., Morley, J.F.: Comparing self-reported and objective monitoring of physical activity in Parkinson disease. Parkinsonism Relat. Disord. **67**, 56–59 (2019)
30. Prodoehl, J., et al.: Two-year exercise program improves physical function in Parkinson's disease: the PRET-PD randomized clinical trial. Neurorehabilitation Neural Repair **29**, 112–122 (2015)
31. Schenkman, M., Hall, D.A., Baron, A.E., Schwartz, R.S., Mettler, P., Kohrt, W.M.: Exercise for people in early- or mid- stage Parkinson disease: a 16-month randomized controlled trial. Phys. Ther. **92**, 1395–1410 (2012)
32. Rovini, E., Fiorini, L., Esposito, D., Maremmani, C., Cavallo, F.: Fine motor assessment with unsupervised learning for personalized rehabilitation in Parkinson disease. In: IEEE International Conference on Rehabilitation Robotics, vol. 2019-June, pp. 1167–1172. IEEE Computer Society, June 2019
33. Post, B., Van Den Heuvel, L., Van Prooije, T., Van Ruissen, X., Van De Warrenburg, B., Nonnekes, J.: Young onset Parkinson's disease: a modern and tailored approach, January 2020
34. Templeton, J.M., Poellabauer, C., Schneider, S.: Design of a mobile-based neurological assessment tool for aging populations. In: Ye, J., O'Grady, M.J., Civitarese, G., Yordanova, K. (eds.) MobiHealth 2020. LNICST, vol. 362, pp. 166–185. Springer, Cham (2021). https://doi.org/10.1007/978-3-030-70569-5_11
35. Scarpina, F., Tagini, S.: The Stroop color and word test. Front. Psychol. **8**, 557 (2017)

36. Gao, L., Zhang, J., Hou, Y., Hallett, M., Chan, P., Wu, T.: The cerebellum in dual-task performance in Parkinson's disease. Sci. Rep. **7**, 1–11 (2017)
37. Mazzoni, P., Shabbott, B., Cortés, J.C.: Motor control abnormalities in Parkinson's disease. Cold Spring Harbor Perspect. Med. **2**(6) (2012)

Signal/Data Processing and Computing For Health Systems

A Multi-classifier Fusion Approach for Capacitive ECG Signal Quality Assessment

Zhikun Lie[1(✉)], Yonglin Wu[1], Guoqiang Zhu[1], Yang Li[1], Chen Chen[2], and Wei Chen[1,2]

[1] Center for Intelligent Medical Electronics, School of Information Science and Technology, Fudan University, Shanghai 200433, China
{20210720105,w_chen}@fudan.edu.cn

[2] Human Phenome Institute, Fudan University, Shanghai 201203, China

Abstract. Capacitive ECG (cECG), as a contactless solution for measuring ECG, has been extensively explored in existing works. However, the signal quality obtained by cECG can abruptly degrade due to body movement. Hence, it substantially increases the challenge in signal quality assessment of cECG. In this paper, a novel multi-classifier fusion approach is proposed to assess the cECG signal quality. It combines three commonly used classifiers namely, support vector machine (SVM), K-nearest neighbor (KNN) model, and decision tree (DT) and fuse these classifiers with a voting mechanism to provide a robust decision. With the proposed approach, the overall accuracy of 98.32% can be achieved in distinguishing the cECG signal quality into three categories, namely clear ECG signal, blurry ECG signal with clear R peaks, and noisy ECG signal. Experimental results exhibit that the proposed method outperforms existing works. The classification accuracy and F1-Score of this method are better than traditional methods. Meanwhile, the proposed method is expected to be integrated with cECG device for practical long-term heart monitoring.

Keywords: capacitive ECG · Signal quality assessment · Support vector machine · K-nearest neighbor model · Decision tree model

1 Introduction

Cardiovascular diseases (CVDs), as one of the main threat to human health, constitute the leading cause of morbidity and mortality. In China, the average number of sudden deaths caused by heart attacks exceeds 540,000 each year [1]. Early detection and timely treatment are vitally important to provide an early warning of sudden cardiac events or avoid the progressive deterioration of the CVDs [2]. ECG, as a significant tool to monitor cardiac rhythm for diagnosing CVDs, has been extensively used in the hospital and remote healthcare [3]. Figure 1 shows the waveform of the ECG signal in one cycle. A whole cycle includes P wave, QRS complex, T wave, U wave, P-R interval, Q-T interval, and other wavebands. The morphology of ECG contains detailed information about the condition of the heart. So accurately recording details of ECG weighs a lot in clinical settings.

X. Gao et al. (Eds.): MobiHealth 2021, LNICST 440, pp. 259–269, 2022.
https://doi.org/10.1007/978-3-031-06368-8_17

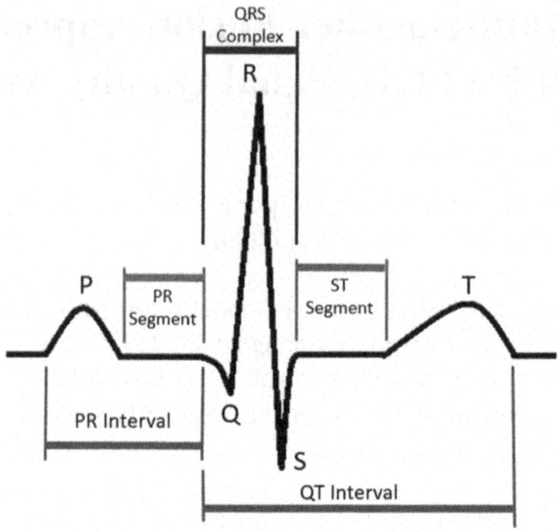

Fig. 1. ECG waveform in one cycle

Nowadays, the traditional method of measuring ECG uses the surface electrodes, such as Ag/AgCl electrodes, to acquire high-quality ECG signals. However, there are several limitations, mainly reflected as follows. Firstly, skin preparation such as removing hair and cuticle from the skin is necessary. Secondly, we need to use alcohol to clean the skin and apply gel to improve the conductibility of the skin. Then stick the electrodes on the patient's skin [4]. Obviously, the traditional measurement method is inconvenient, especially for people whose skin is fragile and sensitive, such as infants and elderly people [5]. Moreover, this method may arouse panic and anxiety of the patient, and then disturb the patient's heart rhythm, thereby raising questions about the authenticity of measurements. Thus, a contactless approach based on capacitively coupled electrodes for ECG monitoring has been proposed. According to Peng's article, it uses a non-contact ECG measurement device based on capacitively coupled electrodes and this device allows patients to take measurements with clothes in a comfortable way. The device uses a real-time denoising algorithm and stores the ECG signal automatically. This measurement method overcomes the limitations of traditional methods and provides possibilities for telemedicine and home health care. However, both contact measurement and non-contact measurement have noise and interference [6], which makes partial signals useless for clinical purposes. Especially for non-contact measurement methods, it is more sensitive to noise, such as power line interference, myoelectric signal, body movements, baseline drift, and so on. Therefore, it is necessary for us to assess the quality of the collected ECG signal in an automated way.

Currently, there are many machine learning algorithms for ECG signal quality assessment. For example, train an SVM model for classification by extracting multiple feature values of the ECG signal [7], calculate high-dimensional ECG features and use a KNN model based on Euclidean distance metric for classification [8]. Extract several non-benchmark features from the ECG signal and use the binary DT model to classify the signal [9]. ECG classification based on time and frequency domain features using random forests [10]. Different classifiers have different classification standards. The classification accuracy is related to many factors such as the statistical distribution characteristics of the data it classifies, the size of the training data sample, and the structure of the classifier. Meanwhile, noncontact ECG signals is a non-stationary millivolt signal with a low signal-to-noise ratio. And it is easy to be interfered by other signals. Therefore, it is difficult for a single classifier to classify the capacitive ECG signals with high accuracy. In this article, based on the designed voting mechanism, we integrate three classifiers (SVM, KNN, and DT) to form an ECG classification system and achieve a high-precision classification of the cECG signals.

The rest of this article is organized as follows: Sect. 2 introduces the methodology and performance measurement. Section 3 introduces the experimental setup, results and comparison with the existing techniques. Conclusions are drawn in Sect. 4.

2 Methodology

2.1 Algorithm Framework

The whole system consists of the following three parts: signal acquisition, feature extraction, signal quality classification. Through the voting mechanism, the support vector machine (SVM), K-nearest neighbor (KNN) model, and decision tree (DT) model are combined to a fusion classifier and make classification decision together. The fusion model is shown in Fig. 2. It can effectively divide the ECG signal into three categories, namely clear ECG signal (classified as category A), blurry ECG signal with clear R peaks (classified as category B), and noisy ECG signal (classified as category C).

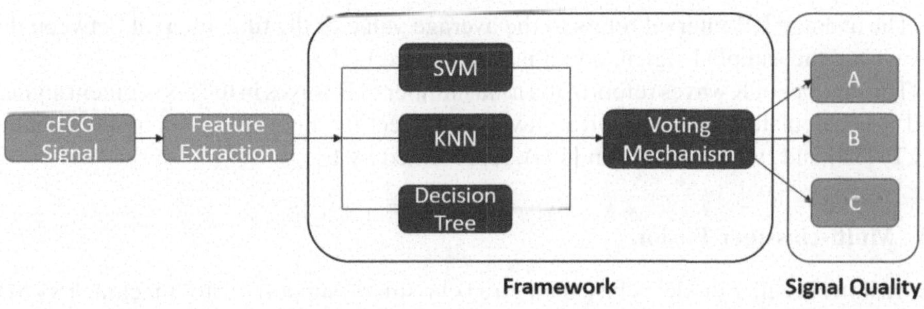

Fig. 2. Fusion classifier model

2.2 Feature Extraction

Six kinds of features of the cECG signal were extracted in total. The details of the features are explained below.

Kurtosis, also known as kurtosis coefficient, is the characteristic number that characterizes the peak height of the probability density distribution curve at the average value [11]. Kurtosis is generally used to describe the statistics of the steepness of the distribution of all values in the population, the calculation formula is as follows:

$$K = \frac{\frac{1}{n}\sum_{i=1}^{n}(x_i - \overline{x})^4}{\left(\frac{1}{n}\sum_{i=1}^{n}(x_i - \overline{x})^2\right)^2} \tag{1}$$

Skewness is a measure of the direction and degree of skewness in the distribution of statistical data. Its calculation formula is as follows:

$$S = \frac{\frac{1}{n}\sum_{i=1}^{n}(x_i - \overline{x})^3}{\left(\frac{1}{n}\sum_{i=1}^{n}(x_i - \overline{x})^2\right)^{\frac{3}{2}}} \tag{2}$$

Range is used to count the difference between the maximum value and the minimum value in the data, which is represented by F_1.

The standard deviation can reflect the degree of dispersion of a data set. Standard deviation is a measure of the degree of data dispersion and is represented as F_2. The calculation formula is as follows:

$$F_2 = \sqrt{\frac{\sum_{i=1}^{n}(x_i - \overline{x})^2}{n}} \tag{3}$$

The average RR interval refers to the average value of the time interval between the R waves in the sampled signal, and it is represented by F_3.

The number of R waves refers to the total number of R waves in the 5-s segment signal. And it is calculated based on QRS waveform detection algorithm (Pan and Tompkins (P&T) [12] and 'wqrs' algorithm [13]), represented by F_4.

2.3 Multi-classifier Fusion

Our fusion classifier model is based on three classifiers, support vector machine (SVM), K-nearest neighbor (KNN), and decision tree (DT). Next, we explain the basic principles of the three classifiers respectively, and then explain the principles and composition of our fusion classifier, as well as the voting mechanism.

The basic model of SVM is to find the linear classifier of separation hyperplane with maximum interval in feature space. We use different kernel functions to improve the performance of the SVM classifier, such as linear, polynomial, and radial basis function (RBF) [14]. The KNN algorithm finds the k records closest to the new data from the training set, and then determines the category of the new data according to their features, and infers its category from the target's neighbors [8]. Decision tree model is a simple and easy-to-use nonparametric classifier and it does not require any prior assumptions about the data. The generation of the decision tree is a recursive process. The calculation speed of the decision tree model is fast, the results are easy to explain, and its robustness is strong [7].

We use 1465 cECG data as the training set and 535 data as the test set. Taking 5 s as a cycle, we calculate six statistical characteristics of each sample signal. Through the voting mechanism, the three classifiers of support vector machine, KNN nearest-neighbor model, and decision tree model are combined to be an overall classification system. After many times of training and 13-fold cross-validation, the signal is divided into three levels: A, B, and C in a high-precision way finally. The voting mechanism is: if two or more classifiers regard signal as a certain level, we are confident to rate this segment of signal as that level. If the classification results of the three classifiers are inconsistent, we randomly select the classification result of one of the classifiers. Three classifier models are integrated through the voting mechanism. When the accuracy of the validation set is 99.1%, we use the 13-fold cross-validation method to determine the hyper-parameters of each classifier. The average classification accuracy obtained by the fusion classifier on the test set data is 98.3%.

2.4 Performance Measurement

Performance evaluation is done using Confusion Matrix. It is a performance measure for Machine Learning classification. To evaluate the trained model, we applied the confusion matrix and calculate the recall (Re), precision (P+), accuracy (Acc), and F1-Score of the fusion classifier model. The confusion matrix is a table that includes three indices represented by true-positive (TP), false-negative (FN), and false-positive (FP). The calculation formula of each index is as follows:

Accuracy (Acc): The fraction of correct predictions to the total predictions.

$$Acc = \frac{2 \times TP}{2 \times TP + FN + FP} \tag{4}$$

Precision (P+): It is the fraction of correct predicted positives to the total predicted positives.

$$P_{+} = \frac{TP}{TP + FP} \tag{5}$$

Recall (Re): It measures the proportion of positives that are correctly identified.

$$\mathrm{Re} = \frac{TP}{TP + FN} \tag{6}$$

F1-Score: It gives a way to merge the Recall and Precision into a single quantity that captures both the properties [15].

$$F_1 - Score = \frac{2 \times Re \times P_{+}}{Re + P_{+}} \tag{7}$$

3 Experimental Setup and Results

This section firstly introduces the experimental process and data acquisition method. And then we explain the classification performance of the fusion classifier model through a confusion matrix, and measure the performance of the model through the method proposed in Sect. 2.4. Finally, we compare with the existing common methods such as SVM, KNN, DT, Random Forest.

3.1 Experimental Setup

The data of this article is collected by a non-contact cECG measurement system published in article [4]. The ECG acquisition device is jointly developed by the author's laboratory team. The cECG measurement system is based on capacitively coupled electrode and it can acquire ECG signal both in contact with skin and through clothes with real-time denoising algorithm and automatically store ECG data for later analysis.

Thirty volunteers (15 men and 15 women, average age 30 $\pm$ 10), were enrolled in this study. All subjects have good health and no history of cardiovascular disease. And all of them signed the informed consent. The cECG signals were measured at a sampling frequency of 500 Hz for 2 h. The collected signals were divided into five-second segments. 2000 of sampled signal with obvious statistical characteristics were selected. Each segment was la-belled as A, B, or C type by well-trained researchers according to its quality. We randomly select 1465 cases as the training set and 535 cases as the test set, including 172 cases of class A data, 183 cases of class B data and 180 cases of class C data.

The ECG signals are divided into three categories according to the needs of medical diagnosis. Especially for cECG signals, it is necessary for us to decide whether the piece of signal is useful or not for further data processing [16]. Through manual labeling, the ECG signals can be divided into the following three categories. 1) Type A: clear ECG signal which is clear enough for medical diagnosis, as shown in Fig. 3; 2) Type B: blurry ECG signal with clear R peaks and a little bit of noise, which needs further processing before further medical usage, as shown in Fig. 4; 3) Type C: noisy ECG signal with obvious noise and unobvious ECG waves, which is useless from a medical perspective, as shown in Fig. 5.

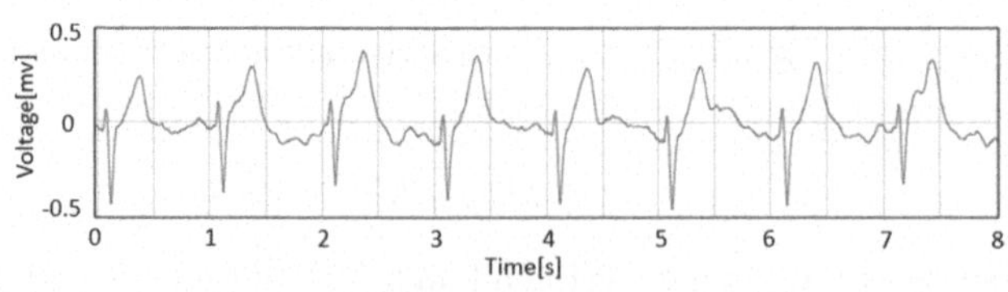

Fig. 3. Type A signal waveform

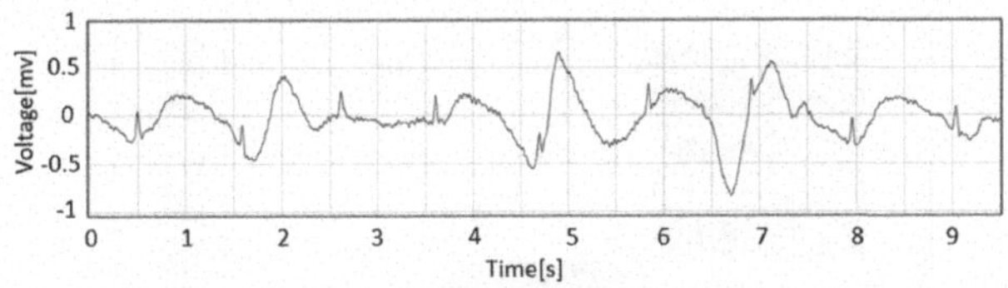

Fig. 4. Type B signal waveform

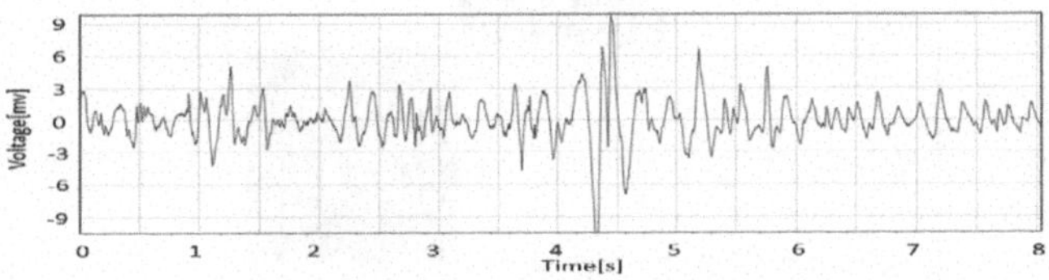

Fig. 5. Type C signal waveform

3.2 Result

Based on the 6 feature values obtained in Sect. 2.2, we establish the feature matrix: $\vec{F} = [K, S, F_1, F_2, F_3, F_4]$ and each set of data has a level label corresponding to it. The range of the six characteristic values of the three types ECG signals are shown in Table 1.

Table 1. A/B/C signal quality characteristics distribution (mean ± standard deviation)

Feature	A	B	C
K	0.36 ± 0.32	0.15 ± 0.28	0.42 ± 1.86
S	0.45 ± 0.98	−0.23 ± 0.82	2.12 ± 1.25
F_1	0.82 ± 0.20	1.40 ± 0.34	8.25 ± 4.35
F_2	0.22 ± 0.20	0.52 ± 0.47	1.59 ± 2.23
F_3	0.60 ± 0.21	0.90 ± 0.45	1.52 ± 2.21
F_4	8.00 ± 2.00	5.00 ± 2.00	3.00 ± 2.00

We use the fusion classifier to classify the cECG signals on the test set and the confusion matrix of the classification results are shown in Fig. 6.

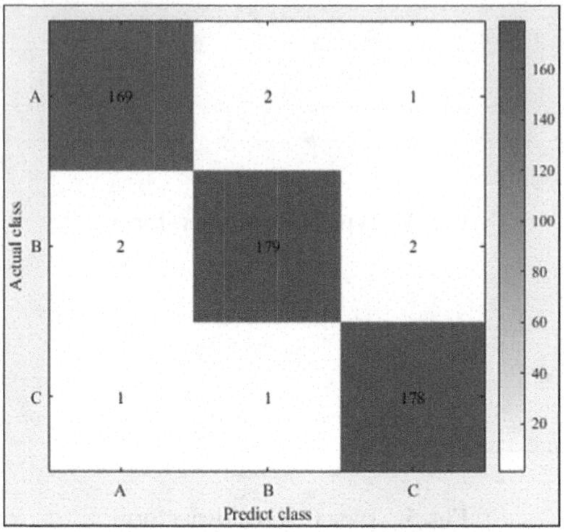

Fig. 6. Confusion matrix of the fusion classifier

It can be known from the confusion matrix that in the 535 test set data, the fusion classifier model can accurately identify 526 sample data, and there are only 9 prediction errors. For our cECG test set data, the fusion classifier model can achieve 98.3% classification accuracy. This method has higher classification accuracy and better performance than the conventional single classifier [9]. Especially for noise-sensitive ECG signal, the fusion model can achieve more stable and reliable results.

According to the statistical analysis of the confusion matrix results, we can calculate the P_+ value of type A is 98.26%, and the value of Re is 98.26%; the P_+ value of type B is 98.35% and the value of Re is 97.81%; the P_+ value of type C is 98.34% and the value of Re 98.89%; The F1-Score of A, B, and C are: 98.26%, 98.08%, 98.61%. The average classification accuracy obtained by the fusion classifier on the test set data is 98.32%. The performance measure is shown in Table 2.

Table 2. Performance measures

Type	Acc	P_+	Re	F1-Score
A	98.26%	98.26%	98.26%	98.26%
B	97.81%	98.35%	97.81%	98.08%
C	98.89%	98.34%	98.89%	98.61%
Average	98.32%	98.32%	98.32%	98.32%

3.3 Comparison with the Single Classifier

Compared to existing classifiers and methodologies, the fusion classifier has given better accuracy, whereas Ö. Özaltın et al., [17] have used SVM to classify ECG signals that were converted into two-dimensional images using continuous wavelet transform and got an accuracy of 95%. In contrast, P.Michael Infant Lincy et al., [18] extracted ECG signal features and used KNN to classify the signal and obtained an accuracy of 93.40%. B. B.U. Demirel et al., [9] used DT algorithm to classify ECG signals on the PhysioNet/Computing in Cardiology Challenge 2011 database and obtained an accuracy of 94.70%, Li Xiaolin et al., [19] used the CNN algorithm on the Physionet MIT-BIH database to classify the arrhythmia of the ECG signal and got an accuracy of 98.12. But the proposed model can achieve the accuracy, Recall, F1-score, and precision of 98.32%, 98.32%, 98.32%, and 98.32% respectively. Because the data sets are different, it is less rigorous to directly compare the results of the method proposed in this article with the results of traditional methods. However, we can still know from Table 3 that the fusion classifier model has higher classification accuracy than traditional methods in classifying the quality of capacitive ECG signals. Meanwhile, we can know from Table 3 that the fusion classifier model has higher classification accuracy than traditional methods in classifying the quality of capacitive ECG signals, and the fusion model has higher stability and stronger robustness.

Table 3. Comparison with existing techniques

Author	Algorithm	Performance metrics			
		Recall (%)	Precision (%)	F1-score (%)	Accuracy (%)
Ö. Özaltın [17]	SVM	95.00	83.33	89.76	89.17
P. M. Infant Lincy [18]	KNN	**99.59**	88.32	93.62	93.40
B. B.U. Demirel [9]	DT	93.30	**99.00**	96.07	94.70
X. L. Li [19]	CNN	98.07	92.33	95.04	98.12
The proposed method	fusion classifier	98.32	98.32	**98.32**	**98.32**

4 Conclusion

Owing to the non-contact measurement, cECG shows great potential in long-term monitoring. However, it also causes critical issues that the signal quality is unstable due to body movement. To promote the use of cECG, an effective and robust multi-classifier fusion model for cECG signal quality classification is proposed in this paper. The model consists of three commonly used classifiers (SVM, KNN, and DT) and fuse these classifiers with a voting mechanism to achieve the three-classes classification (Type A, Type B, and Type C) of cECG signal quality. Firstly, 6 features of the ECG signal are extracted in the time domain and non-linear domain. Secondly, 1465 ECG signal are randomly selected as the training set and 535 samples as the test set. Finally, a classification accuracy of 98.32% is obtained after many times of training and validation. Comparative results demonstrate the superior performance of this multi-classifier fusion model over traditional methods. As a potential field, the proposed method can be incorporated with cECG device for practical long-term heart monitoring and may help with the noninvasive detection of CVDs.

Acknowledgment. This work was supported in part by Shanghai Municipal Science and Technology International R&D Collaboration Project (Grant No. 20510710500) in part by the National Natural Science Foundation of China under Grant No. 62001118, and in part by the Shanghai Committee of Science and Technology under Grant No. 20S31903900.

References

1. Zhu, H. (ed.): Sudden Death: Advances in Diagnosis and Treatment. Springer, Heidelberg (2020)
2. Mensah, G.A., Sampson, U.K., Roth, G.A., et al.: Mortality from cardiovascular diseases in sub-Saharan Africa, 1990–2013: a systematic analysis of data from the Global Burden of Disease Study 2013. Cardiovasc. J. Afr. **26**(2 Suppl 1), S6 (2015)
3. Benjamin: Heart Disease and stroke statistics-2018 update: a report from the american heart association, vol. 137, p. e67 (2018)
4. Peng, S., Bao, S., Chen, W.: Capacitive coupled electrodes based non-contact ECG measurement system with real-time wavelet denoising algorithm. In: 2019 41st Annual International Conference of the IEEE Engineering in Medicine & Biology Society (EMBC). IEEE (2019). Author, F., Author, S.: Title of a proceedings paper. In: Editor, F., Editor, S. (eds.) CONFERENCE 2016, LNCS, vol. 9999, pp. 1–13. Springer, Heidelberg (2016)
5. Sharma, M., Ritchie, P., Ghirmai, T., Cao, H., Lau, M.P.H.: Unobtrusive acquisition and extraction of fetal and maternal ECG in the home setting. IEEE Sens. **2017**, 1–3 (2017). https://doi.org/10.1109/ICSENS.2017.8234188
6. Satija, U., Ramkumar, B., Manikandan, M.S.: Automated ECG noise detection and classification system for unsupervised healthcare monitoring. IEEE J. Bio-Med. Health Inform. **22**(3), 722–732 (2018). https://doi.org/10.1109/JBHI.2017.2686436
7. Ge, Z., Zhu, Z., Feng, P., Zhang, S., Wang, J., Zhou, B.: ECG-signal classification using SVM with multi-feature. In: 2019 8th International Symposium on Next Generation Electronics (ISNE), pp. 1–3 (2019). https://doi.org/10.1109/ISNE.2019.8896430
8. Prabhakararao, E., Dandapat, S.: Automatic quality estimation of 12-lead ECG for remote healthcare monitoring systems. In: 2018 IEEE-EMBS Conference on Biomedical Engineering and Sciences (IECBES), pp. 554–559 (2018). https://doi.org/10.1109/IECBES.2018.8626686
9. Demirel, B.U., Serinağaoğlu, Y.: Quality assessment of ECG signals based on support vector machines and binary decision trees. In: 2020 28th Signal Processing and Communications Applications Conference (SIU), pp. 1–4 (2020). https://doi.org/10.1109/SIU49456.2020.930 2262.

10. Kropf, M., Hayn, D., Schreier, G.: ECG classification based on time and frequency do-main features using random forests. In: 2017 Computing in Cardiology (CinC), pp. 1–4 (2017). https://doi.org/10.22489/CinC.2017.168-168
11. Yao, W., Wu, M., Wang, J.: RobustICA, Kurtosis- and negentropy-based FastICA in maternal-Fetal ECG separation. In: 2018 11th International Congress on Image and Signal Processing, BioMedical Engineering and Informatics (CISP-BMEI), 2018, pp. 1–5. https://doi.org/10.1109/CISP-BMEI.2018.8633123.
12. Thakor, N.V., Webster, J.G., Tompkins, W.J.: Estimation of QRS complex power spectra for design of a QRS filter. IEEE Trans. Biomed. Eng. **BME-31**(11), 702–706 (1984). https://doi.org/10.1109/TBME.1984.325393
13. Balachandran, A., Ganesan, M., Sumesh, E.P.: Daubechies algorithm for highly accurate ECG feature extraction. In: 2014 International Conference on Green Computing Communication and Electrical Engineering (ICGCCEE), pp. 1–5 (2014). https://doi.org/10.1109/ICGCCEE.2014.6922266
14. Xia, Y., Jia, H.: ECG quality assessment based on multi-feature fusion. In: 2017 13th International Conference on Natural Computation, Fuzzy Systems and Knowledge Discovery (ICNC-FSKD), pp. 672–676 (2017). https://doi.org/10.1109/FSKD.2017.8393352.
15. Medapati, B., Rajani Kumari, L.V.: KNN based sleep Apnea detection using ECG signals. In: 2021 2nd International Conference for Emerging Technology (INCET), pp. 1–5 (2021). https://doi.org/10.1109/INCET51464.2021.9456404
16. Healey, J., Logan, B.: Wearable wellness monitoring using ECG and accelerometer data. In: Ninth IEEE International Symposium on Wearable Computers (ISWC 2005), pp. 220–221 (2005). https://doi.org/10.1109/ISWC.2005.59
17. Özaltın, Ö., Yeniay, Ö.: ECG classification performing feature extraction automatically using a hybrid CNN-SVM algorithm. In: 2021 3rd International Congress on Human-Computer Interaction, Optimization and Robotic Applications (HORA), pp. 1–5 (2021). https://doi.org/10.1109/HORA52670.2021.9461295
18. Infant Lincy, P.M., Santhi, D., Geetha, A.: A proficient evalution with the pre-term birth classification in ECG signal using KNN. In: 2020 International Conference on Inventive Computation Technologies (ICICT), pp. 276–282 (2020). https://doi.org/10.1109/ICICT48043.2020.9112448
19. Xiaolin, L., Cardiff, B., John, D.: A 1D convolutional neural network for heartbeat classification from single lead ECG. In: 2020 27th IEEE International Conference on Electronics, Circuits and Systems (ICECS), pp. 1–2 (2020). https://doi.org/10.1109/ICECS49266.2020.9294838

A Pilot mHealth Project for Monitoring Vital Body Signals and Skin Conditions

Rodrigue B. Tchema, Georgios Tzavellas, Marios Nestoros, and Anastasis C. Polycarpou(✉)

Department of Engineering, University of Nicosia, 1700 Nicosia, Cyprus
polycarpou.a@unic.ac.cy
http://www.unic.ac.cy

Abstract. In this paper, we present a pilot project on mobile health (mHealth) which is designed to monitor on a continuous basis the health condition of individuals using a mobile device such as a smartphone or a tablet. The objectives of this pilot project include highly accurate calculation of heart-beat rate using either a smartphone camera or an autonomous, self-powered mini-device which communicates measurement data to the mobile device through Bluetooth or Wi-Fi. In addition, we aim at detecting potentially dangerous skin conditions at an early stage using the smartphone camera and machine learning (ML) or deep learning (DL) algorithms. The trained algorithm will be able to detect malignant cases of skin conditions by searching through various built-in categories of commonly found skin disorders.

Keywords: Heart-beat rate detection · Skin disorder diagnosis · Deep learning algorithms

1 Introduction

As the human life expectancy is increasing, it is extremely important to limit heart diseases and other life-threatening health conditions, and help people maintain a healthy lifestyle. Unambiguously, the early detection of abnormalities in the health of individuals using existing technological tools will have a direct economic and social benefits. Mobile devices (like smartphones and tablets) have sensing elements (e.g., microphones, cameras, accelerometers, etc.) that can be effectively used to monitor vital signs of the human body. This sensor information can be further processed and communicated to the user or a healthcare professional through secured and fast communication channels, mobile applications, and cloud services allowing early intervention which can prevent health complications. The recent ubiquitous penetration of wearable sensors into the healthcare market, and their compatibility with mobile devices and software, allowed widespread use of mHealth monitoring and tracking.

The accuracy, sensitivity and reliability of these apps are often questionable by the majority of their users. Some wearables claim to provide a higher degree of

X. Gao et al. (Eds.): MobiHealth 2021, LNICST 440, pp. 270–280, 2022.
https://doi.org/10.1007/978-3-031-06368-8_18

accuracy in counting steps or pulse rate, and these come in the form of a watch, a wristband, or a strap around the chest. A recent study [1] on the accuracy of tracking apps and wearable devices has revealed that wearables provide a higher degree of accuracy with a maximum error rate equal to 5%. Apps, which depend on the smartphone's built-in accelerometer, are in general less accurate, and therefore, less reliable for professional use in sports.

The work described in this article concerns the use of a smartphone either as a gateway for transferring vital signals from a wearable or peripheral device to the cloud (for analysis and post-processing) or as a sensing device for recording and communicating health monitoring signals directly to the cloud server. At first, we present a prototype design of a compact and lightweight electronic circuit able to accurately extract the heart-beat rate based on the Photo-PlethysmoGraphy (PPG) technique. Then, we investigate the idea of using the smartphone's camera to capture a short video of the finger tip on top of the camera's lens, and use this information to obtain the pulse rate through suitable video processing and signal analysis. At last, we employ machine/deep learning algorithms on images taken using the smartphone's camera for early detection of skin malignancies such as cherry angioma and squamous cell carcinoma.

2 Project Activities

2.1 Heart-Beat Detection Using a Wireless Peripheral Mini-Device

For a daily monitor of someone's health, it is highly important that a reliable device is used to accurately calculate the heart-beat rate at a given moment. Not only that but the measurement data should be transferred to the cloud, post-processed, and compared with historical data thus providing mobile users important information on their health and well-being. Artificial intelligence (AI) algorithms could be employed in order to extract more meaningful results and predictions based on the overall picture of one's health.

In this project, we aim at designing a peripheral mini-device capable of detecting accurately the heart-beat rate of an individual under different body conditions (resting, sleeping, walking or running). For this purpose, we designed an electronic circuit to detect the weak pulse of the finger vein and convert that into a noise-free, amplified signal as a function of time. The technique we used is called Photo-PlethysmoGraphy (PPG) [2,3], which is based on the use of a monochromatic infrared (IR) light emitted by an IR-LED (Light Emitting Diode). This technique could be used in the reflection mode or the transmission mode (see Fig. 1). For example, in the transmission mode, an emitting diode is used on the front side of the finger and a photodiode or phototransistor is used on the back side as a detector. As the volume of the blood that flows through the veins is not constant as a function of time, the transmittance - at that particular wavelength - varies with time. This response is highly correlated with the heart beat. Similar observations are recorded for the reflection mode. Either approach is equally implemented in such applications. In our project, we used the reflection mode, therefore, both the emitting LED and phototransistor are positioned on the front side of the finger.

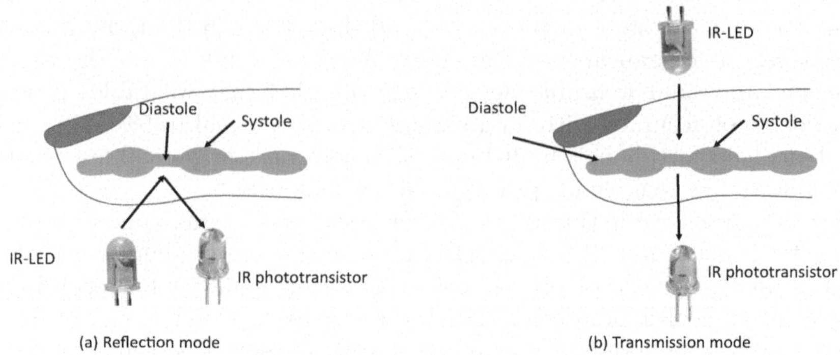

Fig. 1. Implementation of the Photo-PlethysmoGraphy (PPG) technique using the reflection and transmission modes.

A schematic diagram of the IR sensor electronic circuit augmented by active filtering and amplification is depicted in Fig. 2. The part on the left hand side corresponds to the IR sensor made of the IR-LED and the phototransistor. The wavelength emitted by the IR-LED is 940 nm. A band-pass filter (BPF) was designed to filter out unwanted noise and similar type of interference from sources other than the pulsating volume of blood in the finger. The filter was built to operate in a bandwidth of 40 bpm (beats per minute) to 200 bpm where 1 bpm corresponds to 1/60 Hz. In order to achieve a satisfactory level of filtering, two inverting active BPFs were used in conjunction with two inverting active amplifiers, as clearly shown in Fig. 2.

Circuit analysis of the proposed design results in an overall voltage amplification gain approximately equal to $A_v \approx 270$ and cut-off frequencies that define an operating bandwidth from 0.589 Hz to 3.386 Hz and a center frequency of 1.412 Hz. The frequency bandwidth corresponds to a heart-beat rate bandwidth between 35 bpm to 203 bpm with a peak rate at 85 bpm.

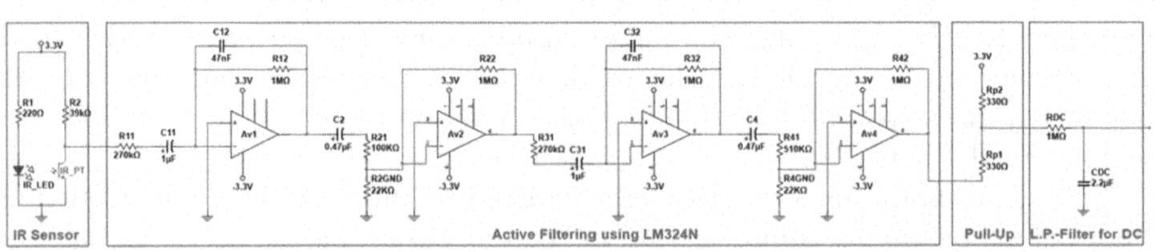

Fig. 2. Electronic circuit design of the heart-beat rate detection, filtering and amplification.

Revisiting the circuit in Fig. 2, two stages of active filtering and two stages of amplification were implemented in the final design. Initially, we started the design with a single active filter and a single amplification stage. However, it was observed that the signal output, especially at low frequencies, had a significant interference from ambient light and other surrounding electromagnetic sources. In addition, the input signal from the IR sensor was too weak hence the need to improve the signal-to-noise ratio (SNR) was necessary. Therefore, two stages of filtering and amplification, using four concatenated Op-Amps, were implemented in order to resolve the aforementioned problem. In addition, two capacitors in between amplifiers and two grounded resistors were used in order to filter out the DC component and improve the SNR. The slight increase in power consumption due to the use of additional components was not considered problematic at this stage of the project.

The complete circuit, which was initially implemented on a breadboard, is shown in Fig. 3. As seen, there are two separate power supplies on the left bottom corner of the board. Specifically, there is a 5-V stabilizer that powers the microcontroller unit and the external SD-board along with the Real-Clock module, and one step-down power supply at 3.3 V that only powers the negative terminal of the quad Op-Amp. The positive terminal of electronic components such as filters, LEDs, and buzzers is attached to the 3.3 V step-down pin of the microcontroller board. The two-stage amplifier-filtering circuit appears in the center of the breadboard. Looking at the top left corner, there exist three optocouplers to be used at a later stage for switching on/off the Op-Amp, the 3.3 V step-down power supply, and the IR sensor. Although the SD-board and Real-Clock board are not essential for the key operations of the project, they are important for data storage in case there is loss of connection between the microcontroller and the Bluetooth receiver (e.g., computer, smartphone). In addition, LED indicators are used for possible debugging and component failure identification.

The circuit shown in Fig. 3 was tested in the lab and several PPG signals were obtained under different physical conditions. An example is shown in Fig. 4 clearly illustrating the systolic and diastolic phases of the heart pumping blood through the veins reaching all the way down to the finger tip. The signal shown in this figure corresponds to processed data which have been smoothed by software written on Python. Specifically, after the microcontroller sends the data sequence in a CSV text file, the software checks on the validity of the data and stores these values in memory. Then, with user's commands, the code implements smoothing and then plots the data as shown in Fig. 4. Data smoothing is based on the Savitzky-Golay filter library. This filter is implemented based on moving average and linear regression concepts. Two parameters are important to note. The first one is the window size that specifies the number of points used in the smoothing, whereas the second one is the degree of the polynomial implemented for curve fitting within the chosen window. In our case, the measurement window is 10 s, whereas the time it takes to transmit and save the data is approximately 5 s.

The heart-beat rate can be subsequently calculated by correctly identifying the extrema of the PPG signal. The maxima and minima of the signal can be easily calculated using a simple three-point algorithm. It simply checks the points before and after the current point. If their values are smaller than the current value, then the point is called a maximum. On the other hand, if their values

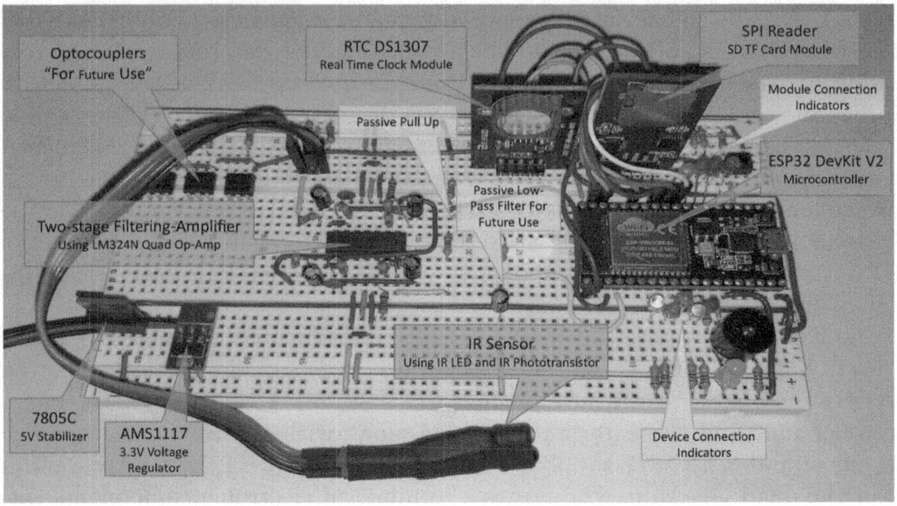

Fig. 3. Picture of the designed circuit implemented on a breadboard.

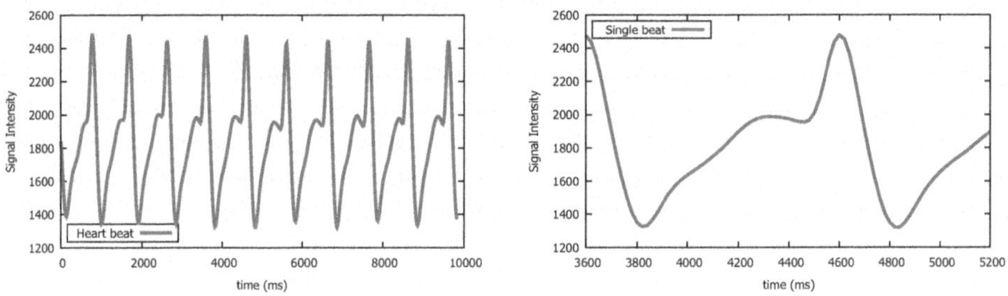

Fig. 4. Recorded heart beat pulses using the peripheral wireless mini-device: train of pulses (left); single pulse (right).

are larger than the current value, then the point is called a minimum. However, from the signal, it is easilly seen that we have additional local extrema. Thus, we save all extrema in two different arrays: one for local maxima and one for local minima. Then, the algorithm calculates the average value for each array and selects the values that are higher than the maxima average or lower than the minima average. Specifically, the heart-beat rate is calculated based on both maxima and minima, thus providing two estimates. If the deviation between the two estimates is larger than 2 bpm, then those estimates are discarded.

The accuracy of the prototype circuit was assessed by testing several users under resting and exercising conditions. Specifically, we tested six healthy individuals by recording their pulse rate when at rest and after performing minor exercise (10 or 20 push-ups). The recorded measurement was compared against the benchmark value obtained by pressing the index and middle fingers of the right hand on the opposite wrist and recording the number of beats manually in

60 s. As seen from Table 1, the two sets of data are in very close agreement. Specifically, the maximum percent deviation obtained was 3.61%, which is deemed to be satisfactory for the initial phase of the project. Further investigations will be performed with an increased number of subjects where the benchmark measurements will be recorded using an approved medical device.

Table 1. PPG circuit measurements and comparison with benchmark records.

User under test	Body activity*	Benchmark	Device	Percent deviation
User 'A'	Rest	67	66	1.52%
User 'A'	Ex-10	78	77	1.30%
User 'B'	Rest	72	71	1.41%
User 'B'	Ex-20	97	99	2.02%
User 'C'	Rest	64	62	3.23%
User 'C'	Ex-10	77	78	1.28%
User 'D'	Rest	86	73	3.61%
User 'E'	Rest	77	78	1.28%
User 'F'	Rest	73	72	1.39%

*Ex-10: After 10 push-ups; Ex-20: After 20 push-ups.

2.2 Heart-Beat Detection Using a Smartphone Built-In Camera

One of the main objectives of the project is to investigate the possibility of using the smartphone camera [4–6] to obtain accurate and reliable measurements of the pulse rate, as well as the oxygen concentration in blood. The smartphone camera is used to take a video of the finger tip which is directly attached to the lens. The flash light of the camera is always on during the recording time. The captured video files (.mp4 or .avi) from the camera will then be transferred to the cloud for further analysis and video processing, thereby allowing calculation of the heart-beat rate. At this point, our goal is to implement image processing techniques and dedicated algorithms that will provide accurate extraction of pulse rate first, and in the future, blood oxygen concentration. This is an alternative approach to calculating the pulse rate, as compared to the wireless circuit approach described in the previous section, aiming at providing a quick but accurate estimate of vital body signals when the user does not have access to the wearable peripheral device introduced earlier.

Our initial experimental data consists of approximately 40-seconds long videos of the index finger while in contact with the rear camera of the smartphone having the flashlight (LED) on. As light from the LED travels through tissue, it suffers absorption and scattering and its intensity is modulated by the pulsating flow of blood according to the PPG principle. The reflected light is then recorded by the camera at 30 fps and the video is stored in the phone. The recording is then reduced into its frames and each frame is subsequently analysed into its three spectral components (Red, Green, Blue). For each component, we calculate the mean value of brightness per frame, and then, we apply a moving average filter in order to smooth the measurement data.

The next step is to identify the peaks in the signal and count their number in a given window. Knowing the number of peaks and the time span of the window, the pulse rate can be easily calculated. The peaks are identified by calculating the gradient (slope) at nearby points to the left and the right of the current evaluation point. This process takes place on data produced by the moving average filter, thus the data are smooth and free of high-frequency noise. A particular data point is identified as a peak (e.g., maximum) if the gradient is positive at three consecutive points before the peak and negative at three consecutive points following the peak. Taking three points before and after improves the calculation of the heart-beat rate by 5–10% as compared to taking a single point before and after. In our code, we experimented with a moving average based on the past 7 samples.

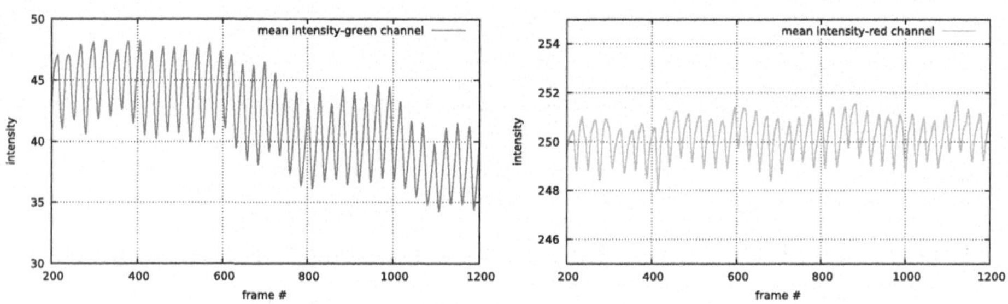

Fig. 5. Mean pixel intensity vs frame number as recorded at 30 fps from a rear smartphone camera: green channel (left); red channel (right). (Color figure online)

Once the video is recorded using the smartphone, the .mp4/.avi file is then transferred to a personal computer where all steps on video/image processing and data analysis are done using MATLAB codes. Figure 5 illustrates the GREEN and RED signal obtained from the smartphone camera after post-processing and smoothing. It is quite evident that both GREEN and RED signals present an oscillatory behavior as a result of the pulsating blood through the finger veins. As mentioned previously, the heart-beat rate can be calculated by counting the number of peaks within a given time window. At this point, it is worth noting that our near-term goal is to use available data from all three components (e.g., RED, GREEN, and BLUE) to also estimate oxygen concentration in blood.

The underlined method was tested against healthy people who belong to a wide range of age (17–52 years old). The recordings were performed under ambient light in the laboratory. The measurements are tabulated in Table 2. The results are compared against the pulse rate measured using the traditional benchmark approach described earlier. Specifically, we used two types of smartphone: one based on iOS and another one based on ANDROID. From this exercise, it was observed that the percent deviation is relatively high in some cases reaching a value of up to 11.7%. Note that the BLUE component was excluded from the measurements because of its low correlation with pulse-rate calculation. Our observation is that the results are susceptible to slight movements of the finger, ambient light conditions, or even the charging level of the smartphone's battery. Consequently, it is highly important that, in the near future, all these effects be carefully filtered out from the individual RGB signals thus providing the ground for more accurate PR calculations.

Table 2. Pulse rate (PR) in bpm measured using a smartphone camera.

User	Device	PR - GREEN	PR - RED	Benchmark	Percent deviation
1	IOS	54	59	56	3.57% (G) : 5.36% (R)
2	IOS	64	65	66	3.03% (G) : 1.52% (R)
3	IOS	54	59	56	3.57% (G) : 5.36% (R)
4	IOS	86	83	83	3.61% (G) : 0.00% (R)
5	ANDROID	53	56	60	11.7% (G) : 6.67% (R)
6	ANDROID	62	62	67	7.46% (G) : 7.46% (R)
7	ANDROID	62	62	61	1.64% (G) : 1.64% (R)
8	ANDROID	62	60	65	4.62% (G) : 7.69% (R)

2.3 Deep Learning for Early Detection of Serious Skin Disorders

In this part of the project, we are using Deep Learning (DL) algorithms [7] to detect at an early stage possible health-threatening skin conditions in humans. We strongly believe that such an automated diagnosis system could be complementary to the work of experienced physicians, thereby increasing confidence in the results. In fact, there is enough evidence in the literature [8] that deep learning algorithms currently investigated in the area of medical diagnostics are equivalent in terms of performance to that of health-care professionals.

Health-threatening conditions may include categories of skin cancer some of which might be classified as malignant and life threatening. The smartphone camera is used to take a picture of the affected skin area, which is then uploaded to the cloud for processing and classification. The objective of this work is to implement codes based on DL algorithms able to identify with high success rate the type of skin condition. In this effort, we implemented YOLO v.4 (You Only Look Once) which is considered as the state-of-art algorithm in object detection due to its high accuracy and superb speed. The methodology used in implementing this particular algorithm include the following: (a) Data collection; (b) Data processing which involves sorting, labeling, and dataset augmentation; (c) Classification.

Our first task was to collect images from different repositories available to the public or researchers. Initially, we chose to work with only four classes of skin conditions namely angioma cherry, squamous cell carcinoma, varicella, and normal skin. Once we collected a number of images from different sites, we started the pre-processing of images from which we excluded repeated ones and those with very bad resolution. Eventually, we ended up with a balanced dataset containing 120 images per class (480 images for the four classes in total). At this stage, we performed four simulations, each one with a different number of training sets. In other words, the training dataset was constantly modified but the testing dataset was kept fixed to a set of 60 images for all simulations. In order to test our approach in terms of performance accuracy, we restricted the number of classes to just two (angioma cherry and squamous cell carcinoma). For data augmentation, we used a MATLAB code. Particularly, images were flipped, rotated and cropped. For annotation, we used an open-source software called *LabelImg* which has the option of saving data into YOLO format.

For the first simulation, we implemented data augmentation on the 120 images per class, thus raising the total number of images per class to 200. For the two classes in hand, we had 400 images to use for training. In order to annotate the images, we used a bounding box around the most pronounced lesion in a given image, as shown in Fig. 6. Upon the completion of the training process, a total of 60 images per class were used for the testing phase. The result was 96.7% accuracy for the case of angioma cherry and 10% accuracy for the case of squamous cell carcinoma. Specifically, out of 60 images for each class, 58 images were correctly classified as angioma cherry and only 6 images for squamous cell carcinoma. This indicates very good performance on the classification of angioma cherry but very poor performance on the classification of squamous cell carcinoma.

In an attempt to improve the above results, a second simulation was performed. As the YOLO algorithm is used for classification instead of detection, the labeling technique was altered. Instead of labeling only the more pronounced lesions on an image (as shown in Fig. 6), we chose to label the entire image. In addition, a third class of training data was added which is the normal skin (image without any abnormality). A total of 120 images for all three classes was initially trained. The corresponding results in terms of success rate include 76.7% for angioma cherry, 53.3% for squamous cell carcinoma, and 100% for normal skin. For further improvement of the results, we repeated the simulation with a training dataset of 360 images (120 images per class). In this case, the achieved success rate was 90.0% for angioma cherry, 73.3% for squamous cell carcinoma, and 100% for normal skin. At last, the dataset was increased to a total of 1800 images (600 images per class). This increase in the training set resulted in a significant improvement in the success rate. Specifically, the obtained success rate for angioma cherry was 98.3%, for squamous cell carcinoma was 76.0%, and for

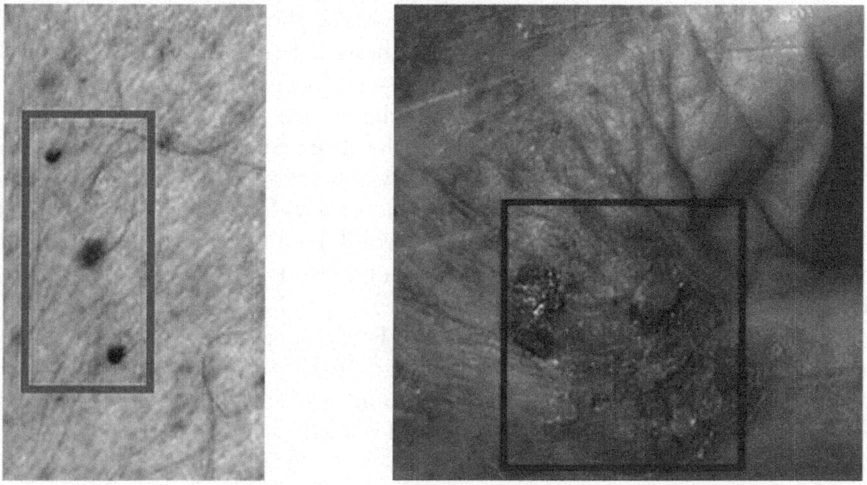

Fig. 6. Assigning bounding box around most pronounced lesion in an image: angioma cherry (left); Squamous cell carcinoma (right).

normal skin was 100%. The increase in the number of images per simulation was achieved by flipping an image, rotating an image, or by adding Gaussian noise. Consequently, we generate additional images from the initial group of images obtained from available repositories. The results are collectively tabulated in Table 3.

Table 3. Success rate of classification based on different size of training sets.

Size of training set	Angioma cherry	Squamous cell carcinoma	Normal skin
120	76.7%	53.3%	100%
360	90.0%	73.3%	100%
1800	98.3%	76.0%	100%

3 Conclusions

In this paper, we presented preliminary results obtained in the context of a recently launched pilot project on mobile health. The results sought are quite promising providing a solid ground for further investigation and improvement of the techniques utilized in this work. As already indicated, our primary goal is to enhance currently used techniques in order to provide accurate estimates of vital health signals or even to use newly introduced methods, such as machine learning or similar algorithms, in order to increase the probability of accurately identifying harmful skin conditions for the human being. As illustrated in this paper, a newly proposed electronic circuit used as a peripheral device was developed illustrating accurate extraction of the heart beat rate. This circuit will be augmented in the near term to calculate blood oxygen saturation as well. We also demonstrated a MATLAB algorithm which provides accurate calculation of heart beat rate based on image processing of a video of one's finger directly attached to the lens of a smartphone camera. This algorithm will be extended soon to also calculate the blood oxygen saturation. It was also illustrated that machine learning algorithms could be used as a tool for potential diagnosis of harmful skin conditions at an early stage. For a successful implementation of these algorithms and improved outcome, it is highly important that data are judiciously prepared based on certain rules and criteria before they are eventually fed to these algorithms for training and testing.

Acknowledgments. The authors would like to thank the University of Nicosia for their financial support of the project.

References

1. Stavropoulos, T.G., Andreadis, S., Mpaltadoros, L., Nikolopoulos, S., Kompatsiaris, I.: Wearable sensors and smartphone apps as pedometers in eHealth: a comparative accuracy, reliability and user evaluation. In: 2020 IEEE International Conference on Human-Machine Systems (ICHMS), Rome, pp. 1–6 (2020)
2. Daimiwal, N., Sundhararajan, M., Shriram, R.: Respiratory rate, heart rate and continuous measurement of BP using PPG. In: International Conference on Communication and Signal Processing, Melmaruvathur, India, pp. 999–1002 (2014)
3. Fujita, D., Suzuki, A.: Evaluation of the possible use of PPG waveform features measured at low sampling rate. IEEE Access **7**, 58361–58367 (2019)
4. Grimaldi, D., Kurylyak, Y., Lamonaca, F., Nastro, A.: Photoplethysmography detection by smartphone's videocamera. In: 6th IEEE International Conference on Intelligent Data Acquisition and Advanced Computing Systems, Prague, pp. 15–17 (2011)
5. Holz, C., Ofek, E.: Doubling the signal quality of smartphone camera pulse oximetry using the display screen as a controllable selective light source. In: 40th Annual International Conference of the IEEE Engineering in Medicine and Biology, Honolulu, pp. 1–4 (2018)
6. Pelegris, P., Banitsas, K., Orbach, T., Marias, K.: A novel method to detect heart beat rate using a mobile phone. In: 32nd Annual International Conference of the IEEE EMBS Buenos Aires, Argentina, pp. 5488–5491 (2010)
7. Winkler, J.K., et al.: Melanoma recognition by a deep learning convolutional neural network performance in different melanoma subtypes and localisations. Eur. J. Cancer **127**, 21–29 (2020)
8. Liu, X., et al.: A comparison of deep learning performance against health-care professionals in detecting diseases from medical imaging: a systematic review and meta-analysis. Lancet Digit. Health **1**(6), e271–e297 (2019)

Automatic Subject Identification Using Scale-Based Ballistocardiogram Signals

Beren Semiz[1(✉)], M. Emre Gursoy[2], Md Mobashir Hasan Shandhi[3], Lara Orlandic[4], Vincent J. Mooney[5], and Omer T. Inan[5]

[1] Electrical and Electronics Engineering, Koc University, Istanbul, Turkey
besemiz@ku.edu.tr

[2] Computer Engineering, Koc University, Istanbul, Turkey
emregursoy@ku.edu.tr

[3] Biomedical Engineering, Duke University, Durham, NC, USA
mobashir.shandhi@duke.edu

[4] Electrical Engineering, Ecole Polytechnique Fédérale de Lausanne, Lausanne, Switzerland
lara.orlandic@epfl.ch

[5] Electrical and Computer Engineering, Georgia Institute of Technology, Atlanta, GA, USA
{mooney,omer.inan}@ece.gatech.edu

Abstract. Many electronic devices such as weighing scales, fitness equipment and medical devices are nowadays shared by multiple users. In such devices, automatic identification of device users becomes an important step towards improved user convenience and personalized service. In this paper, we propose a novel approach for subject identification using ballistocardiogram (BCG) signals collected unobtrusively from a modified weighing scale. Our approach first segments BCG signals into heartbeats using signal filtering and beat detection techniques, and averages beats to obtain smoother ensemble averaged BCG frames that are more robust to noise. Second, it extracts features related to subjects' cardiovascular performance and musculoskeletal system from their BCG frames. Finally, it trains a machine learning model for predicting the owner of an unlabeled BCG recording based on its features. We evaluated our approach through a pilot experimental study with subjects' BCG signals recorded at rest and following different physiological modulation. Our approach achieves up to 97% identification accuracy at rest conditions and incurs a 15–20% accuracy drop on average under physiological modulation.

Keywords: Subject identification · Ballistocardiography · Biometrics · Machine learning

X. Gao et al. (Eds.): MobiHealth 2021, LNICST 440, pp. 281–292, 2022.
https://doi.org/10.1007/978-3-031-06368-8_19

1 Introduction

Recent advancements have made it possible to embed various sensors into electronic devices such as electronic scales, fitness equipment, and hospital equipment, which enable unobtrusive and non-invasive collection of physiological signals. These devices are often shared by multiple users such as members of a family, athletes in a sports team, or patients in a hospital. It becomes desirable that these shared devices can automatically identify their users (subjects) based on collected signals, for improved user convenience, personalization of devices and services, as well as enabling safer and more secure systems through biometric authentication [6,13].

Currently, subject identification in most smart household devices such as smart scales rely either on simple biometrics such as weight and heart rate, or require the user to manually introduce themselves by entering their ID or pairing with a third party device (e.g., smartphone) at each time of use [4,5,21]. The main drawback of the state-of-the-art is that biometrics such as weight or heart rate are not subject-specific, i.e., they can change over time and different users may have similar weights. The drawback of the latter is its inconvenience, e.g., the user has to carry their smartphone or enter their ID to the smart scale every time. In contrast, automatic subject identification using physiological signals alleviates both drawbacks – physiological signals are naturally present in living individuals at all times and they often contain subject-specific features.

In this paper, we study subject identification using ballistocardiography (BCG), an important physiological signal that measures the recoil forces of the body in reaction to cardiac ejection of blood into the vascular tree [20]. With advances in sensor technology (e.g. accelerometers), it has become easier to measure BCG signals using pervasive accessories such as weighing scales, beds, chairs, and wearables [9,12,16]. In particular, we use a modified weighing scale in our setup, which has two main advantages. First is the popularity of weighing scales – more than 80% of American households own a scale, and emerging smart scales leverage advanced capabilities [11]. Second, subjects naturally stand up when using a scale, which ensures that the BCG measurements are completely longitudinal.

Our system for identifying scale users from their BCG signals has many practical applications in the real world. One pervasive application is in smart scales which are already equipped with sensors with capabilities exceeding weight measurement. As these devices nowadays support multiple users, e.g., the QardioBase 2 supports up to 5 users [2], Withings WS-50 and Aria 2 support up to 8 users [1,4] and Garmin Index Smart Scale supports up to 16 users [3], reliable subject identification methods other than manual subject selection, phone pairing or weight biometrics would be beneficial.

While there has been prior work in identifying subjects using certain physiological signals such as electrocardiogram (ECG), electroencephalogram (EEG) and photoplethysmogram (PPG) [14,17,23], subject identification with BCG signals has been less studied. Recent studies using BCG for subject identification suffer from certain limitations [8,9,16,22], which we aim to circumvent in this

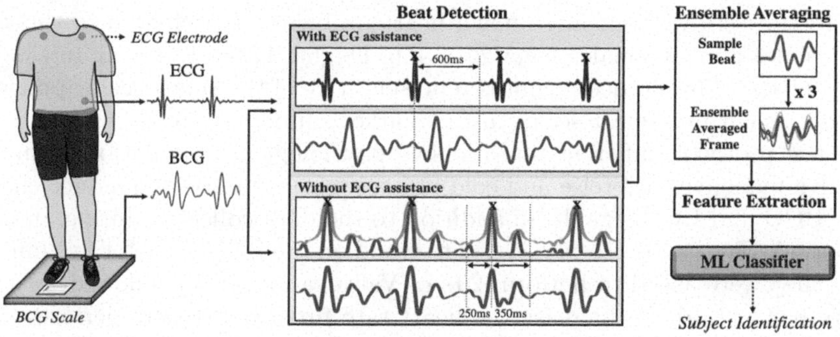

Fig. 1. Overview and steps of our approach

work. First, in most studies a wearable device (head-mounted or wrist-mounted) is needed to record the BCG signals [8,9,16,22], which may cause inconvenience to the user. In contrast, we rely on BCG signals collected from a modified weighing scale, without requiring wearables. Second, sensors on wearable devices only capture the local vibrations at specific locations in the body (head or wrist), whereas our scale can capture the longitudinal whole-body motions. Third, in existing studies BCG signals are collected while subjects are motionless in a specific posture without any external force or physiological modulation [8,22]. In contrast, we also study the effect of various physiological modulations such as Valsalva maneuver, exercise, and cold pressor. Finally, as discussed by Hernandez et al. [9], most studies require simultaneous electrocardiogram (ECG) recordings along with the BCG recordings [22], which can make it difficult to measure the effectiveness of BCG signals for subject identification in isolation. We propose and implement both ECG-assisted and non-assisted versions of our system, where the ECG-assisted version employs the simultaneous ECG signal only to improve beat detection and segmentation of BCG signals.

2 Methods

2.1 Hardware Setup

The overview of our study is provided in Fig. 1. Two types of physiological signals are recorded using our hardware setup: BCG and ECG. BCG signals are recorded using a modified weighing scale, the function of which was previously validated in [12]. The output of the scale is connected to the MP150 data acquisition system (BIOPAC System, Inc., Goleta, CA). ECG signals are recorded concurrently using BN-EL50 module (BIOPAC System, Inc., Goleta, CA) and transmitted wirelessly to the MP150. All signals are sampled at 2 kHz.

2.2 Experimental Protocol

This study was conducted under a protocol approved by the Georgia Institute of Technology Institutional Review Board and all subjects provided written consent. 10 subjects without any known heart problems participated in the study (five females and five males, age: 22 ± 0.6, height: 172.3 ± 9.8 cm and weight: 65.4 ± 9.9 kg). This subject count is representative of the smart scale application scenario, as current smart scales in the market support up to 5–16 users.[1]

In the protocol, different non-invasive physiological modulation techniques (Valsalva maneuver, exercise and cold pressor test) were used to induce changes in the BCG and ECG signals, in addition to the data collected during an initial rest period. First, subjects were asked to stand on the BCG scale for five minutes. Then, they were asked to perform 20 s of Valsalva maneuver followed by a two-minute rest period. To increase the heart rate further, subjects performed two minutes of walking exercise on a treadmill at 4.8 km per hour (kph). This walking exercise was followed by 90 s of squatting exercise. Subjects were then asked to stand on the BCG scale again for five minutes. At the end of this recovery period, each subject's left hand was immersed into 4 °C water for 15 s, followed by two minutes of a final rest period. Physiological signals were collected throughout the protocol. In total, we collected 14 min of data from each subject: five minutes of initial rest, two minutes after the Valsalva maneuver, five minutes after exercise, and two minutes after the cold pressor.

2.3 Pre-processing and Beat Detection

After BCG and ECG signals are collected, they are filtered with finite impulse response (FIR) Kaiser-window band-pass filters (0.5–20 Hz and 0.5–40 Hz, respectively). We propose two options for beat detection (Fig. 1): with ECG assistance and without ECG assistance, one of which is chosen depending on whether simultaneously recorded ECG signals are available. If a simultaneous ECG signal is available, for each BCG-ECG pair, R-peaks are detected on the ECG signal and the BCG is segmented into beats using the R-peak locations. The beat length is determined to be 600ms as previously done in [19]. These BCG beats are then ensemble averaged to remove noise and reduce the impact of outlier beats. The moving window size is determined to be 3 beats/frame with an overlap of 2 beats between consecutive ensemble averaged frames. We empirically observed that larger window sizes are not desirable, as they decrease the total number of ensemble averaged frames in each recording.

If a simultaneously recorded ECG signal is not available, we use the J-peaks of the BCG signals as our reference points. J-peaks are the points having the highest amplitude and occurring approximately 250 ms after the beginning of each beat [12]. To detect J-peaks, the BCG portion where amplitude is greater than zero is taken on the BCG signal and the upper envelope is constructed. The local maxima points in this envelope correspond to the J-peaks, which are detected from the enveloped signal. A minimum distance of 400 ms between consecutive peaks is enforced to detect the local maxima, which corresponds to a heart rate of 150 beats/min [9]. This strategy minimizes the risk of missing beats even if the subject's heart rate is high. Also, using an envelope function

[1] Examples: QardioBase 2, Fitbit Aria 2, Garmin Index Smart Scale.

flattens the actual BCG signal by covering the less prominent smaller peaks and makes the J-peaks more explicit, so that misdetections are prevented. Once the J-peaks are located, we take the BCG signal segments that are 250 ms before and 350 ms after each J-peak location on the BCG recording (600 ms in total). We keep the portion before the J-peak shorter than the portion after it, since the J-peak typically occurs around 250 ms [9]. The detected beats are ensemble averaged into frames using a moving average window size of 3 beats/frame, identical to the above.

2.4 Feature Extraction

Following the formation of ensemble averaged BCG frames as explained in the previous section, our system extracts relevant features from these frames. In particular, we focus on the I-J-K waves of the frames, which have previously been found clinically useful in cardiovascular performance assessment [10]. These features are also driven by the underlying anatomical structure of the heart, vasculature, and musculoskeletal system for the person, and thus exhibit more inter-subject variability compared to intra-subject variability, even in the presence of changing cardiovascular health.

Our system extracts a total of 12 features from each ensemble averaged frame, including the amplitudes and locations of I, J, K-waves; the durations of I-J, J-K and I-J-K segments; the RMS power of the I-J-K complex; and the amplitudes of I-J and J-K waves. As a typical J-wave occurs approximately 250 ms after the beginning of a beat [15,24], it can be detected by taking the peak with the largest amplitude in between 150–400 ms of the frame. The I and K-waves are determined as the valleys before and after the J-wave, respectively. For consistency, the same features are extracted regardless of whether ECG recordings are available, i.e., no ECG-related feature (such as R-R interval) is included in our feature set.

2.5 Classifier Training and Prediction

We pose the subject identification problem as a multi-class classification task that can be solved via supervised machine learning. Let D denote the training data. Each instance in the training data corresponds to an ensemble averaged BCG frame, and is of the form: $(\mathbf{x}_i, y_i)$, where $\mathbf{x}_i = (x_{i,1}, x_{i,2}, ..., x_{i,12})$ are the 12 features extracted as described in the previous section, and y_i is the label equal to the unique subject identifier of the subject that the frame belongs to. The training dataset D is used to build a classifier denoted $\mathcal{M}$ that learns to predict the subject identifier of a frame usings its features, i.e., $\mathcal{M} : \mathbf{x} \rightarrow$ subject ID.

We use Support Vector Machine (SVM) to train our classifier model $\mathcal{M}$, which is a popular supervised learning method in biometrics and bioinformatics due to its accuracy, flexibility, and ability to deal with high-dimensional feature spaces [25], as well as high performance in physiological signal analysis [9,26]. SVM aims to construct a hyperplane or set of hyperplanes that separates points from different classes with largest margins. In addition to linear margins, SVM can enforce non-linear margins through kernel functions [7,18] for capturing linear and non-linear relationships in the feature space. As such, we implemented SVM with *grid search* to automatically search for optimal hyperparameters, including the kernel function (linear or RBF), kernel coefficient γ (options ranging from 0.0001 to 1 in multiples of 10), and penalty parameter C (options ranging from 0.01 to 100 in multiples of 10). Our model supports multi-class classification through the one-vs-all strategy.

At prediction (test) time, an unlabeled BCG recording is provided to the system. This recording goes through the pre-processing, beat detection, ensemble averaging, and feature extraction process. At the end of the process, a set of *unlabeled* feature vectors are obtained: $\mathbf{X}^u = (\mathbf{x}_1^u, \mathbf{x}_2^u, ..., \mathbf{x}_n^u)$, where n is the number of ensemble averaged frames in the unlabeled recording. Each of the unlabeled feature vectors are provided to $\mathcal{M}$, and $\mathcal{M}$ predicts a label for each vector, collectively denoted by: $Y^u = (y_1^u, y_2^u, ..., y_n^u)$. Finally, our system predicts the subject of the whole test BCG recording using the label that is observed most number of times in Y^u. We denote this final output prediction by y_{pred}.

2.6 Confidence Measurement and Threshold

In our system, each prediction is associated with a *confidence* value, denoting how confident our system is in predicting that y_{pred} is the true subject ID of a test BCG recording. Prediction confidence is measured as:

$$\text{Confidence} = \frac{\#\text{ of occurrences of } y_{pred} \text{ in } Y^u}{|Y^u|} \tag{1}$$

We use a threshold τ such that for a test recording with confidence $< \tau$, our system outputs that subject identification was unsuccessful for that recording (i.e., "subject could not be found"), instead of making an unconfident prediction which has higher risk of being incorrect. If confidence $\geq \tau$, the system outputs y_{pred} as usual.

Our confidence-based thresholding approach has multiple advantages. When using a smart scale, if the scale is not sufficiently confident who the user is, it could be preferable that the user manually tells the scale who the user is, instead of the scale carrying a higher risk of misidentifying the user. Misidentifications may allow one scale user to view another user's data which could be sensitive (e.g., pregnant housemember), or misidentified user's readings may be saved under another user's name which may cause problems in long-term health tracking. Furthermore, in future BCG-based biometric authentication systems that grant access to classified environments, mispredictions and false positives should be avoided since they may grant access to unauthorized users. On the other hand, finding an appropriate value for the threshold parameter τ is worthy of investigation. By definition, $\tau \in [0, 1]$. Having a large τ has the desirable outcome that we prevent incorrect predictions, since incorrect predictions typically have lower confidence. However, if τ is too large, some correct predictions (true positives) which do not have as large confidence might be lost. We empirically study the impact of different τ in a variety of settings in Sect. 3.2.

3 Evaluation and Results

In the experiments, we operate in multiples of 20 s since it is a reasonable amount of time to stand on a smart scale for BMI, vital signs, and fat and water percentage measurement. To do so, we divide the continuous BCG and ECG signals into 20-s long segments to obtain multiple non-overlapping recordings per subject. We use leave-k-recordings-out cross-validation (LkRO-CV), i.e., we run multiple iterations where in each iteration we leave out k recordings of each subject (out of n total recordings per subject) from the training data. These k recordings constitute the test data, whereas the remaining $n-k$ recordings constitute the training data.

3.1 Subject Identification Accuracy

We measure the subject identification accuracy of our approach under two scenarios. First, we keep the test recording durations fixed and vary the total training data duration for each subject. Note here that training data does not need to be collected in one session; data from multiple sessions can be concatenated. Second, we keep the total training data duration fixed and vary the test recording durations for each subject. We report the results in Figs. 2a and 2b.

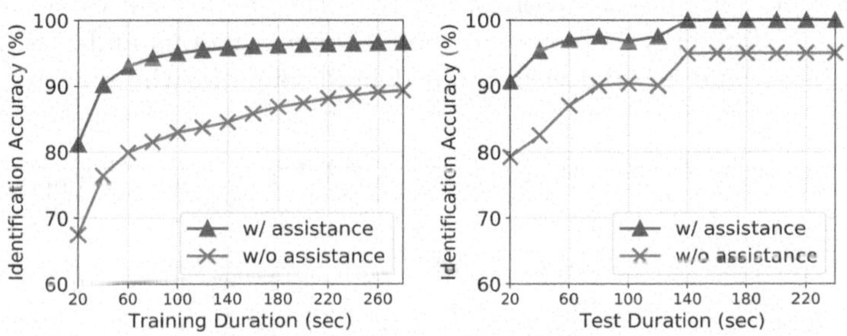

(a) Varying training duration (b) Varying test duration

Fig. 2. Subject identification accuracy of our approach with and without ECG assistance in beat detection. In (a), test recording duration is fixed to 20 s. In (b), total training data duration per subject is fixed to 1 min.

In Fig. 2a, the test recording duration is fixed to 20 s and we experiment with total training duration varying between 20 s and 280 s. Overall, we observe that ECG assistance in beat detection improves the subject identification accuracy of our system. Although the accuracy difference between the assisted and non-assisted versions is 14% when training durations are short (e.g., 20 s), the difference decreases as longer training data becomes available and becomes less than 7% when total training data duration is 4 min or longer. Furthermore, 1 min of training data is sufficient for our system to achieve 80% and 93% subject identification accuracy in the non-assisted and assisted cases, respectively.

This training data can be collected in 3 initial sessions of scale usage. Note that the accuracy of random prediction is only 10% (since we have 10 test subjects). Having more training data clearly improves accuracy, as shown by the accuracy becoming 97% with 4 min or more training data.

In Fig. 2b, the total training data duration is fixed to 1 min per subject and we experiment with test recording durations varying between 20 s and 240 s. We observe that subject identification is accurate even for 20 s of test recordings: 80% and 91% for non-assisted and assisted versions of our system. Accuracy increases substantially with longer test recordings and our system achieves 95% and 100% accuracy for the non-assisted and assisted cases, when test recordings are longer than 2 min.

3.2 Prediction Confidence

We vary the confidence threshold τ between 0 and 1 in increments of 0.1 and measure the mispredictions prevented as well as the correct predictions lost under different τ values. We report the results in Fig. 3 for three different training durations: 20 s, 1 min, and 4 min. In each setting, two lines are plotted: the ratio of mispredictions prevented and the ratio of correct predictions lost (due to a correct prediction not having sufficiently high confidence to meet τ). We observe that $\tau \leq 0.3$ causes little or no loss in correct predictions while being able to prevent some mispredictions. On the other hand, the value of τ which maximizes the difference between prevented mispredictions and loss of correct predictions is around $\tau \cong 0.6$ or 0.7 (our default value for the reported results).

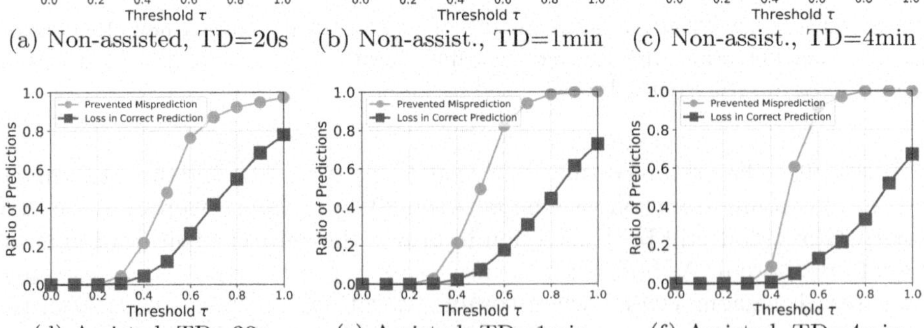

(a) Non-assisted, TD=20s (b) Non-assist., TD=1min (c) Non-assist., TD=4min

(d) Assisted, TD=20s (e) Assisted, TD=1min (f) Assisted, TD=4min

Fig. 3. Impact of confidence threshold parameter τ under different total training data durations, with and without ECG assistance. (TD = Training Duration)

In addition, longer training durations not only increase confidence in correct predictions but also decrease confidence in mispredictions. For example, with $\tau = 0.6$, the loss in correct predictions is 0.26 in Fig. 3d, it is 0.18 in Fig. 3e, and 0.13 in Fig. 3f. The confidence values for correct predictions must have increased to lose fewer predictions under the same τ. Furthermore, in Fig. 3d the prevented misprediction ratio is 0.76, in Fig. 3e it is 0.82, and in Fig. 3f it is 0.91. Confidence values for mispredictions must have decreased to prevent more mispredictions under the same τ. Hence, we conclude that longer training durations have a dual positive impact on prediction confidence.

3.3 Experiments on Physiologically Modulated Signals

In the experiments so far, we trained and tested our system using BCG signals from subjects' fully rested (sedentary) conditions. While we expect this to be the common setting, in some cases it is also possible that subjects are involved in some form of physiological exercise before they step on the scale, which increases their heart rate and results in non-traditional BCG and ECG signals. These are called physiological modulations. Recalling Sect. 2.2, we collected data with three types of modulations: Valsalva maneuver, walking and squats exercise, and cold pressor. To evaluate the generalizability of our approach, we also measure subject identification under physiological modulation. We perform training using either 1 min or 4 min of rest data and measure accuracy using modulated BCG recordings as test data. Results are provided in Table 1.

Comparing Table 1 with Fig. 2, we observe that on average, the accuracy of modulated recordings is 15–20% lower than rest recordings. This drop is expected, considering that the training data does not contain any modulation, hence our model is not acquainted with modulated signals with different feature values. In particular, we would expect the location (duration) features to have different values depending on the existence of modulation, due to increased heart rates and shortened R-R intervals resulting from modulation. Note that the type of modulation is also important; for example, exercise and cold pressor typically cause higher accuracy loss than the Valsalva maneuver. On the other hand, considering that the accuracy of random prediction is 10%, our results in Table 1 show that our approach still has substantial identification ability.

Table 1. Impact of physiological modulation on accuracy.

	Train data	Test data	Accuracy
Our approach w/ECG assistance	Rest (1 min)	Valsalva	0.820
		Exercise	0.708
		Cold pressor	0.721
	Rest (4 min)	Valsalva	0.863
		Exercise	0.773
		Cold pressor	0.779
Our approach w/o ECG assistance	Rest (1 min)	Valsalva	0.696
		Exercise	0.632
		Cold pressor	0.623
	Rest (4 min)	Valsalva	0.717
		Exercise	0.697
		Cold pressor	0.638

4 Conclusion and Future Work

In this paper, we studied subject identification using BCG signals collected from a weighing scale. In future work, we will consider its applicability to bed-, chair-, and wearable-based BCG sensors; as well as fitness equipment for identifying athletes in sports teams and medical equipment for patient monitoring in hospitals and long-term care facilities. We will also focus on validating our approach with larger datasets with more subjects, as well as customize our system according to the detected modulation impact to render the overall approach less susceptible to modulation-related accuracy loss.

Acknowledgements. Research reported in this publication was supported in part by the National Heart, Lung and Blood Institute under R01HL130619. The content is solely the responsibility of the authors and does not necessarily represent the official views of the National Institutes of Health.

References

1. Fitbit aria 2 review & rating, pcmag.com (2017). https://www.pcmag.com/review/357402/fitbit-aria-2
2. Qardiobase 2 review & rating, pcmag.com (2017). https://www.pcmag.com/review/357255/qardiobase-2
3. Garmin index smart scale (2019). https://buy.garmin.com/en-US/US/p/530464
4. Smart body analyzer (ws-50) (2019). https://support.withings.com/hc/en-us/articles/201490007-Smart-Body-Analyzer-WS-50-Setting-up-the-scale-for-multiple-users
5. User guide for smart weigh digital BMI body fat bathroom scale (2019). https://www.betterbasics.com/guide/SW-SBS500

6. Bolle, R.M., Connell, J.H., Pankanti, S., Ratha, N.K., Senior, A.W.: Guide to Biometrics. Springer, Heidelberg (2013)
7. Cortes, C., Vapnik, V.: Support-vector networks. Mach. Learn. **20**(3), 273–297 (1995)
8. Hebert, J., Lewis, B., Cai, H., Venkatasubramanian, K.K., Provost, M., Charlebois, K.: Ballistocardiogram-based authentication using convolutional neural networks. arXiv preprint arXiv:1807.03216 (2018)
9. Hernandez, J., McDuff, D.J., Picard, R.W.: Bioinsights: extracting personal data from "still" wearable motion sensors. In: 2015 IEEE 12th International Conference on Wearable and Implantable Body Sensor Networks (BSN), pp. 1–6. IEEE (2015)
10. Inan, O.T., Etemadi, M., Wiard, R.M., Kovacs, G.T., Giovangrandi, L.: Non-invasive measurement of valsalva-induced hemodynamic changes on a bathroom scale ballistocardiograph. In: 2008 30th Annual International Conference of the IEEE Engineering in Medicine and Biology Society, pp. 674–677. IEEE (2008)
11. Inan, O.T., et al.: Ballistocardiography and seismocardiography: a review of recent advances. IEEE J. Biomed. Health Inform. **19**(4), 1414–1427 (2015)
12. Inan, O., Etemadi, M., Wiard, R., Giovangrandi, L., Kovacs, G.: Robust ballistocardiogram acquisition for home monitoring. Physiol. Meas. **30**(2), 169 (2009)
13. Jain, A.K., Bolle, R., Pankanti, S.: Biometrics: Personal Identification in Networked Society, vol. 479. Springer, Heidelberg (2006)
14. Karimian, N., Tehranipoor, M., Forte, D.: Non-fiducial ppg-based authentication for healthcare application. In: 2017 IEEE EMBS International Conference on Biomedical & Health Informatics (BHI), pp. 429–432. IEEE (2017)
15. Lindqvist, A., Pihlajamäki, K., Jalonen, J., Laaksonen, V., Alihanka, J.: Static-charge-sensitive bed ballistocardiography in cardiovascular monitoring. Clin. Physiol. **16**(1), 23–30 (1996)
16. McConville, R., Santos-Rodriguez, R., Twomey, N.: Person identification and discovery with wrist worn accelerometer data. In: Proceedings of the European Symposium on Artificial Neural Networks, Computational Intelligence and Machine Learning (2018)
17. Odinaka, I., Lai, P.H., Kaplan, A.D., O'Sullivan, J.A., Sirevaag, E.J., Rohrbaugh, J.W.: ECG biometric recognition: a comparative analysis. IEEE Trans. Inf. Forensics Secur. **7**(6), 1812–1824 (2012)
18. Schölkopf, B., Smola, A.J., Bach, F., et al.: Learning with Kernels: Support Vector Machines, Regularization, Optimization, and Beyond. MIT Press, Cambridge (2002)
19. Shandhi, M.M.H., Semiz, B., Hersek, S., Goller, N., Ayazi, F., Inan, O.: Performance analysis of gyroscope and accelerometer sensors for seismocardiography-based wearable pre-ejection period estimation. IEEE J. Biomed. Health Inf. **23**, 2365–2374 (2019)
20. Starr, I., Rawson, A., Schroeder, H., Joseph, N.: Studies on the estimation of cardiac ouptut in man, and of abnormalities in cardiac function, from the heart's recoil and the blood's impacts; the ballistocardiogram. Am. J. Physiol.-Legacy Content **127**(1), 1–28 (1939)
21. Vhaduri, S., Poellabauer, C.: Multi-modal biometric-based implicit authentication of wearable device users. IEEE Trans. Inf. Forensics Secur. **14**, 3116–3125 (2019)
22. Vural, E., Simske, S., Schuckers, S.: Verification of individuals from accelerometer measures of cardiac chest movements. In: 2013 International Conference of the BIOSIG Special Interest Group (BIOSIG), pp. 1–8. IEEE (2013)

23. Wang, M., El-Fiqi, H., Hu, J., Abbass, H.A.: Convolutional neural networks using dynamic functional connectivity for EEG-based person identification in diverse human states. IEEE Trans. Inf. Forensics Secur. **14**, 3259–3272 (2019)
24. Wiens, A., Etemadi, M., Klein, L., Roy, S., Inan, O.T.: Wearable ballistocardiography: preliminary methods for mapping surface vibration measurements to whole body forces. In: 2014 36th Annual International Conference of the IEEE Engineering in Medicine and Biology Society, pp. 5172–5175. IEEE (2014)
25. Witten, I.H., Frank, E., Hall, M.A., Pal, C.J.: Data Mining: Practical Machine Learning Tools and Techniques. Morgan Kaufmann (2016)
26. Zakeri, V., Akhbardeh, A., Alamdari, N., Fazel-Rezai, R., Paukkunen, M., Tavakolian, K.: Analyzing seismocardiogram cycles to identify the respiratory phases. IEEE Trans. Biomed. Eng. **64**(8), 1786–1792 (2017)

Detection of Multiple Small Moving Targets Against Complex Ground Background

Junhua Yan[1,2](✉), Jingchun Qi[2], Xuyang Cai[2], Yin Zhang[1,2], Kun Zhang[2], and Yue Ma[2]

[1] Key Laboratory of Space Photoelectric Detection and Perception (Nanjing University of Aeronautics and Astronautics), Ministry of Industry and Information Technology, No. 29 Yudao Street, Nanjing 210016, China
yjh9758@126.com

[2] College of Astronautics, Nanjing University of Aeronautics and Astronautics, Nanjing 210016, Jiangsu, China

Abstract. To tackle the problem that it is difficult to detect small moving targets accurately against complex ground background, a target detection algorithm that combines target motion information and trajectory association is proposed. To tackle the problem of small target size, firstly, background motion compensation is performed to obtain the background motion parameters. Then, forward and backward motion history maps are calculated to fuse continuous difference images for enhanced motion information of small targets. Finally, morphology processing is used to obtain the area of small moving targets. To tackle the problem of complex background, the Kalman predictor is used to predict the target position, and the Hungarian matching algorithm is used to correlate targets to obtain the target trajectory. Then, based on the target trajectory, targets missed by detection are supplemented to improve the target recall rate and false alarm targets are filtered out to improve the target precision rate. Experimental results show that the proposed algorithm has good detection performance, with the recall rate higher than 93%, the precision rate higher than 92%, and the F-measure higher than 93%.

Keywords: Small target detection · Complex background · Target motion information · Trajectory association · Trajectory feature

1 Introduction

In this paper, we aim to investigate the detection of multiple small moving targets, such as flying UAVs (Unmanned Aerial Vehicle), against complex ground background. When the altitude of the photodetector platform is far above that of UAVs, the targets in the image have few pixels, making them small targets that lack morphology information. When UAVs and the photodetector platform fly above a terrain with complex features, the obtained images may have a complex background. In this paper, we focus on the above difficulties in order to accurately detect multiple small moving targets against complex ground background.

X. Gao et al. (Eds.): MobiHealth 2021, LNICST 440, pp. 293–315, 2022.
https://doi.org/10.1007/978-3-031-06368-8_20

Small moving target detection against complex background has always been a challenging issue, which have drawn extensive research attention.

In 2012, M. Hofmann et al. [1] proposed a method following a non-parametric background modeling paradigm, which adjusted foreground judgment threshold and model update rate according to background complexity. This method performs well when the background is steady but performs badly when targets are small. Siam M et al. [2] extracted FAST (Features from accelerated segment test) corners, and classified targets' optical flow through a clustering algorithm - DBSCAN (Density based spatial clustering of applications with noise) to detect moving targets. This method has difficulty extracting corner points and easily misses targets when the targets are small.

In 2013, Kwang Moo Yi et al. [3] proposed a pixel-based method modeling the background through dual-mode single Gaussian model (SGM) and compensating the motion of the camera by mixing neighboring models. This method is able to detect small targets, but the false alarm rate was high when background is complex. Shen Hao et al. [4] proposed a novel hierarchical moving target detection method based on spatiotemporal saliency. Temporal saliency based on Forward-Backward Motion History Image and spatial saliency is combined to get refined detection results. When the background is complex, the method is prone to miss detection, because the spatial saliency of the target is not significant.

In 2014, Shakeri M et al. [5] applied a two-level registration to estimate the effect of camera motion for motion compensation, extracted target pixels by Gaussian mixture model, refined noisy results using component-based and pixel-based methods, and improved the detection accuracy through the temporal coherence of foreground motion. This method performs well in complex environments, but it easily misses small targets. Sadeghitehran et al. [6] extracted BRISK [7] (Binary Robust Invariant Scalable Key points) corner optical flow features and classified targets' optical flow through ELM (Evolving Local Means) algorithm to detect moving targets. The method can adapt to complex backgrounds, but the detection effect is poor when lacking target texture information.

In 2015, Wang Z et al. [8] computed the 2-dimensional histogram of entropy flow field to estimate background motion, obtained the difference image through background motion compensation, and detected targets by spatial-temporal association. This method omits targets easily when targets are small. Wei Liu et al. [9] used an improved Oriented FAST and Rotated BRIEF (Binary Robust Independent Elementary Features) algorithm to achieve an accurate background moving model and then detected small moving targets in aerial video by multiplying four continuous difference images with morphology processing. The method has good real-time performance, but the detection results depend on the accuracy of the ORB (Oriented FAST and Rotated BRIEF) feature matching results. The target detection effect is poor when the background is complex. Artem Rozantsev et al. [10] used boosted trees algorithm for motion compensation, obtained spatio-temporal image cubes by stacking motion-stabilized image windows over several consecutive frames and detected targets in spatio-temporal image cubes through AdaBoost classifier. In 2017, they substituted CNN (Convolutional Neural Networks) [11] for boosted trees to better adapt to complex background. This method has difficulty obtaining accurate detection results when targets are small.

In 2016, Junhua Yan et al. [12] proposed a detection algorithm for small moving targets based on adaptive threshold segmentation. In this method, the background motion was compensated by pyramid Lucas-Kanade optical flow of feature points, so the difference images were binary segmented using an adaptive segmentation threshold to detect moving targets. This method has poor detection performance in case of complicated background because it is difficult to accurately compensate for background motion. Meng Yi et al. [13] proposed a detection algorithm for small moving targets based on multi-view aerial registration system. This method extracted global Harris feature points, then compensated for background motion through Delaunay triangulation match and accumulated motion energy to detect small targets. The disadvantage of this method is that background noise is easily mis-detected as moving targets in complex background. Yang T et al. [14] obtained target motion information by background model, built the motion heat map by target motion accumulation, and detected targets in the hot regions based on saliency-based background model. Although this method is suitable for small targets, it has high false alarm rate in complex background. Li Y et al. [15] proposed a novel spatio-temporal saliency approach, which calculated the spatial saliency map and the temporal saliency map on the spatial domain and the temporal domain, depicted the motion consistency characteristic of the moving target by continuous multi-frame video sequence, and obtained spatio-temporal saliency map by fusing them to detect moving targets. However, it is difficult for this method to detect targets in complex background.

In 2017, Lou J et al. [16] raised an approach for small targets detection through region stability and saliency. The stability map was generated by a set of locally stable regions derived from sequential Boolean maps. The saliency map was obtained by comparing the color vector of each pixel with its Gaussian blurred version. Both the stability and saliency maps were integrated in a pixel-wise multiplication manner for small targets detection. This method has high false alarm rate and bad detection performance when the targets are inconspicuous in complex background. Yan J et al. [17] put forward a moving target detection algorithm, which obtained background compensated images based on a nonlinear transformation model. This method can cope with image distortion caused by severe rotation of the detection platform and realize the detection of slowly moving targets in complex rotating background. However, the miss detection rats of this method is high when target size is small. Gao J et al. [18] proposed a method to detect small targets, which combined the self-correlation features of backgrounds and the commonality features of targets in the spatio-temporal domain. The method proposed a dense target extraction model based on nonlinear weights, and a sparse target extraction model based on entry-wise weighted robust principal component analysis to detect small targets, and suppressed background clutters based on target trajectory to improve the detection precision. This method has good detection result for infrared images, but the detection effect is poor for visible light images, where it is difficult to distinguish small targets from the background.

In 2018, Zhang Z et al. [19] proposed a novel flying target detection algorithm based on the spatial and temporal context. This method used multi-frame video sequences to calculate forward and backward motion history maps to extract temporal context information, used conditional random fields to extract spatial contexts, then fused spatial context and temporal context to detect flying targets. This method has poor detection results in complex background, where it is difficult to extract spatial contexts, resulting in low recall rate. Yan D et al. [20] used the ORB operator to extract global feature points, compensated the global motion model through affine transformation and calculated the difference image, then accumulated the multi-frame difference images to obtain the target motion energy map to accurately detect small moving targets in UVA videos. This method accumulates motion energy and has good detection result for small targets, but the false alarm rate is high in the case of complex background.

In 2019, Yi et al. [21] raised a method for fast small moving target detection guided by visual saliency (TDGS), which extracted visual salient regions including small targets according to the differences in global features between the targets and the background, and detected small targets through their temporal relativity in multi-frames. This method has difficulty detecting targets when the color texture of the small targets resembles that of the complex background, resulting in low recall rate.

Therefore, this paper focuses on solving the problem of small target size and complex ground background. To tackle the problem of small target size, firstly, background motion compensation is performed to obtain the background motion parameters. Then, forward and backward motion history maps are calculated to fuse continuous difference images for enhanced motion information of small targets. Finally, morphology processing is used to obtain the area of small moving targets. To solve the problem of complex background, the Kalman predictor is used to predict the target position, and the Hungarian matching algorithm is used to correlate targets to obtain the target trajectory. Then, based on the target trajectory, targets missed by detection are supplemented to improve the target recall rate and false alarm targets are filtered out to improve the target precision rate. The block diagram of the proposed algorithm is shown in Fig. 1:

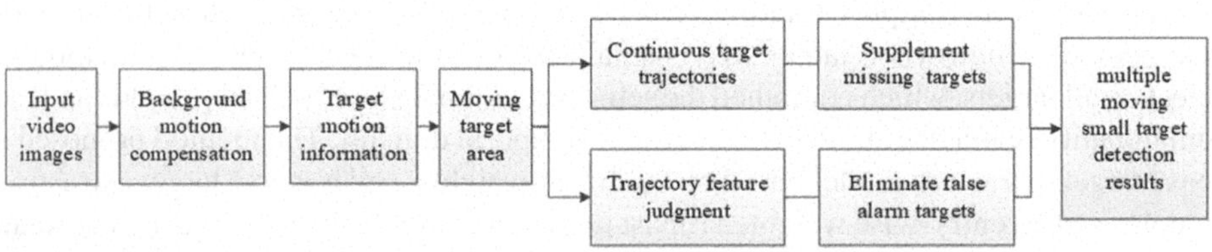

Fig. 1. Block diagram of the algorithm for multiple small moving target detection in complex ground background

2 Detection of Multiple Small Moving Targets

Small targets have a few pixels and lack shape information. Therefore, the motion information of small targets is used for detection, which are more suitable for small targets in the scene.

2.1 Background Motion Compensation

In this paper, regional random points and the Lucas–Kanade (LK) optical flow method [22] are used to obtain random optical flow tracking points. Regional random points can well represent regional characteristics and do not require much gradient calculations. Regional random points are uniformly extracted from the image I(t), and corresponding random optical flow tracking points are obtained from the image using the LK optical flow method, as shown in Fig. 2.

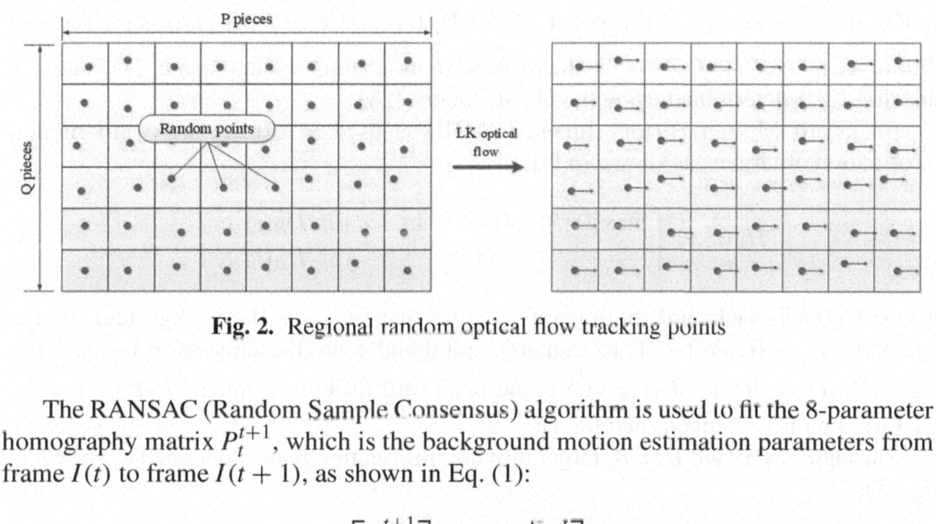

Fig. 2. Regional random optical flow tracking points

The RANSAC (Random Sample Consensus) algorithm is used to fit the 8-parameter homography matrix P_t^{t+1}, which is the background motion estimation parameters from frame $I(t)$ to frame $I(t+1)$, as shown in Eq. (1):

$$\begin{bmatrix} x_i^{t+1} \\ y_i^{t+1} \\ 1 \end{bmatrix} = P_t^{t+1} \begin{bmatrix} x_i^t \\ y_i^t \\ 1 \end{bmatrix} \tag{1}$$

where (x_i^t, y_i^t) is the coordinate of the regional random point in frame $I(t)$, and (x_i^{t+1}, y_i^{t+1}) is the coordinate of the corresponding optical flow tracking point. Background motion compensation is done based on background motion parameter P, as shown in Eq. (2):

$$I'(t \mp 1) = P_{t\mp 1}^t I(t \mp 1) \tag{2}$$

where I′ is the motion compensated image, "−" means forward motion compensation and "+" means backward motion compensation.

2.2 Target Motion Information

In order to enhance the motion information of small targets, the Forward Backward Motion History Image (FBMHI [23]) is used to fuse continuous difference images with background motion compensation in order to obtain the complete motion information of small targets.

Forward Motion History Image (FMHI) is used to extract forward motion information of targets, as shown in Eq. (3):

$$H_F(t) = \begin{cases} \max\left(0, P_{t-1}^t H_F(t-1) - d\right) & \textit{if } D_F(t) < T \\ 255 & \textit{if } D_F(t) \geq T \end{cases} \tag{3}$$

where $H_F(t)$ is forward motion information map, P_{t-1}^t is the background motion parameter from frame(t − 1) to frame(t), d is attenuation parameter ranged from 0 to 255. In order to form the span of pixel intensity values within continuous L frames, d is set as 255/L. L represents the effective number of layers of forward moving images within the FMHI, and L is set as 3 in this paper. $D_F(t)(D_F(t) = \left|I(t) - I'(t-1)\right|)$ is the forward difference image, and $I'(t-1)$ is the forward motion compensated image. The adaptive threshold T is determined using the OTSU theory [24].

Backward Motion History Image (BMHI) is used to extract backward motion information of targets, as shown in Eq. (4):

$$H_B(t) = \begin{cases} \max\left(0, P_{t+1}^t H_B(t+1) - d\right) & \textit{if } D_B(t) < T \\ 255 & \textit{if } D_B(t) \geq T \end{cases} \tag{4}$$

where $H_B(t)$ is backward motion information map, P_{t+1}^t is the background motion parameter from frame(t + 1) to frame(t), and d and T are the same as in formula (3). $D_B(t)(D_B(t) = \left|I(t) - I'(t+1)\right|)$ is the backward difference image, $I'(t+1)$ is the backward motion compensated image.

Through FMHI and BMHI, target moving information map is obtained as shown in Eq. (5):

$$H_{FB}(t) = \min(blur(H_F(t)), blur(H_B(t))) \tag{5}$$

where $blur(\bullet)$ is a smoothing filter which effectively reduces the impact of background noise. $\min(\bullet)$ operation can effectively suppress the trail of the motion history map to guarantee that the detected pixels are those within the boundary of moving targets. The target motion information map $H_{FB}(t)$ is shown in Fig. 3.

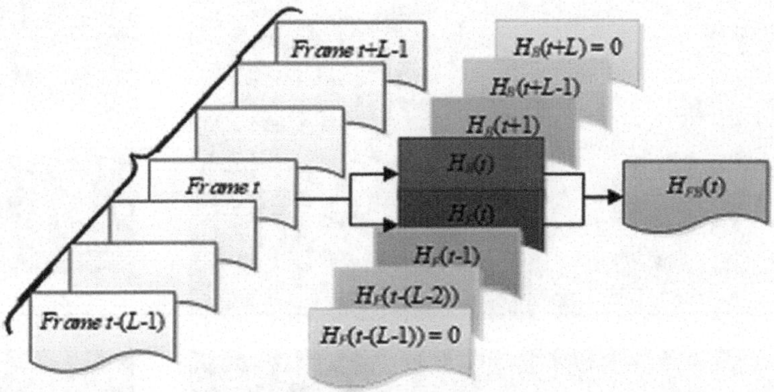

Fig. 3. Target motion information extraction

2.3 Extraction of Moving Target Area

Double thresholds are calculated on the target motion information map $H_{FB}(t)$ with the Otsu method, and the lower threshold δ is used to retain the recall rate of targets. $H_{FB}(t)$ is binarized to get the binary map $M_{FB}(t)$, as shown in Eq. (6).

$$M_{FB}(t) = \begin{cases} 255 & H_{FB}(t) > \delta \\ 0 & H_{FB}(t) \leq \delta \end{cases} \tag{6}$$

One erosion and two dilation operations are performed on the binary map $M_{FB}(t)$ to get the moving target area map $M_{RGE}(t)$, as shown in Fig. 4.

$$M_{REG}(t) = ((M_{FB}(t) \ominus b_{erode}) \oplus b_{dilate}) \oplus b_{dilate} \tag{7}$$

where $\ominus$ and $\oplus$ respectively represents erosion and dilation operation, and b_{erode} and b_{dilate} respectively represents rhombus structure element whose R = 1 and R = 3, with R being the radius.

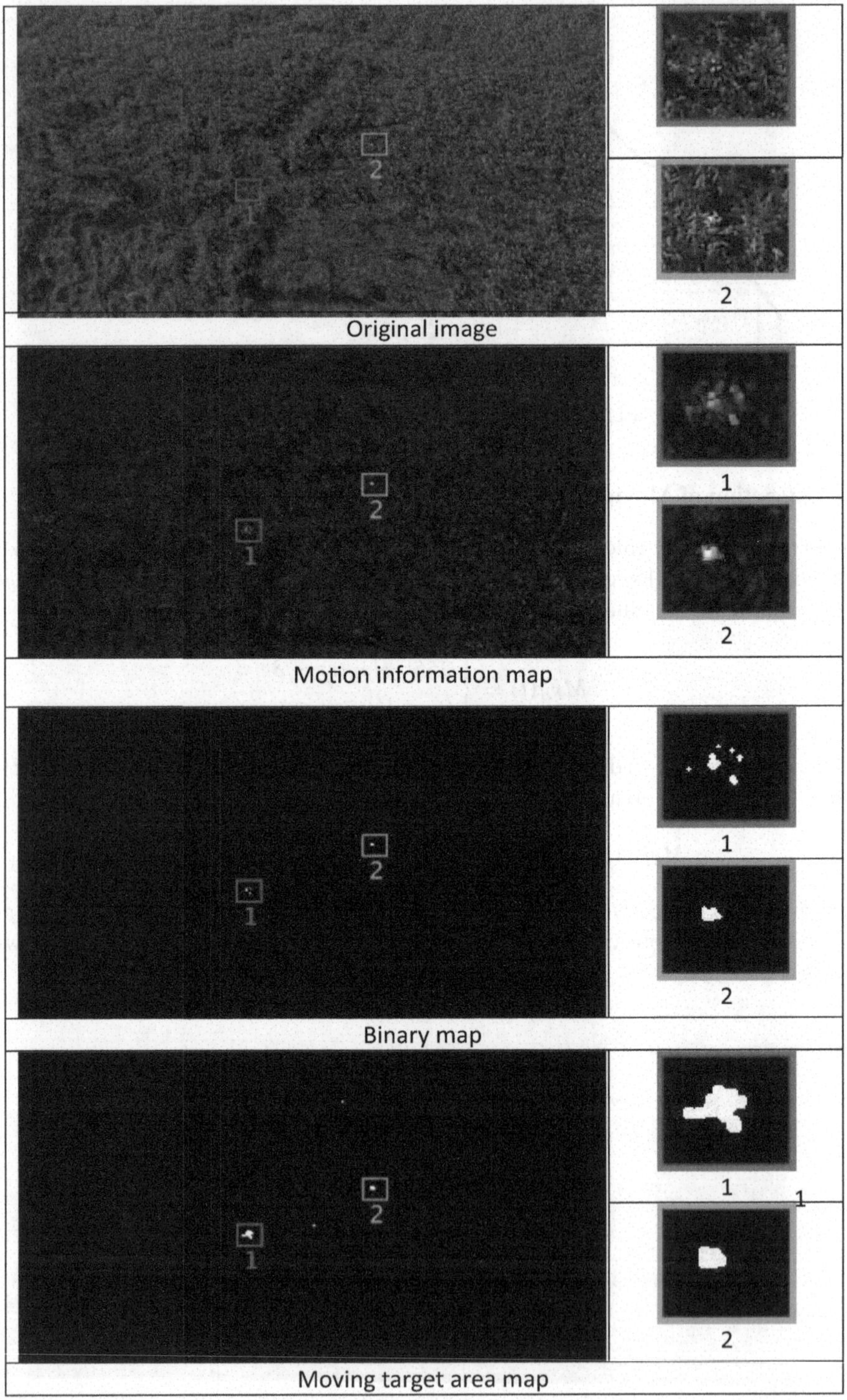

Fig. 4. Moving target area map extraction

3 Detection of Multiple Small Moving Targets Against Complex Ground Background

There are some missed detections and false alarms in the moving target area map $M_{RGE}(t)$. When the background is complex, the false alarm rate increases, and the contrast between small targets and the background is inconspicuous, making it difficult to detect small targets. The Kalman predictor is used to predict each target's position. Based on the Euclidean distance between the detected target position and the predicted target position, the Hungarian matching algorithm is used to correlate targets to obtain multiple target trajectories. If no detected target has the position that matches the predicted target position, which indicates missed detection, then the missed target is supplemented at the predicted target position to improve the recall rate. If the false alarm trajectory features are different from the target trajectory features, then the trajectory features are used to filter out false alarm target trajectories to improve precision rate.

3.1 Target Trajectories Association

Within the moving target area map $M_{RGE}(t)$, the target's location in the next frame $M_{RGE}(t+1)$ can be predicted. Based on the Euclidean distance between the detected target position and the predicted target position, corresponding targets are associated to form multiple target trajectories.

1) Predict targets. Eight-connected domain algorithm is used to detect targets and their locations, then the Kalman predictor is used to predict each target's position in the next frame $M_{RGE}(t+1)$.
2) Detect targets. Eight-connected Domain algorithm is used to detect targets and their locations in $M_{RGE}(t+1)$.
3) Associate targets. In $M_{RGE}(t+1)$, the detected position and the predicted position of each target is matched. If the detected position of the target matches the predicted position, they are associated as the same target. If the predicted position of the target matches none of the detected positions, which indicates missed detection, then the missed target is supplemented at the predicted position in $M_{RGE}(t+1)$. If the detected position of the target matches none of the predicted positions, then this indicates that a new target appears.
4) Determine target trajectory. All the associated targets are determined as target trajectories, if the target in one trajectory is supplemented at the predicted position for five consecutive frames, the target is considered to have disappeared, and the trajectory will be deleted. Then the target trajectories are determined, as shown in Fig. 5.

In Fig. 5, the targets which are associated in the 1st, 2nd and 3rd frames are determined as three target trajectories. Their labels are ID1, ID2 and ID3. A new target appears in the 4th frame and is labeled as ID4. In the consecutive 5th, 6th, 7th, 8th and 9th frames, the target trajectory ID3P is supplemented at the predicted position, which suggests that the target has disappeared, so the target ID3 is deleted from the 5th frame. In the 11th frame, the target ID1 is supplemented at the predicted position, which is marked as ID1P. In the 12th frame, the missed target ID1P is associated as ID1 again.

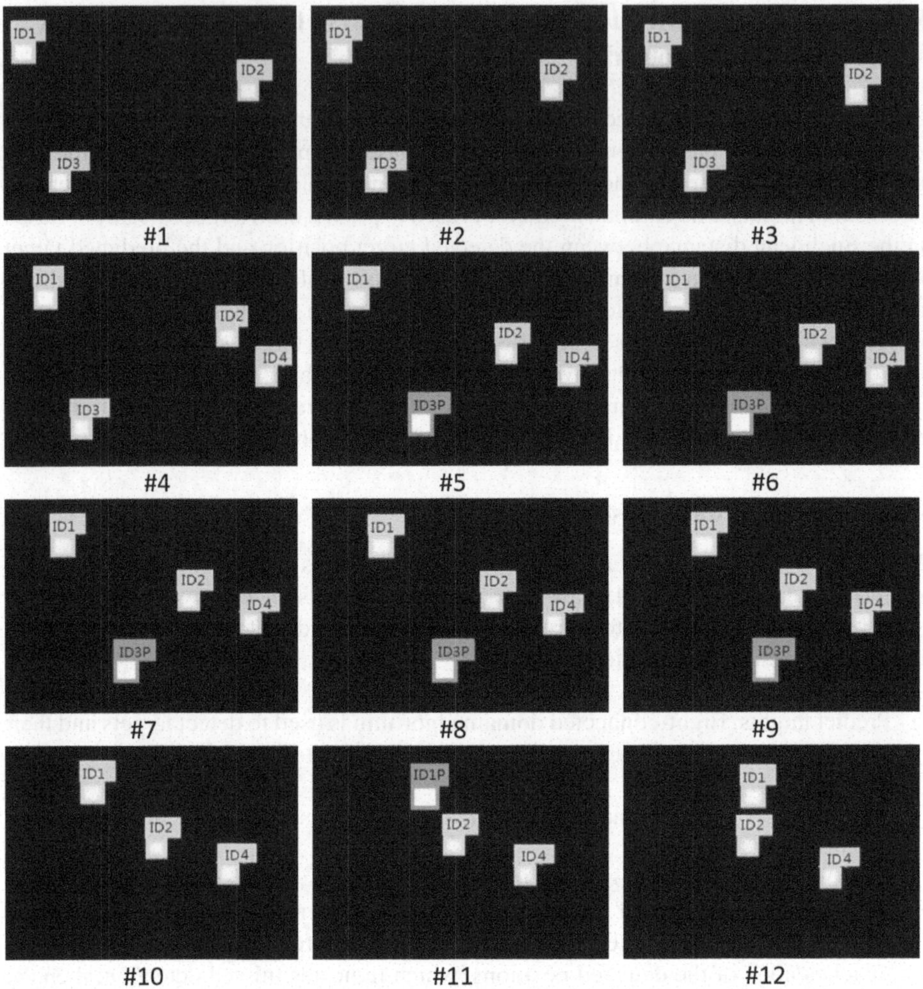

Fig. 5. Result of target trajectory correlation

3.2 Extraction of Target Trajectory Features

The trajectory features of the real targets are different from that of the false alarm targets, hence the trajectory features can be used to filter out the false alarm target trajectories. The target trajectory features include target area feature A, target position feature V and target movement direction feature D. The mean square error of the target area in the target trajectory is calculated to obtain the target area feature A. The target's area in the real trajectory changes little, so the value of A is small, while the target's area in the false alarm target trajectory changes greatly, giving a large A value. The mean square error of the moving pixels of the targets between adjacent frames in the target trajectories is calculated to obtain the target position feature V. The target's position in the real target trajectory changes little, so the value of V is small, while the target's position in the false alarm target trajectory changes greatly, giving a large V value. The mean square error of the angle between the target movement direction and the vertical direction in the target trajectory is calculated to obtain the target movement direction feature D. The target's movement direction is ordered in the real target trajectory, so the value of D is small, the target moving direction is disordered in the false alarm target trajectory, giving a large D value.

Due to the movement of the target, the target trajectory features change greatly during the existence of trajectories. Therefore, the target trajectories need to be segmented. Target trajectory features in each segment change little, which can improve the accuracy of false alarm target trajectories filtration. In this paper, 10 consecutive frames are used as a segment to extract the target trajectory features. As shown in Eq. (8–10), 'area' represents the size of the target area, 'speed' represents the moving pixels between adjacent frames, and 'direction' represents the angle between the direction of the target's movement direction and the vertical direction.

$$A = Var(area_t, area_{t+1}, \ldots, area_{t+9}) \tag{8}$$

$$V = Var(speed_t, speed_{t+1}, \ldots, speed_{t+9}) \tag{9}$$

$$D = Var(direction_t, direction_{t+1}, \ldots, direction_{t+9}) \tag{10}$$

Combining the target area feature A, target position feature V, and target movement direction feature D, the target trajectory feature vector S = [A,V,D] is obtained.

3.3 Filtration of False Alarm Target Trajectories Based on the Trajectory Feature Vector

In the trajectory feature vector S, when A, V, and D are less than the corresponding threshold, the trajectory is determined to be a real target trajectory; otherwise, it is determined to be the false alarm target trajectory, as shown in Eq. (11).

$$flag = \begin{cases} 1 \;\; if\ A < m\_area, V < m\_speed, D < m\_direction \\ 0 \;\; otherwise \end{cases} \tag{11}$$

where m_area, m_speed, and m_direction are thresholds corresponding to A, V, and D, which are related to the target motion in the video. The mean square errors of A, V, and D values are normalized to get the minimum values of A, V, and D. The thresholds corresponding to A, V, and D are determined by experiments to be double the minimum values. If flag is 1, the trajectory is determined to be the real target trajectory, otherwise, the trajectory is determined to be the false alarm target trajectory, as shown in Fig. 6.In Fig. 6, there are four target trajectories from the 1st frame to the 10th frame, which are respectively labeled as ID1, ID2, ID3, and ID4. The changes in area, position, and movement direction of the target ID1 are small from the 1st frame to the 10th frame. A, V, and D are all smaller than the corresponding thresholds, so ID1 is determined to be a real target trajectory. The change in the area of the target ID2 is large from the 1st frame

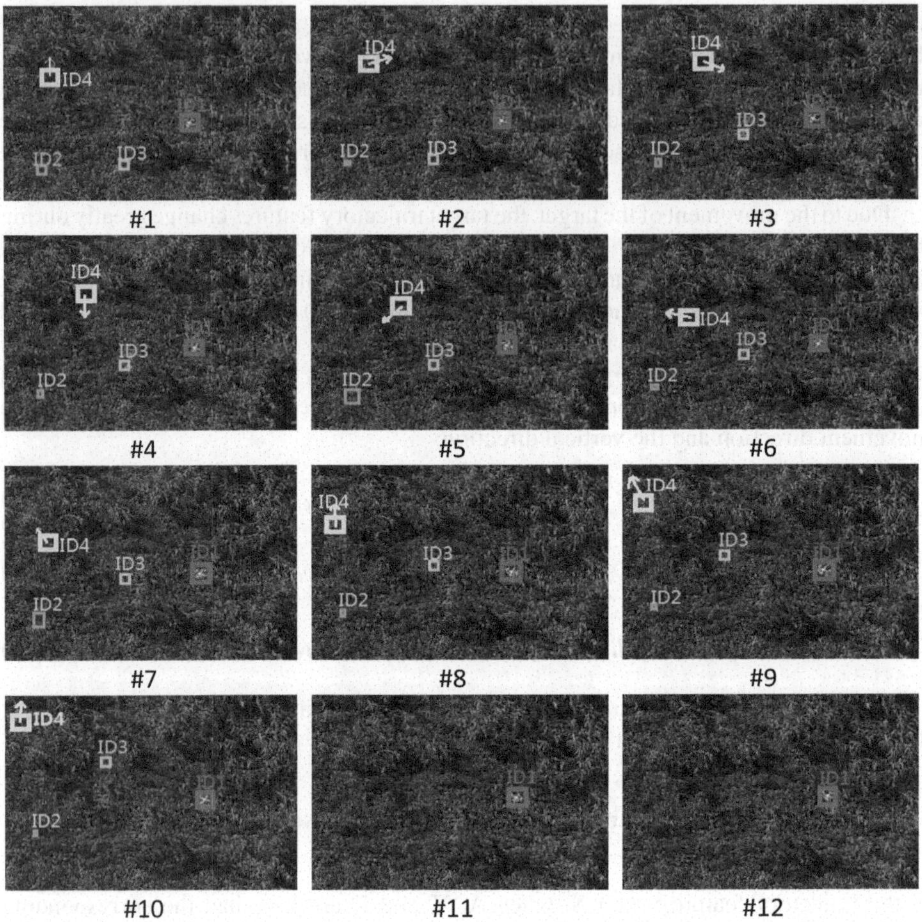

Fig. 6. Target trajectories

to the 10th frame. The minimum area is about 9 pixels in the 2nd frame and the maximum area is about 200 pixels in the 5th frame. A is greater than the corresponding threshold, so ID2 is determined to be a false alarm target trajectory. The change in position of the target ID3 is large from the 1st frame to the 10th frame. The target moves about 2 pixels from the 3rd frame to the 4th frame, and it moves about 30 pixels from the 9th frame to the 10th frame. V is greater than the corresponding threshold, so ID3 is determined to be a false alarm target trajectory. The change in movement direction of the target ID4 is large from the 1st frame to the 10th frame. The target movement direction is to the right in the 2nd frame, downward in the 4th frame and to the left in the 6th frame. D is greater than the corresponding threshold, so ID3 is determined to be a false alarm target trajectory. Therefore, ID2, ID3, and ID4 are filtered out.

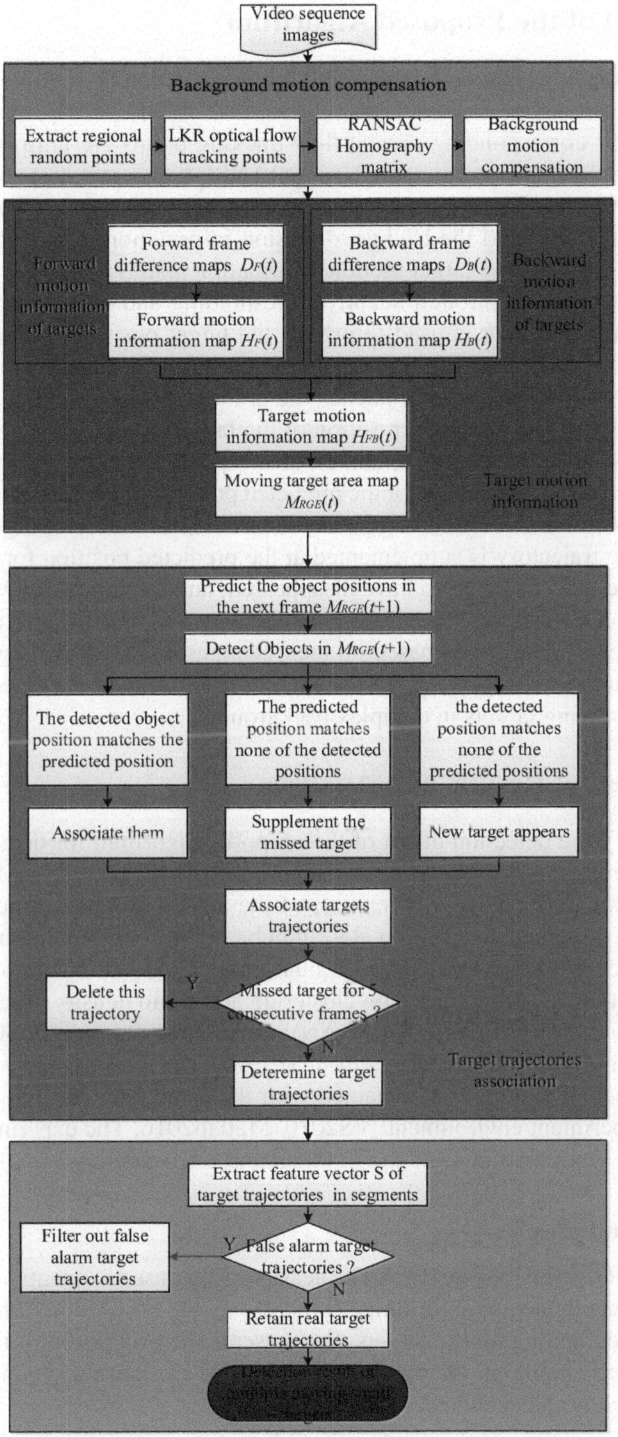

Fig. 7. Flow chart of multiple small moving target detection algorithm in complex ground background

4 Flowchart of the Proposed Algorithm

Figure 7 shows the flowchart of the algorithm for the detection of multiple small moving targets against complex ground background (DMSMT-CGB). Firstly, random points in the area and their corresponding optical flow tracking points are uniformly extracted, and the homography matrix is calculated using RANSCA to compensate for background motion. Secondly, multiple difference images are used to extract the forward motion information map $H_F(t)$ and the backward motion information map $H_B(t)$. $H_F(t)$ and $H_B(t)$ are fused to obtain the target motion information map $H_{FB}(t)$, and the target area map $M_{REG}(t)$ is obtained through adaptive thresholding and morphology processing. Then, the Kalman predictor is used to predict the target position in $M_{REG}(t+1)$, and targets are detected. The Hungarian matching algorithm is used to correlate targets. If the detected position of the target matches the predicted position, they are associated as the same target; If the predicted position of the target matches none of the detected positions, a missed target is supplemented at the predicted position. If the detected position of the target matches none of the predicted positions, it is determined that a new target appears. All the associated targets are determined as multiple target trajectories. If a target in one trajectory is supplemented at the predicted position for 5 consecutive frames, the target is considered to have disappeared, and the trajectory will be deleted. Finally, the trajectory features are extracted in segments, and whether they are false alarm target trajectories is determined based on their changes. False alarm target trajectories are filtered out and true target trajectories are retained to obtain the detection result of multiple small moving targets in complex background.

5 Experimental Results and Analysis

In order to verify the detection effect of the proposed algorithm for detecting multiple small moving targets in complex ground background. The algorithm DMSMT-CGB in this paper is compared with four other state-of-the-art algorithms for multiple moving target detection, which are a detection algorithm based on spatio-temporal saliency (ST saliency), a detection algorithm based on dual-mode Gaussian background modeling (DGM), a detection algorithm based on clustering algorithm density based spatial clustering of applications with noise (DBSCAN) and a detection algorithm based on the clustering algorithm evolutionary local mean (ELM).

All experimental results were obtained with the same data and initialization conditions. The experiment environment: VS2010, Matlab2016. The experiment platform: 3.60 Ghz-Intel i7 processor, 64-bit win7 system and 8 GB memory.

5.1 Evaluation Index

The recall rate (R), precision rate (P) and F-measure (F) are used to quantitatively evaluate the multiple target detection algorithms. R represents the proportion of targets that are correctly detected among all the targets. P represents the proportion of targets that are correctly detected among all the detection results. F is the harmonic weighted average of the two, which is calculated is as follows:

$$R = TP\Big/(TP + FN) \tag{12}$$

$$P = TP/(TP + FP) \tag{13}$$

$$F = \frac{(1 + \beta^2) \times P \times R}{\beta^2 \times P + R} \tag{14}$$

where TP represents the number of targets that are correctly detected as targets, FN represents the number of targets that are incorrectly detected as background, and FP represents the number of backgrounds that are incorrectly detected as targets. β determines the relative significance of the recall and precision rate. $\beta = 1$ means that the significance is equal. $\beta > 1$ means that the recall rate is more significant, $\beta < 1$ means that the precision rate is more (significant). After overall consideration of recall and precision rate, in this paper β is set to 1.

5.2 Experimental Data

For the purpose of the current experiment, the experimental video has to satisfy a number of conditions, such as background motion, small target scale, weak contrast, and complex background. It is difficult to obtain an experimental video that meets all the conditions above. In this paper, we obtained three experimental videos by field shooting.

The first experimental video (Translational grass background) contains 2000 frames of images with the image size of 1920 × 1080 pixels. The background of the images is grass, and the targets include a small white quad-rotor UAV (Unmanned Aerial Vehicle) and a black one flying in a straight line close to the ground from near to far. The camera platform is set on another UAV during shooting, which follows the two targets in translation motion. From the whole video, 500 consecutive images containing the target are selected to obtain the experimental video VD1.

The second experimental video (Rotational road background) contains 2400 frames of images with the image size of 1920 × 1080 pixels. The background of the images is city roads. The targets include a small white quad-rotor UAV and a black one slowly flying in a curve close to the ground. The camera platform is set on another UAV during shooting, which follows the two targets in rotation motion. From the whole video, 500 consecutive images containing the targets are selected to obtain the experimental video VD2.

The third experimental video (Pitching road background) contains 1000 frames of images with the image size of 1920 × 1080 pixels. The background of the images is city roads, and the targets include a small white quad-rotor UAV and a black one flying in a straight line close to the ground from far to near. The camera platform is set on another UAV during shooting, which is in pitching movement. From the whole video, 200 consecutive images containing the targets are selected to obtain the experimental video VD3.

In the above three experimental videos, the black UAV is the key target because it is similar in color to the background, and has a small size, which makes it easily obscured by the background. The characteristics and main detection difficulties of each video are shown in Table 1.

Table 1. Experiment videos

Video	Frame	Resolution (pixels)	Minimum target size (pixels)	Major detection difficulties
VD1	500	1920 × 1080	6 × 5	Translational background, scene motion, small target scale, weak contrast, black UAV obscured by background
VD2	500	1920 × 1080	20 × 15	Rotational background, complex background, black UAV obscured by background, the white and the black UAVs' slow relative motion to background
VD3	200	1920 × 1080	20 × 15	Pitching Background, complex background, black UAV obscured by background

5.3 Result Analysis

The proposed algorithm and other comparison algorithms are tested on the three experimental videos to compare the detection performance. Experimental results are compared and analyzed using the aforementioned evaluation indicators.

Detection of Multiple Moving Targets Against the Translational Grass Background. The performance of the proposed algorithm for detecting multiple moving targets against the translational grass background is verified on VD1. Experimental results of the proposed algorithm and other comparison algorithms are shown in Table 2.

Table 2 shows that the proposed algorithm has the highest TP, the lowest FP, the most correctly detected targets and the lowest false alarm rate, indicating superiority over the other four algorithms. The DBSCAN algorithm and the ELM algorithm are based on target feature points. In VD1, the small target size makes it difficult to extract feature points, hence the two algorithms fail to detect targets.

Detection of Multiple Moving Targets Against the Rotating Road Background. The performance of the proposed algorithm for detecting multiple moving targets against the rotating road background is verified on VD2. Experimental results of the proposed algorithm and other comparison algorithms are shown in Table 3.

Table 3 shows that the proposed algorithm has the highest TP, and the most correctly detected targets. Although the DBSCAN algorithm and the ELM algorithm have lower FP, the TP of these two algorithms are both very low, which means a large number

Table 2. Results of multiple moving target detection in the translational grass background

Algorithm	135th frame (2 moving targets)		385th frame (2 moving targets)		Whole video
ST saliency	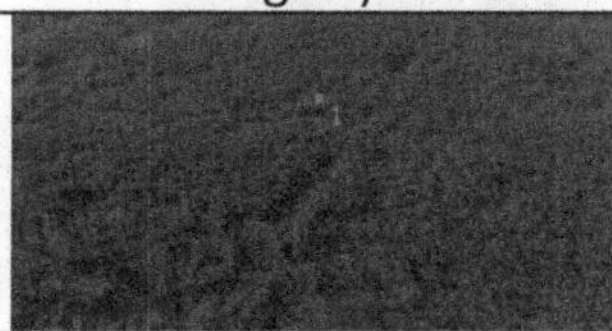		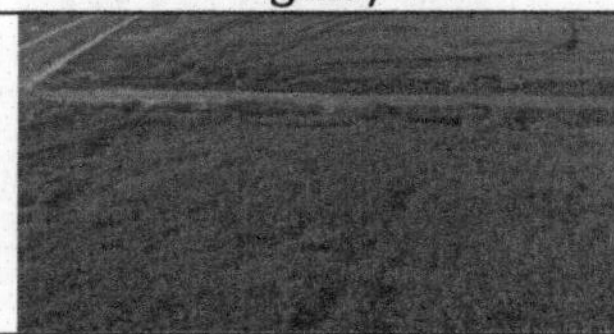		TP=488 FP=122
	1	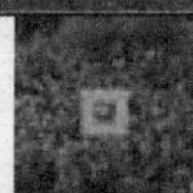	1		
DGM			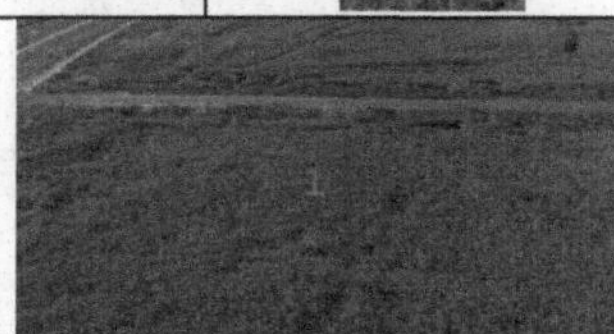		TP=388 FP=5581
	1	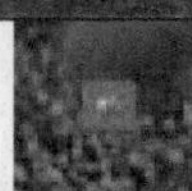	1	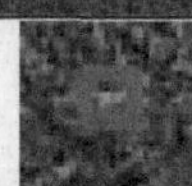	
DBSCAN			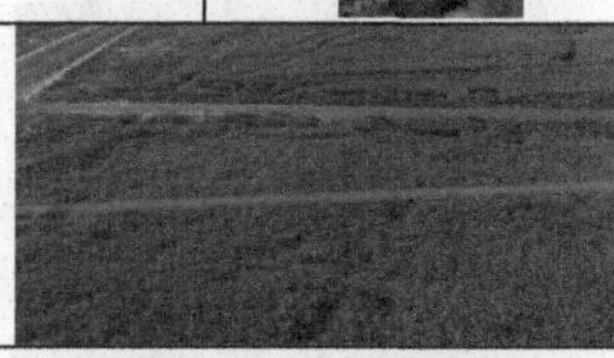		TP=0
	Undetected targets		Undetected targets		
ELM	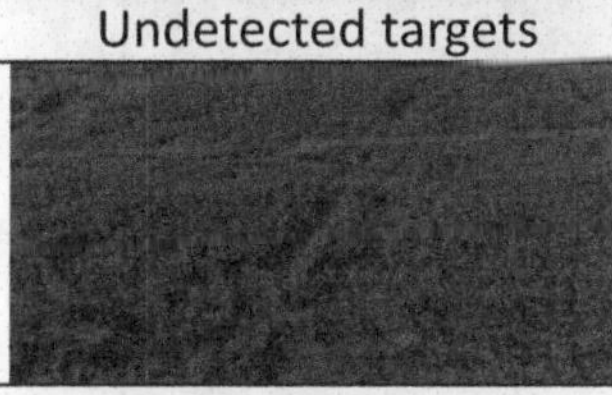		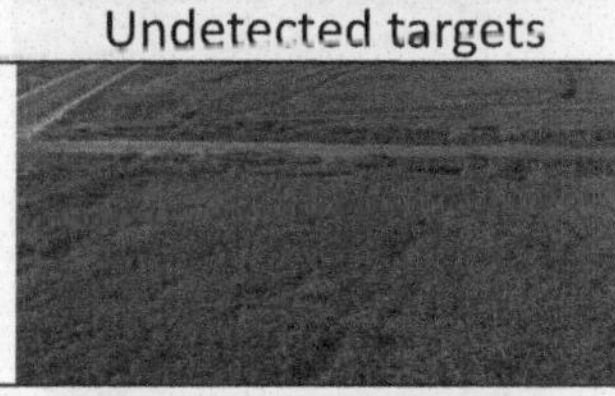		TP=0
	Undetected targets		Undetected targets		
DMSMT-CGB（OURS）	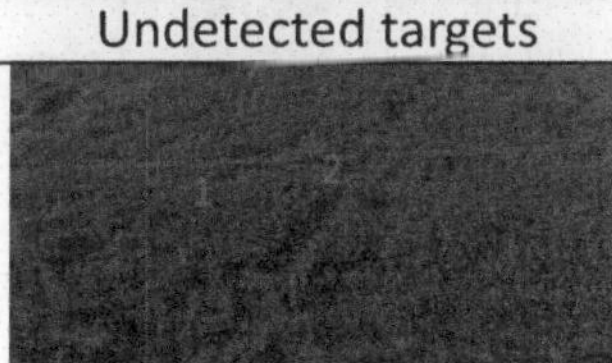		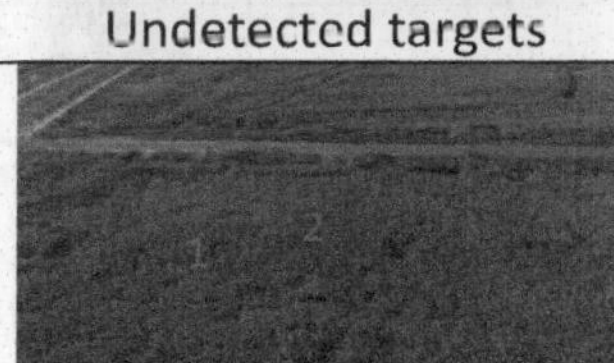		TP=933 FP=70
	1	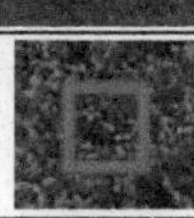	1		
	2	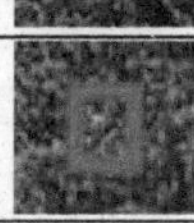	2		

Table 3. Results of multiple moving target detection in the rotating road background

Algorithm	15th frame (3 moving targets)		220th frame (2 moving targets)		Whole video
ST saliency	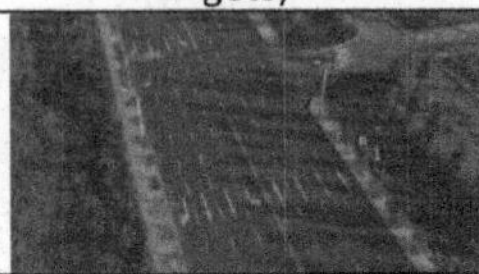		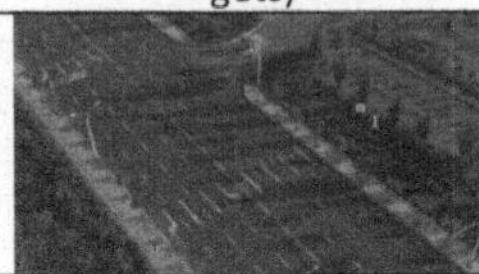		TP=518 FP=745
	1	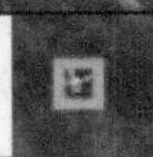	1	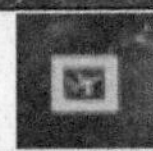	
DGM	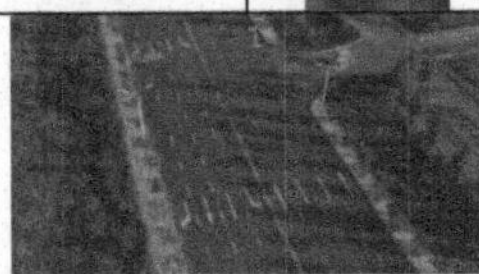		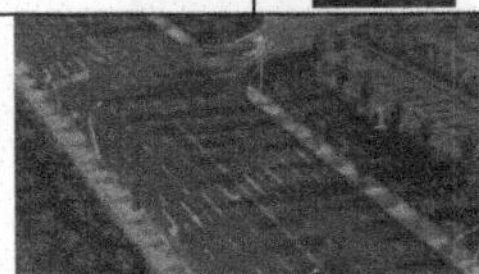		TP=509 FP=385
	1	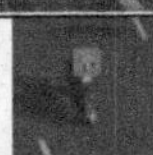	1	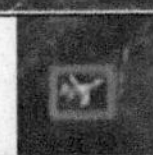	
DBSCAN	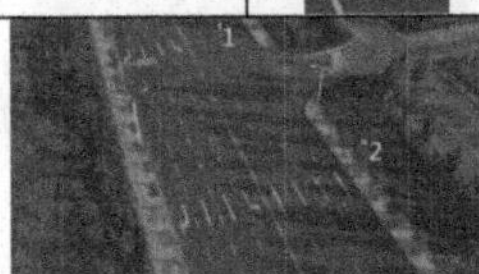		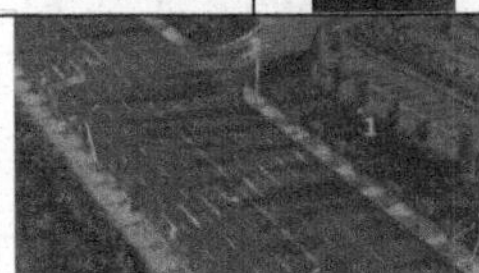		TP=309 FP=12
	1	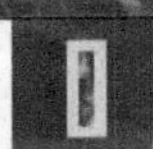	1	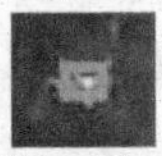	
	2	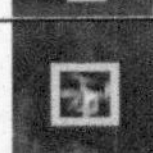			
ELM	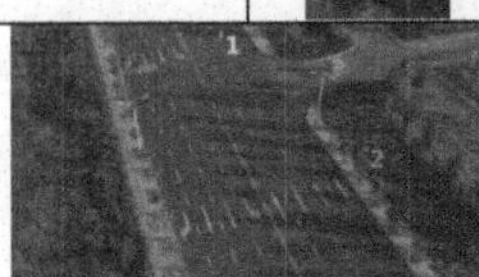		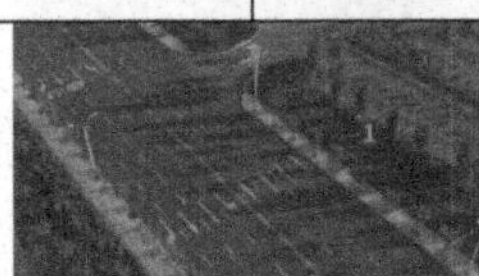		TP=324 FP=10
	1	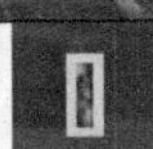	1	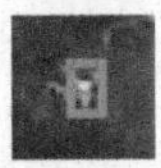	
	2	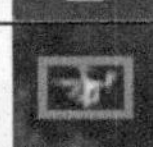			
DMSMT-CGB (OURS)	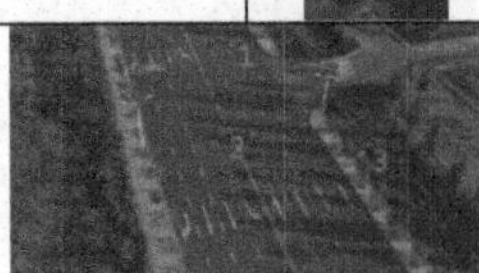				TP=1098 FP=89
	1	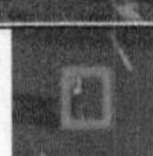	1	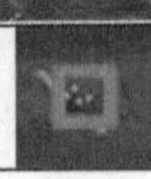	
	2	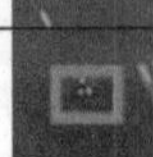	2	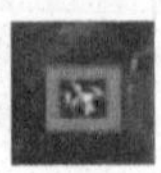	
	3	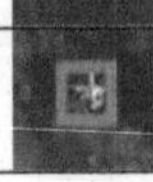			

of missed detections. The proposed algorithm has lower FP while ensuring the highest TP, which which means that the most number of targets are correctly detecting while ensuring few false alarms. Therefore, the performance of the proposed algorithm is better than the other four algorithms.

Detection of Multiple Moving Targets Against the Pitching Road Background. The performance of the proposed algorithm for detecting multiple moving targets against the pitching road background is verified on VD3. Experimental results of the proposed algorithm and other comparison algorithms are shown in Table 4.

Table 4 shows that the proposed algorithm has the highest TP and the most correctly detected targets. Although the FP of the ST saliency algorithm, the DBSCAN algorithm and the ELM algorithm are lower than that of the current algorithm, the TP of these three algorithms are very low, which means a large number of missed detections. The proposed algorithm has lower FP while ensuring the highest TP, which means that the most number of targets are correctly detected while ensuring the least number of missed detections and few false alarms. Therefore, the performance of the proposed algorithm is better than the other four algorithms.

Performance Comparison Among Multiple Moving Target Detection Algorithms. The performance of the proposed DMSMT-CGB algorithm is compared with the other four multiple target detection algorithms, and their performance is evaluated by recall rate (R), precision rate (P), and F measure (F) indicators. Experimental results are shown in Table 5.

Table 5 shows that the proposed algorithm has the highest recall rate R and F, indicating that our algorithm performs better than the other four algorithms. It is observed that in the experimental video VD2 and VD3, the precision rate P of the ELM algorithm is higher than that of the proposed algorithm by 4.5% and 3.4% respectively, and that the precision rate P of the DBSCAN algorithm is higher than that of the proposed algorithm by 3.8% and 2.6% respectively. However, the recall rate R of the ELM algorithm is 27.8% in VD2 and 46.5% in VD3, which is much lower than that of the proposed algorithm. Likewise, the recall rate R of the DBSCAN algorithm is 26.2% in VD2 and 50.5% in VD3, which is much lower than that of the proposed algorithm. In VD1, the DBSCAN algorithm and the ELM algorithm cannot detect the targets, so that the recall rate (R), precision rate (P), and F-measure (F) are all 0. Experimental results show that the proposed algorithm has the best detection performance for detecting multiple small moving targets against complex ground background.

Table 4. Results of multiple moving target detection in the pitching road background

Algorithm	10th frame (2 moving targets)		136th frame (2 moving targets)		Whole video
ST saliency	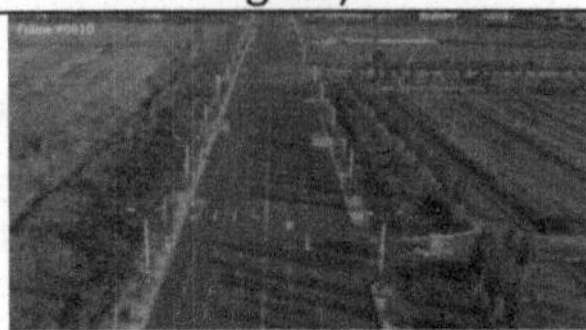		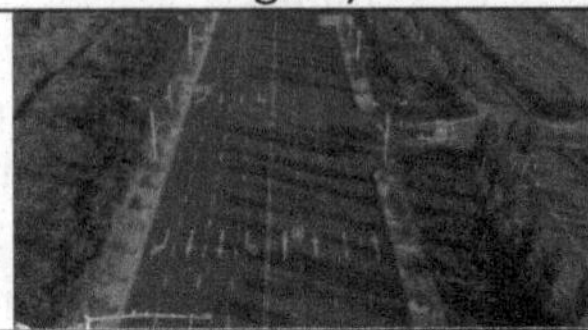		TP=236 FP=14
	1	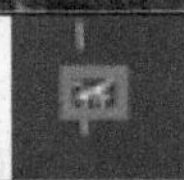	1	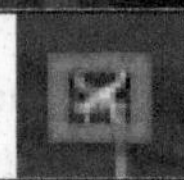	
DGM	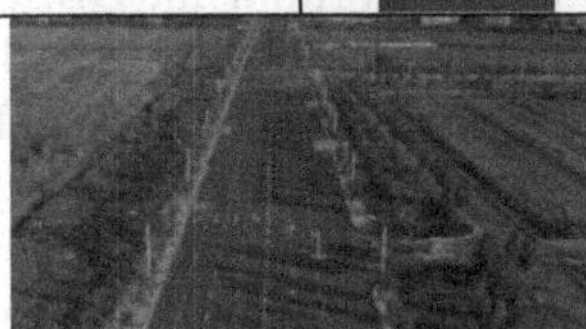		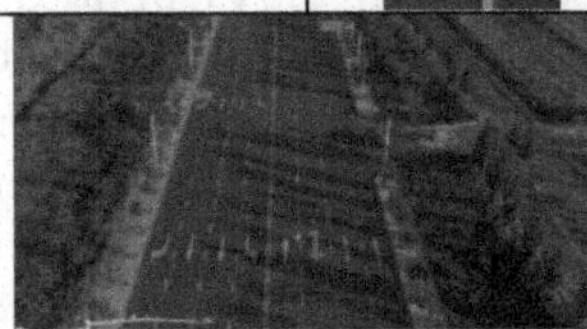		TP=350 FP=186
	1	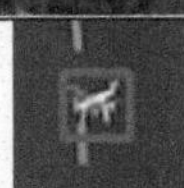	1	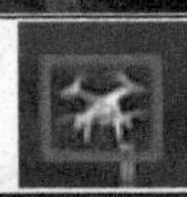	
DBSCAN	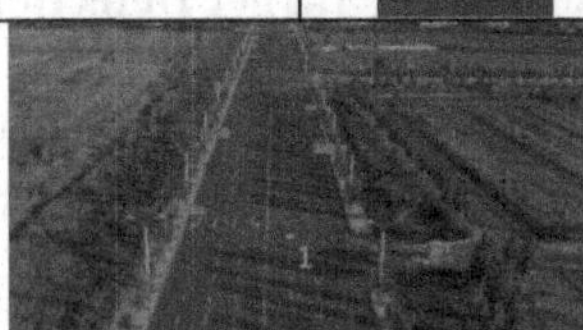		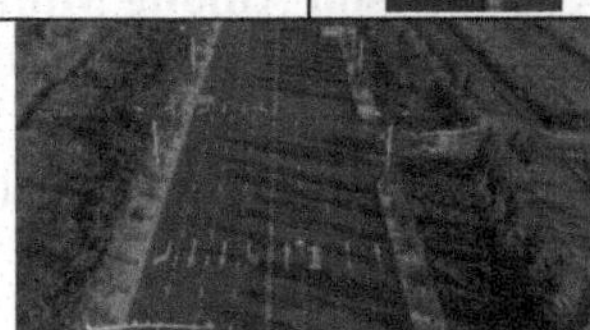		TP=202 FP=4
	1	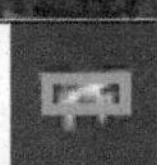	1	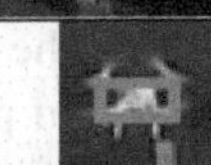	
ELM	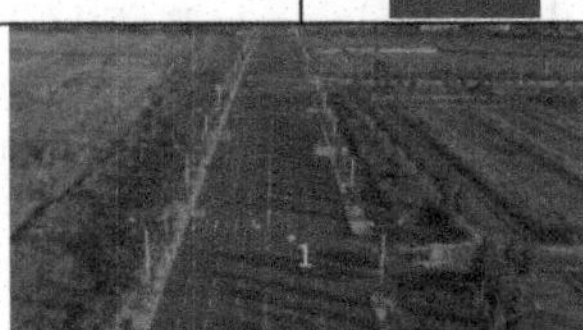		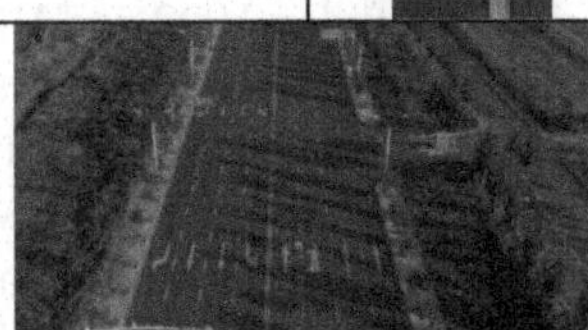		TP=186 FP=2
	1	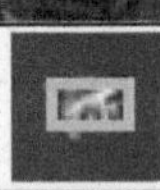	1	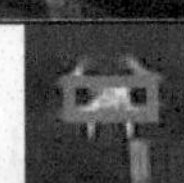	
DMSMT-CGB（OURS）	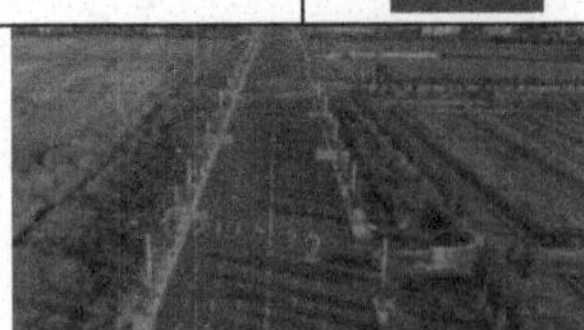		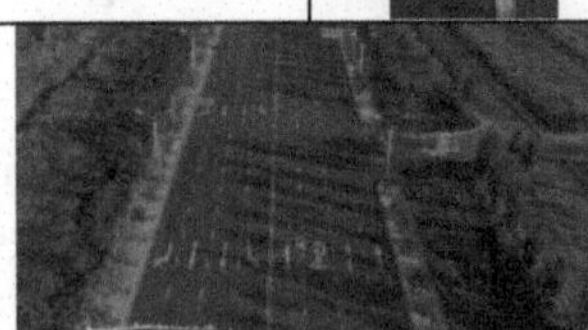		TP=389 FP=18
	1	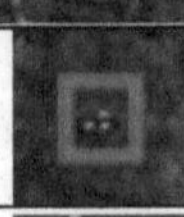	1	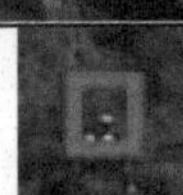	
	2	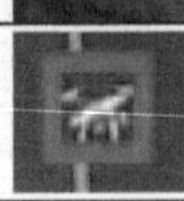	2	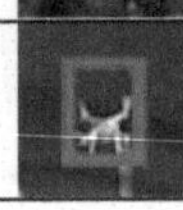	

Table 5. Performance evaluation of multiple small moving target detection algorithms in complex ground background)

	Algorithm	*R*	*P*	*F*
VD1	ST saliency	48.8	80.0	60.6
	DGM	38.8	6.5	11.1
	DBSCAN	0	0	0
	ELM	0	0	0
	DMSMT-CGB (OURS)	93.3	93.0	93.2
VD2	ST saliency	44.5	41.0	42.7
	DGM	43.7	56.9	49.4
	DBSCAN	26.2	96.3	41.2
	ELM	27.8	97.0	43.2
	DMSMT-CGB (OURS)	94.2	92.5	93.4
VD3	ST saliency	59.0	94.3	72.8
	DGM	87.5	65.3	74.8
	DBSCAN	50.5	98.1	66.7
	ELM	46.5	98.9	63.3
	DMSMT-CGB (OURS)	96.7	95.5	96.1

6 Conclusion

This paper proposes a multiple small moving target detection algorithm against complex ground background, which solves the problem of small targets, which have few pixels and lack topographical information, making them difficult to be accurately detected against complex background. In the proposed algorithm, multiple forward-backward target motion information is fused based on the FBMHI algorithm to improve the recall rate. Target trajectories are correlated to supplement missed targets at the predicted position and reduce missed targets. Target trajectory features are extracted in segment to filter out false alarm target trajectories, further reducing the false alarm rate. Experimental results show that the proposed algorithm has higher recall rate, precision rate and F-measure. Future research will be focused on conducting in-depth research on the detection of multiple small moving targets against severe rotational background, which will help solve the problem of accurately detecting targets by the photodetector platform under large-range UAV movement.

Acknowledgments. This work was supported by the National Natural Science Foundation of China (61471194 and 61705104), the Fundamental Research Funds for the Central Universities (NJ2020021, NT2020022), the Natural Science Foundation of Jiangsu Province (BK20170804), and National Defense Science and Technology Special Innovation Zone Project.

References

1. Hofmann, M., Tiefenbacher, P., Rigoll, G.: Background segmentation with feedback: the pixel-based adaptive segmenter. In: 2012 IEEE Computer Society Conference on Computer Vision and Pattern Recognition Workshops, pp. 38–43. IEEE (2012)
2. Siam, M., ElSayed, R., ElHelw, M.: On-board multiple target detection and tracking on camera-equipped aerial vehicles. In: 2012 IEEE International Conference on Robotics and Biomimetics (ROBIO), pp. 2399–2405. IEEE (2012)
3. Moo Yi, K., Yun, K., Wan Kim, S., Jin Chang, H., Young Choi, J.: Detection of moving objects with non-stationary cameras in 5.8 ms: bringing motion detection to your mobile device. In: Proceedings of the IEEE Conference on Computer Vision and Pattern Recognition Workshops, pp. 27–34 (2013)
4. Shen, H., Li, S., Zhu, C., Chang, H., Zhang, J.: Moving object detection in aerial video based on spatiotemporal saliency. Chin. J. Aeronaut. **26**(5), 1211–1217 (2013)
5. Shakeri, M., Zhang, H.: Detection of small moving targets using a moving camera. In: 2014 IEEE/RSJ International Conference on Intelligent Robots and Systems (IROS 2014), pp. 2777–2782. IEEE (2014)
6. Sadeghi-Tehran, P., Clarke, C., Angelov, P.: A real-time approach for autonomous detection and tracking of moving objects from UAV. In: 2014 IEEE Symposium on Evolving and Autonomous Learning Systems (EALS), pp. 43–49. IEEE (2014)
7. Leutenegger, S., Chli, M., Siegwart, R.Y.: BRISK: binary robust invariant scalable keypoints. In: 2011 International Conference on Computer Vision, pp. 2548–2555. IEEE (2011)
8. Wang, Z., Wang, C., Huang, F., Liu, J.: Based on spatial-temporal multiframe association infrared target detection. In: MIPPR 2015: Automatic Target Recognition and Navigation, vol. 9812, p. 98121A. International Society for Optics and Photonics (2015)
9. Wei, L., Weijie, Z., Cheng, L., Zhonglin, X., Kaiqiao, T.: Small moving object detection based on the improved ORB feature matching method. Optoelectron. Eng. **42**(10), 13–20 (2015)
10. Rozantsev, A., Lepetit, V., Fua, P.: Flying objects detection from a single moving camera. In: Proceedings of the IEEE Conference on Computer Vision and Pattern Recognition, pp. 4128–4136 (2015)
11. Rozantsev, A., Lepetit, V., Fua, P.: Detecting flying objects using a single moving camera. IEEE Trans. Pattern Anal. Mach. Intell. **39**(5), 879–892 (2016)
12. Junhua, Y., He, D., Qianqian, X., Yong, Y.: Slowly moving small object detection in complex moving background based on adaptive threshold segmentation. Electron. Des. Eng. **24**(06), 77–80+84 (2016)
13. Meng, Y., Yan, C.: Detection and tracking of small moving objects based on multi-view aerial photography registration. Comput. Eng. Appl. **52**(14), 27–31 (2016)
14. Yang, T., et al.: Small moving vehicle detection in a satellite video of an urban area. Sensors **16**(9), 1528 (2016)
15. Li, Y., Zhang, Y., Yu, J.G., Tan, Y., Tian, J., Ma, J.: A novel spatio-temporal saliency approach for robust dim moving target detection from airborne infrared image sequences. Inf. Sci. **369**, 548–563 (2016)
16. Lou, J., Zhu, W., Wang, H., Ren, M.: Small target detection combining regional stability and saliency in a color image. Multimed. Tools. Appl. **76**(13), 14781–14798 (2017).
17. Yan, J., Xu, Q., Duan, H., Yang, Y., Xiao, Y.: Slow ground moving object detection in rotating complex background. J. Imaging Sci. Technol. **61**(2), 20507–20511 (2017)
18. Gao, J., Wen, C., Liu, M.: Robust small target co-detection from airborne infrared image sequences. Sensors **17**(10), 2242 (2017)
19. Zhang, Z., Cao, Y., Ding, M., Zhuang, L., Wang, Z.: Spatial and temporal context information fusion based flying objects detection for autonomous sense and avoid. In: 2018 International Conference on Unmanned Aircraft Systems (ICUAS), pp. 569–578. IEEE (2018)

20. Yan, D., Sun, W.: Small moving object detection based on sequence confidence method in UAV video. In: Krömer, P., Zhang, H., Liang, Y., Pan, J.-S. (eds.) ECC 2018. AISC, vol. 891, pp. 676–683. Springer, Cham (2019). https://doi.org/10.1007/978-3-030-03766-6_76
21. Yi, X., Wang, B., Zhou, H., Qin, H.: Dim and small infrared target fast detection guided by visual saliency. Infrared Phys. Technol. **97**, 6–14 (2019)
22. Lucas, B.D.: An iterative image registoration techniques with an application to stereo vision. Proc. IJCAI **81**(3), 674–679 (1981)
23. Yin, Z., Collins, R.: Moving object localization in thermal imagery by forward-backward MHI. In: 2006 Conference on Computer Vision and Pattern Recognition Workshop (CVPRW 2006), p. 133. IEEE (2006)
24. Otsu, N.: A threshold selection method from gray-level histograms. IEEE Trans. Syst. Man Cybern. **9**(1), 62–66 (1979)

A Two-Stream Model Combining ResNet and Bi-LSTM Networks for Non-contact Dynamic Electrocardiogram Signal Quality Assessment

Guoqiang Zhu[1], Yang Li[1], Yonglin Wu[1], Zhikun Lie[1], Chen Chen[2], and Wei Chen[1,2](✉)

[1] Center for Intelligent Medical Electronics, School of Information Science and Technology, Fudan University, Shanghai 200433, China
{20210720211,w_chen}@fudan.edu.cn

[2] Human Phenome Institute, Fudan University, Shanghai 201203, China

Abstract. With the rapid advancement of monitoring without contact electrocardiogram (ECG), dynamic and real-time signal quality assessment (SQA) becoming a practical problem. In this paper, a two-stream structure that combines residual network (ResNet) and bidirectional long short-term memory (Bi-LSTM) for dynamic ECG (dECG) signals quality assessment is proposed. The ResNet stream is dedicated to extracting spatial features using time-frequency spectrum images as inputs. Meanwhile, the Bi-LSTM stream is devoted to exploring the temporal features using the ECG time series as the input. Then, these two streams are fused using a decision fusion mechanism and the performance is significantly boosted. As compared to the single stream-based approach, the proposed structure can compensate for either temporal or spatial information effectively. The overall accuracy of 99.69% can be achieved in distinguishing the dECG signal quality into three categories, namely clear ECG signal with clear R waves, blurry ECG signal without clear R waves, and noisy ECG signal with motion artifact. Experimental results show that this method demonstrates superior accuracy in determining the quality of dECG signals measured by the noncontact device. Therefore, the proposed model is expected to be a promising solution for non-contact dECG signal quality assessment in a practical ECG diagnosis.

Keywords: Non-contact ECG · Signal quality assessment · Convolutional neural network (CNN) · Recurrent neural network (RNN)

1 Introduction

With the fast-developing sensing technologies, the progress in non-contact electrocardiogram (ECG) monitoring is significantly promoted [1]. It's an important tool to detect cardiovascular diseases (CVDs) early [2]. However, noncontact measurement methods

X. Gao et al. (Eds.): MobiHealth 2021, LNICST 440, pp. 316–328, 2022.
https://doi.org/10.1007/978-3-031-06368-8_21

are sensitive to noise. These include baseline drift, electromagnetic signals, motion artifacts, etc. Poor signal quality affects reliable manual or automatic ECG analysis; a lack of signal quality makes it difficult to understand the correct diagnosis information [3], raises the probability of false alerts [4], and increases the assignment of doctors [5]. Therefore, it's important to use automatic signal quality assessment (SQA) methods. A reliable SQA method helps to give suggestions of re-take recording when signal quality isn't good [6], to improve the efficiency of information transmission by rejecting signals of bad quality [7], and to deliver reliable cardiac recordings for CVDs scanning [8].

Many studies have been conducted on the quality evaluation of ECG signals in the previous literature. With the development of computer analysis and processing capabilities, the ECG SQA algorithm can be split into three categories approximately: rule-based SQA methods, machine learning-based SQA methods, and deep learning-based SQA methods. Early designed signal algorithms were limited in processing capacity. Thus, low-complexity algorithms were usually designed with rule-based SQA methods combined with waveform and interval features [9, 10]. The accuracy of this method for multi-classification ECG SQA is barely satisfactory. It is also proposed that ECG SQA has been used using classical machine learning (ML) algorithms. However, to identify the available features, such techniques require time-consuming feature engineering. For instance, Y. Zhang [11] input some features from ECG signals into ML models like decision tree (DT) and support vector machine (SVM). Such classical ML models include many intrinsic limitations, such as weak generalization capability and boring feature extraction. Moreover, deep learning [12] doesn't require complicated feature engineering and has been widely applied to many domains such as picture classification [13], voice recognition [14], and Intelligent translation [15]. Non-contact ECG signals are non-stationary millivolt signals with a low signal-to-noise ratio and it is easy to be interfered with by other signals. Therefore, it's hard to classify the dECG signals with high accuracy through a single neural network. In this paper, a dECG classification algorithm based on deep Residual Networks (ResNet) and Bi-directional Long Short-Term Memory (Bi-LSTM) networks is proposed, which achieves a high accuracy three-classes classification of dECG signals.

The rest of the article is on the following: Sect. 2 introduces the Materials and Methods. Section 3 introduces the experimental setup, results, and comparison with other methods. Finally, a conclusion is in Sect. 4.

2 Materials and Methods

In this section, we will introduce the materials and methods involved in our work. Firstly, we introduce the acquisition and annotation of data involved in our work. Secondly, we transform data to time-frequency spectrum images as network input. At last, we propose the SQA method based on ResNet and Bi-LSTM.

2.1 Data Collection and Annotation

The data of this article is collected by a non-contact dECG measurement system published previously by our teammates [16]. Acquisition of dECG is based on the capacitively coupled electrode and it can acquire ECG signal both in contact with skin and through clothes. The system can denoise and store data simultaneously. Forty volunteers (25 men and 15 women, average age 25 ± 10), were enrolled in this study. All subjects have good health and no history of cardiovascular disease. Meanwhile, all of them signed the informed consent. The dECG signals were measured at a sampling frequency of 500 Hz for 4 h. The collected signals were divided into five-second segments. 4859 sampled signals with obvious statistical characteristics were selected. By consulting ECG experts, we define the dECG signal quality categories as follows.

- Level 0 (clean): A good recording with clear R waves.
- Level 1 (noise): A poor recording without clear R waves.
- Level 2 (motion artifact): A high-amplitude noise signal caused by the movement of the testee.

The waveforms of three types of dECG signals are shown in Fig. 1. Four undergraduates of biomedical engineering with training in ECG analysis annotated each segment respectively and an ECG expert reviewed each annotation. Finally, five of them voted to determine the category of dECG signal segments. The number and categories distribution of dECG signal segments taken for the training set, validation set, and test set are shown in Table 1.

2.2 Pre-processing of dECG Signals

Short-time Fourier transform (STFT) [17] is a popular time-frequency analysis tool that explains frequency domain features in a sequence with a fragment of a signal in the time domain. The frequency features of different window functions are different in STFT. So, Time-domain and frequency-domain resolution should all be thought over.

We used the frequency spectrum of our dECG signals into the CNN model in an effort akin to voice classification [18–21]. This study used a symmetric Hamming window for 8 points that decreased spectrum leakage and obtained superior time-frequency particulars after many experiments. Consequently, after STFT, dECG signals (with a dimension of 1×2500) were transformed into the time-frequency spectrum image (with a dimension of $875 \times 656 \times 3$). The time-frequency spectrum images for three categories of dECG signals are shown in Fig. 1.

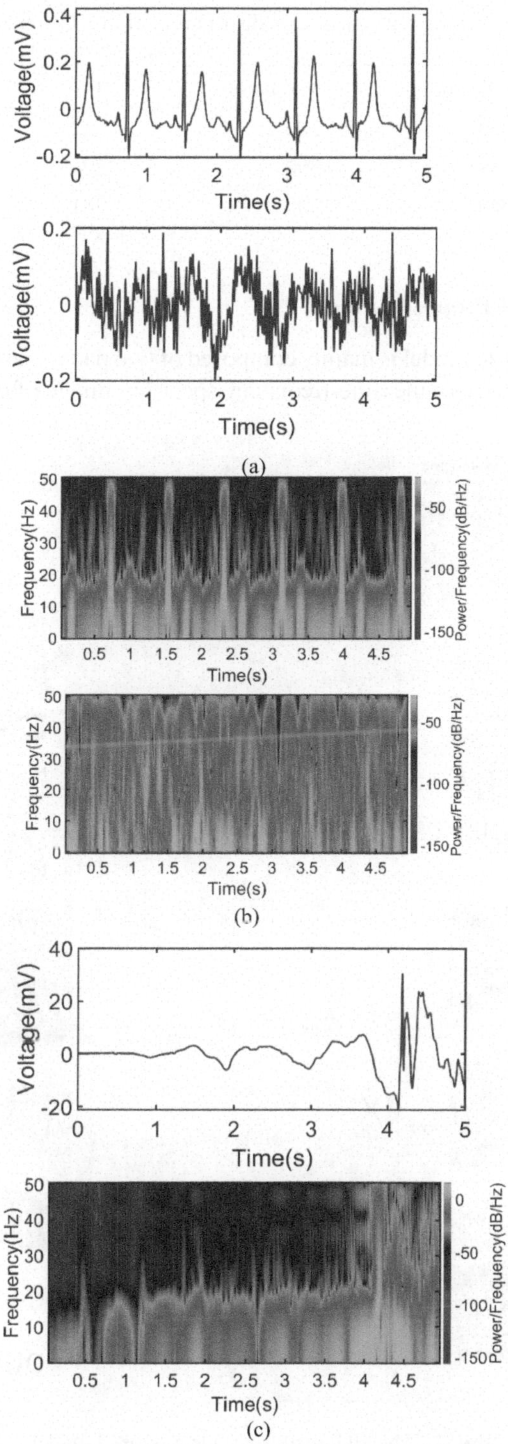

Fig. 1. (a), (b), and (c) show three types of dECG signals and their time-frequency spectrum image respectively

Table 1. The number and categories distribution of dECG signal segments

Category	Training	Validation	Test	Total
Level 0	1000	300	382	1682
Level 1	1000	300	296	1596
Level 2	1000	300	281	1581

2.3 Architecture of Proposed Model

The proposed algorithm model is mainly composed of two parts, one is ResNet, the other is Bi-LSTM. We first resize the time-frequency spectrum image of dECG signals to the

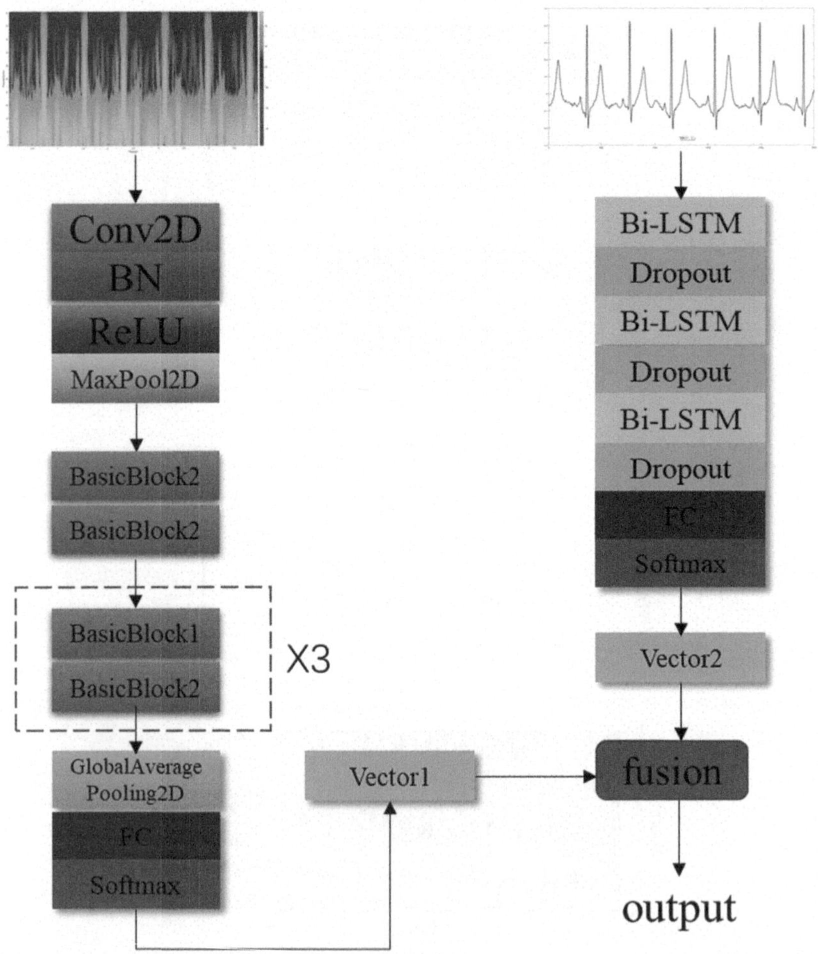

Fig. 2. The architecture of our proposed model.

size of 256 × 256 × 3 by bilinear interpolation and then use them to train the ResNet network. We directly use the dECG signals (with a dimension of 1 × 2500) to train the Bi-LSTM network. When the test set is input to the two trained networks, we take out the output vectors of the softmax layer of the two networks, add them and multiply them by 0.5. In this way, the prediction probability value of each type is obtained. Finally, the category with the largest probability value is taken as the prediction category. The whole framework of the model is shown in Fig. 2. This model is composed of two networks, ResNet and Bi-LSTM, which improve the total accuracy and robustness of the model by using the idea of ensemble learning.

Description of CNN Layers. The time-frequency spectrum images of dECG signals pass through the two-dimensional convolutional layer (Conv2D) and two-dimensional maximum pooling (Maxpool2D) layer and then get into the residual module. The residual module is composed of 8 basic blocks of 2 kinds, as shown in Fig. 3. The kernel dimension of the Conv2D layer in this network was all 3 × 3. The first Conv2D layer had 32 convolution kernels, and the number of kernels for the Conv2D layer among the 8 basic blocks in the latter residual module was taken as 32, 32, 64, 64, 128, 128, 128, 128. When the CNN implemented convolution layer by layer, the acquired characteristics were transformed from particulars to abstractions. The residual module could catch a lot of messages from the characteristics acquired from different Conv2D layers, thus effectively improving features' recognition capabilities and avoiding a substantial increase in network parameters. Moreover, the residual module provided not only characteristic extraction, but also improved gradient flow [22]. ReLU is the activation function of total the Conv2D layers. For better training, we add the BN layer after the convolution layer. Finally, input the output vectors of ResNet to the softmax layer to obtain the vector containing the probability value of each category.

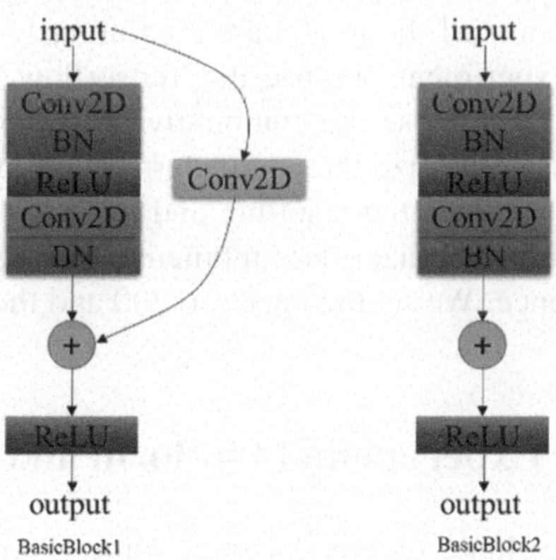

Fig. 3. Structure of two types of residual blocks.

Description of RNN Layers. Because Bi-LSTM has a good effect in processing timing signals, we take the dECG signal as the input of the Bi-LSTM network. Specifically, the module contains 3 Bi-LSTM layers [23], and each layer's size was 64. As seen in Fig. 4, Bi-LSTM, as a particular LSTM, receives information in both forward and backward directions at the same time, which makes the characteristics of time sequence richer, because each signal possesses context message from past and future. In the meantime, In order to prevent overfitting, we add the Dropout layer with a coefficient of 0.5 after each Bi-LSTM layer. Then, the output of the Bi-LSTM was input to the softmax layer to acquire the vectors containing the probability value of each category.

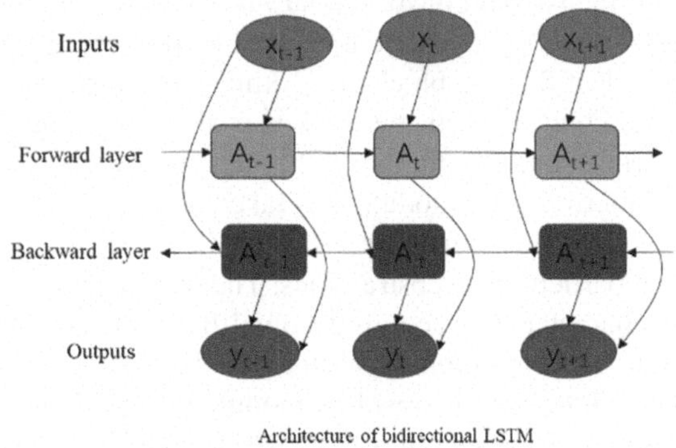

Fig. 4. The architecture of Bi-LSTM.

Training Method. We randomly extract data from the training set in batches to train the model. The weight parameters of the model are continuously updated by the gradient descent method. In this experiment, we use the Tensorflow framework to build and train our network model. We choose the commonly used cross-entropy loss function and Adam optimizer [24] to optimize the parameters. The cross-entropy loss function determines the difference between the resulting and the true values for each round of training samples. The Adam optimizer uses momentum and adaptive learning rate to accelerate model convergence. We set the epoch to 200 and the batch_size to 64.

3 Evaluation Index Experimental Platform and Results

In this section, we first evaluate our model with some evaluation criteria. Then we describe the hardware and software we use to process data and training models. Finally, we discuss the result of our experiments and compare it with some commonly used methods.

3.1 Evaluation Index

We randomly selected 959 segments from 4859 dECG signals as the test set. To evaluate the trained model, we applied the confusion matrix and calculate the sensitivity (Se), precision (P_+), accuracy (ACC), and F-Score of the fusion classifier model. The confusion matrix is a table that includes three indices represented by true-positive (TP), true-negative (TN), false-negative (FN), and false-positive (FP). The calculation formula of each index is as follows:

Accuracy (ACC): The proportion of correct predictions in total predictions.

$$ACC = \frac{TP + TN}{TP + TN + FN + FP} \tag{1}$$

Precision (P_+): The proportion of correct predicted positives to the total predicted positives.

$$P_+ = \frac{TP}{TP + FP} \tag{2}$$

Sensitivity (Se): It is also called Recall. Sensitivity describes the proportion of all positive cases identified in all positive cases.

$$Se = \frac{TP}{TP + FN} \tag{3}$$

F1-Score (F1): It gives a method to merge Sensitivity and Precision.

$$F1 = \frac{2 \times Se \times P_+}{Se + P_+} \tag{4}$$

3.2 Experimental Platform

The proposed network was performed using the Tensorflow framework based on the Python language and MATLAB 2020b was used for data processing. Total experiments were implemented under a Linux OS on a server with CPU Intel(R) Xeon(R) E5-2687 W v4 @ 3.00 GHz, GPU NVIDIA GTX 1080Ti, and 64 GB of RAM.

3.3 Results

Individual ResNet and Bi-LSTM models perform well in the training set, achieving accuracy rates of close to 100% and 95%, respectively. Although their respective accuracy on the validation set is also high, there is a large fluctuation in the accuracy among epochs. The changes of accuracy and loss values of the two networks on the training data and validation data with epoch are shown in Fig. 5. Therefore, we use the idea of ensemble learning to combine the trained ResNet and Bi-LSTM networks to reduce the overall variance of the model and improve the accuracy. The accuracy of using the ResNet model and the Bi-LSTM on the test set was 0.9499 and 0.9541, respectively. The accuracy of using the ResNet + Bi-LSTM model on the test set has been improved to 0.9969. Further comparison of the confusion matrix (ResNet + Bi-LSTM network vs. ResNet, Bi-LSTM) showed that the ResNet + Bi-LSTM network was more robust with higher accuracy (Fig. 6). As shown in Table 2, the ResNet + Bi-LSTM network also performed better on these evaluation indices of precision, sensitivity, and F1 score.

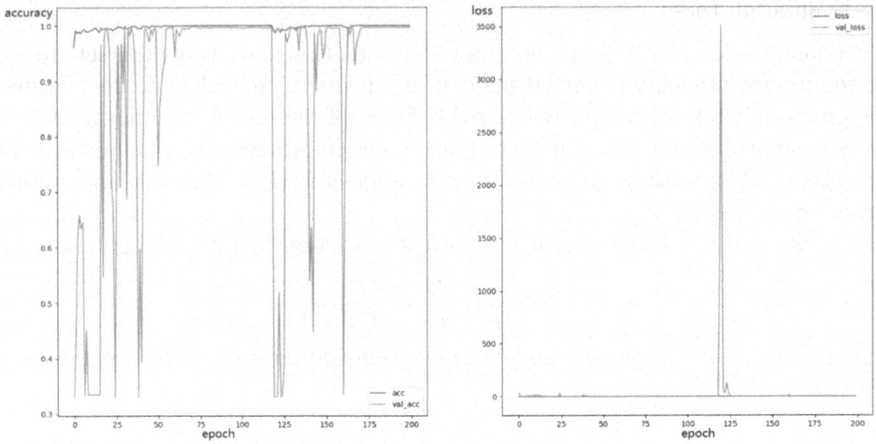

(a)

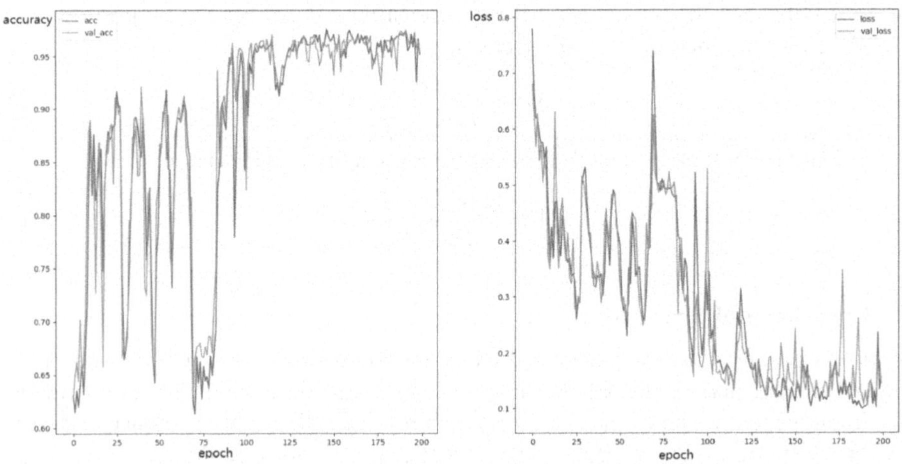

(b)

Fig. 5. (a), (b) the accuracy and loss value of each epoch on the training set and validation set of ResNet and Bi-LSTM networks

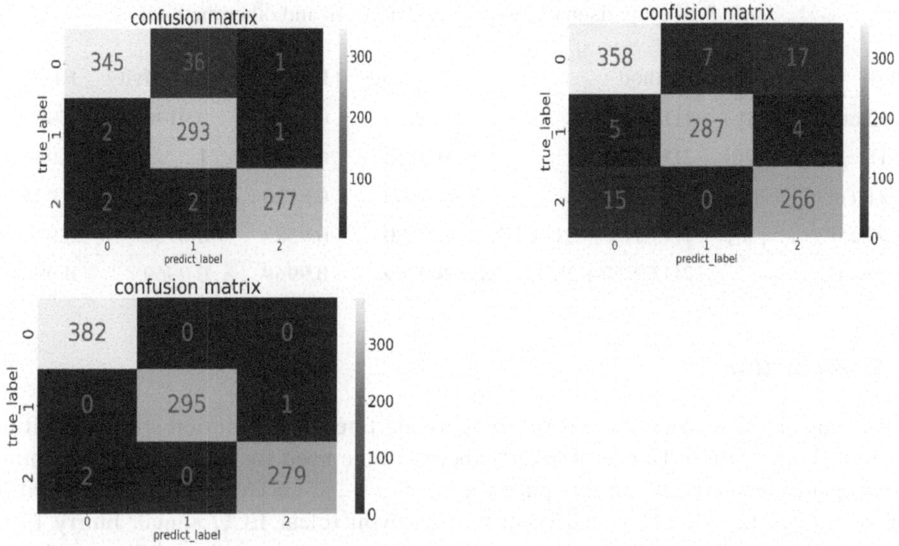

(a) (b) (c)

Fig. 6. (a), (b) and (c) are the confusion matrices of Bi-LSTM, ResNet, and ResNet + Bi-LSTM on the test set respectively

Table 2. Comparison of three methods

Method	Accuracy	Precision	Sensitivity	F1
ResNet	0.9541	0.9579	0.9541	0.9543
Bi-LSTM	0.9499	0.9501	0.9499	0.9499
ResNet + Bi-LSTM	**0.9969**	**0.9969**	**0.9969**	**0.9969**

3.4 Comparison with Methods in Other Papers

Our proposed method improved accuracy in comparison to the existing methods. Xue Zhou et al. [25] used a 1D CNN to classify ECG signals on the database of PhysioNet/Computing in Cardiology Challenge 2011 and the PhysioNet/Computing in Cardiology Challenge 2017 and obtained an accuracy of 94.30%. A. Huerta et al. [26] used 2D CNN to classify ECG signals on the database of PhysioNet/Computing in Cardiology Challenge 2017 and obtained an accuracy of 91.20%. Zeyang Zhu et al. [27] used the Adaboost algorithm to classify ECG signals on the database of PhysioNet/Computing in Cardiology Challenge 2011 and obtained an accuracy of 95.80%. Qifei Zhang et al. [28] used 1D CNN and 2D CNN to classify ECG signals on the MIT-BIH Arrhythmia database and obtained an accuracy of 91.80%. Although we used different datasets, the comparison of these methods is instructive for the evaluation of the model. As shown in Table 3, our algorithm has higher accuracy and robustness.

Table 3. Comparison of the proposed network and other methods

Work	Method	Accuracy	Precision	Sensitivity	F1
X. Zhou et al. [25]	1D CNN	0.9430	0.9550	0.9130	0.9335
A. Huerta et al. [26]	2D CNN	0.9120	0.9030	**1**	0.9490
Z. Zhu et al. [27]	Adaboost	0.9580	0.8720	0.9860	0.9255
Q. Zhang et al. [28]	1D CNN + 2D CNN	0.9180	0.9583	0.8920	0.9240
Our work	2D CNN + Bi-LSTM	**0.9969**	**0.9969**	0.9969	**0.9969**

4 Conclusion

Non-contact ECG measurement is sensitive to interference and motion artifact, limiting its clinical application. Hence, it greatly increases the need for real-time and dynamic signal quality assessment. In this paper, a ResNet + Bi-LSTM model is proposed to realize a three-level ECG signal quality assessment (clear ECG signal, blurry ECG signal, and noisy ECG signal). The ResNet layers can capture spatial features in the ECG sequences while the Bi-LSTM layer can then learn the temporal features. The proposed model achieves 99.69% accuracy, outperforming the single ResNet - based and Bi-LSTM - based approach. The experimental results demonstrate the superior performance of this ResNet + Bi-LSTM model over the existing methods. By automatic ECG quality classification with high accuracy, wide clinical applications of non-contact ECG measurement may be achieved in the future.

References

1. Johannesen, L., Galeotti, L.: Automatic ECG quality scoring methodology: mimicking human annotators. Physiol. Meas. **33**(9), 1479 (2012). https://doi.org/10.1088/0967-3334/33/9/1479
2. Clifford, G.D., Moody, G.B.: Signal quality in cardiorespiratory monitoring. Physiol. Meas. **33**(9), 1–6 (2012). https://doi.org/10.1088/0967-3334/33/9/e01
3. Jekova, I., Krasteva, V., Christov, I., Abächerli, R.: Threshold-based system for noise detection in multilead ECG recordings. Physiol. Meas. **33**(9), 1463–1477 (2012). https://doi.org/10.1088/0967-3334/33/9/1463
4. Liu, C., Li, P., Zhao, L., Liu, F., Wang, R.: Real-time signal quality assessment for ECGs collected using mobile phones. In: Proceedings of the 2011 Computing in Cardiology, Hangzhou, China, pp. 357–360. IEEE (2011)
5. Allen, J., Murray, A.: Assessing ECG signal quality on a coronary care unit. Physiol. Meas. **17**(4), 249–258 (1996)
6. Clifford, G.D., Behar, J., Li, Q., Rezek, I.: Signal quality indices and data fusion for determining clinical acceptability of electrocardiograms. Physiol. Meas. **33**(9), 1419–1433 (2012). https://doi.org/10.1088/0967-3334/33/9/1419
7. Silva, I., Moody, G.B., Celi, L.: Improving the quality of ECGs collected using mobile phones: the physionet/computing in cardiology challenge 2011. In: Proceedings of the 2011 Computing in Cardiology, Hangzhou, China, pp. 273–276. IEEE (2011)
8. Xia, H., Garcia, G.A., Bains, J., Wortham, D.C., Zhao, X.: Matrix of regularity for improving the quality of ECGs. Physiol. Meas. **33**(9), 1535–1548 (2012). https://doi.org/10.1088/0967-3334/33/9/1535

9. Shi, Y., et al.: Robust assessment of ECG signal quality for wearable devices. In: Proceedings of the IEEE International Conference on Healthcare Informatics (ICHI), Xi'an, China, pp. 1–3 (2019)
10. Satija, U., Ramkumar, B., Manikandan, M.S.: Robust cardiac event change detection method for long-term healthcare monitoring applications. Healthc. Technol. Lett. **3**(2), 116–123 (2016)
11. Zhang, Y., Wei, S., Zhang, L., Liu, C.: Comparing the performance of random forest, SVM and their variants for computational and mathematical methods in medicine 11 ECG quality assessment combined with nonlinear features. J. Med. Biol. Eng. **39**(3), 381–392 (2019)
12. LeCun, Y., Bengio, Y., Hinton, G.: Deep learning. Nature **521**(7553), 436–444 (2015)
13. Rawat, W., Wang, Z.: Deep convolutional neural networks for image classification: a comprehensive review. Neural Comput. **29**(9), 2352–2449 (2017)
14. Xiong, W., Wu, L., Alleva, F., Droppo, J., Huang, X., Stolcke, A.: The Microsoft 2017 conversational speech recognition system. In: Proceedings of the 2018 IEEE International Conference on Acoustics, Speech and Signal Processing (ICASSP), Calgary, Canada (2018)
15. Hill, F., Cho, K., Jean, S., Bengio, Y.: The representational geometry of word meanings acquired by neural machine translation models. Mach. Transl. **31**(1–2), 3–18 (2017). https://doi.org/10.1007/s10590-017-9194-2
16. Peng, S., et al.: Flexible electrodes based smart mattress for monitoring physiological signals of heart and autonomic nerves in a non-contact way. IEEE Sensors J. **21**(1), 6–15 (2020)
17. Nawab, S.H., Quatieri, T.F.: Short-time Fourier transform. In: Advanced Topics in Signal Processing, pp. 289–337, Prentice-Hall, Upper Saddle River (1987)
18. Liu, Z., Wu, Z., Li, T., Li, J., Shen, C.: GMM and CNN hybrid method for short utterance speaker recognition. IEEE Trans. Industr. Inform. **14**(7), 3244–3252 (2018)
19. Zhang, H., McLoughlin, I., Song, Y.: Robust sound event recognition using convolutional neural networks. In: Proceedings of the 2015 IEEE International Conference on Acoustics, Speech and Signal Processing (ICASSP), pp. 559–563, South Brisbane, Australia (2015)
20. Fu, S.W., Tsao, Y., Lu, X.: SNR-aware convolutional neural network modeling for speech enhancement. In: Proceedings of the Interspeech 2016, San Francisco, CA, pp. 3768–3772 (2016)
21. Satt, A., Rozenberg, S., Hoory, R.: Efficient emotion recognition from speech using deep learning on spectrograms. In: Proceedings of the Interspeech 2017, Stockholm, Sweden, pp. 1089–1093 (2017)
22. He, K., Zhang, X., Ren, S., Sun, J.: Deep residual learning for image recognition. In: Proceedings of the IEEE Conference on Computer Vision and Pattern Recognition (CVPR), pp. 770–778 (2016)
23. Cui, Z., Ke, R., Pu, Z., Wang, Y.: Deep bidirectional and unidirectional LSTM recurrent neural network for network-wide traffic speed prediction. CoRR arXiv preprint arXiv:1801.02143 (2018)
24. Kingma, D.P., Ba, J.: Adam: a method for stochastic optimization (2014). http://arxiv.org/abs/1412.6980
25. Zhou, X., Zhu, X., Nakamura, K., Mahito, N.: ECG quality assessment using 1D-convolutional neural network. In: 2018 14th IEEE International Conference on Signal Processing (ICSP), pp. 780–784, IEEE (2018). https://doi.org/10.1109/ICSP.2018.8652479
26. Huerta, A., Martínez-Rodrigo, A., González, V.B., Quesada, A., Rieta, J.J., Alcaraz, R.: Quality assessment of very long-term ecg recordings using a convolutional neural network. In: 2019 E-Health and Bioengineering Conference (EHB), pp. 1–4 (2019). https://doi.org/10.1109/EHB47216.2019.8970077

27. Zhu, Z., Liu, W., Yao, Y., Chen, X., Sun, Y., Xu, L.: Adaboost based ECG signal quality evaluation. In: 2019 Computing in Cardiology (CinC), pp. 1–4 (2019). https://doi.org/10.23919/CinC49843.2019.9005515
28. Zhang, Q., Fu, L., Gu, L.: A cascaded convolutional neural network for assessing signal quality of dynamic ECG. Comput. Math. Methods Med. **2019**, 7095137 (2019)

CANet: Compact Attention Network for Automatic Melanoma Segmentation

Yingyan Hou[1(✉)] and Kaichuang Liu[2]

[1] School of Software, Tsinghua University, Beijing 100084, China
hyy20@mails.tsinghua.edu.cn

[2] Department of Automation, Tsinghua University, Beijing 100084, China
liukc20@mails.tsinghua.edu.cn

Abstract. In the study of skin cancer, particularly melanoma, automatic and accurate segmentation as a crucial step in Computer-Aided Diagnosis (CAD) provides a reliable basis for clinical diagnosis efficiency and pathology research. However, due to the variability of skin lesions in texture, shape, and complex boundaries, automatic and accurate segmentation is still an unsolved challenge. In this paper, we propose a new automatic segmentation network for melanoma segmentation named Compact Attention Network (CANet). Based on the fully convolutional networks, the CANet removes down-sampling so as not to reduce the spatial accuracy. The CANet expands the receptive field by the designed atrous convolution, which could avoid the gridding issue. In order to refine the feature map information and make the segmentation edge smoother, we add an attention module after every designed atrous convolution. Finally, our model achieves State-of-the-Art (SOTA) performance in the task of melanoma segmentation compared with U-net, SegNet, FrCN, and so on. We conduct ablation experiments to prove the effectiveness of each element of the network. Our results show that the melanoma segmentation of the CANet is 91.7% in Sensitivity and 90.7% in Dice scores for the International Skin Imaging Collaboration (ISIC) test dataset. The CANet outperforms FrCN, U-Net, SegNet, Mask R-CNN and nnU-Net in Dice by 3.6%, 14.5%, 8.6%, 5.4% and 1.7% respectively, exhibiting better performance than these classic networks. The CANet can perform medical image segmentation more accurately and quickly, provide an important reference for medical workers in diagnosing diseases, and improve diagnosis efficiency.

Keywords: Melanoma segmentation · Atrous convolution · Attention mechanism

1 Introduction

Semantic segmentation of medical images is one of the important steps in artificial intelligence-assisted medical diagnosis and has been widely used in the

Hunan Key Research and Development Program (2019WK2072).

X. Gao et al. (Eds.): MobiHealth 2021, LNICST 440, pp. 329–342, 2022.
https://doi.org/10.1007/978-3-031-06368-8_22

field of medical image analysis. Using medical image segmentation technology to extract human tissues, organs, and lesions, which provides important references for medical workers to diagnose diseases, reduces the misdiagnosis rate, and improves diagnostic efficiency.

Cancer is one of the leading causes of human unnatural death. The World Health Organization (WHO) has published the latest world cancer report for 2020 [1]. The report shows that there were 19.3 million newly diagnosed cancer cases worldwide in 2020, with nearly 10 million deaths. Skin cancer is one of the most common cancers. The majority of skin cancer deaths are caused by melanoma. Melanoma has been reported to grow at an annual rate of 7% at the American Society of Clinical Oncology (ASCO) annual meeting. Early diagnosis and identification of melanoma are increasingly important.

Early symptoms of melanoma are difficult to distinguish from benign skin lesions on the epidermis, leading to the misdiagnosis of melanoma. Melanoma or benign skin lesions have irregular colors and shapes, and manual segmentation is cumbersome and time-consuming. Therefore, it is necessary to study an automatic and accurate method for melanoma segmentation. In recent years, semantically segmented networks have been commonly used for melanoma segmentation. In earlier studies, there have been many traditional image segmentation algorithms to solve this problem. In 2009, Yuan et al. [3] proposed a skin lesion segmentation method based on region fusion and narrowband energy graph partitioning, which can handle topological changes, weak edges, and asymmetric skin lesion areas, and can accurately detect complex outlines of lesion areas. In 2011, Schaefer et al. [4] proposed a technique for extracting skin lesion areas using an iterative measurement of non-lesion pixels and co-operative neural networks. In the same year, Zhou et al. [5] proposed a gradient vector flow algorithm based on the mean drift to extract the contours of skin lesions. Wong et al. [6] proposed an iterative random area merging method to extract lesion areas from conventional macro-skin images. However, traditional image segmentation algorithms can only segment-specific cases, and neither speed nor accuracy is very high.

In recent years, deep learning has made remarkable progress in the field of computer vision. It has been widely applied in the field of image, and its effect is higher than the previous SOTA performance, which provides inspiration for the segmentation of skin lesions. Long et al. [7] proposed a Fully Convolution Network (FCN), which removed the original full connection layer of the convolution neural network and replaces it with transposed convolution layer. FCN has two main points, one is to expand the receptive field through the pooling layer, the other is to expand the size of the image through up-sampling. Ronneberger et al. [8] proposed U-net, which applied the results of the pooling layer to the decoding process and introduces more coding information. The U-net is a very classical medical image segmentation model because it can be trained with a small amount of data. Zhao et al. [9] proposed a pyramid scene analysis network that used a pooling layer, which had a large core to expand the receptive field. He et al. [10] proposed Mask R-CNN based on Fast R-CNN, which can achieve high-quality semantic segmentation. Peng et al. [11] proposed an encoder-decoder architecture with a large convolution core, which used ResNet [12] structure as the encoder and used the graph convolution network [13] as the decoder. Badrinarayanan et al. [14] proposed an encoder-decoder architecture for semantic pixel-wise segmentation termed SegNet, in which the decoder up-samples its lower resolution input feature maps. Chen et al. [15] proposed Atrous Spatial Pyramid Pooling (ASPP), which could combine information of different sizes. Al-Masni et al. [16] proposed FrCN using the full spatial resolution of the input image to reduce the loss of information. Roy et al. [2] improved the Squeeze & Excitation (SE) module [17] in the field of image classification, and proposed the scSE module that matched semantic segmentation, which greatly improved the accuracy of semantic segmentation. Stringer et al. [18] introduced a generalist, deep learning-based segmentation method called Cellpose, which can precisely segment cells from a wide range of image types and does not require model retraining or parameter adjustments. Fabian et al. [19] proposed the nnU-Net, a deep learning-based segmentation method that automatically configures itself, including preprocessing, network architecture, training and post-processing for any new task.

Most semantically segmented networks down-sample the feature maps of the middle layer and use the full convolution network of encoder-decoder to expand the receptive field of the captured image context. Currently, the common improvement directions are enlarging the receptive field by pooling layers and recovering the input quality by up-sampling. However, the pooling layers lose precise location information and reduce accuracy. The up-sampling layer cannot be fully recovered, and it also incurs additional computative costs.

In this paper, we propose a compact attention network architecture without down-sampling, different from common semantic segmentation. This structure adds the atrous convolution to expand the receptive field. We design the rate of atrous convolution to avoid the gridding issue and add scSE module [2] behind the convolution layers to improve the feature map. In order to further improve performance, we use pre-processing methods such as data augmentation, erosion, and dilation. In Sect. 3, we design ablation experiments and compare our network with existing models (such as U-net). Compared with existing classic models, the CANet has the best advanced performance in melanoma segmentation. The proposed method is innovative in the field of medical image segmentation. The CANet can perform medical image segmentation more accurately and quickly, provide an important reference for medical workers in diagnosing diseases, and improve diagnosis efficiency.

2 Methodology

We propose a method for skin lesion segmentation, which integrates the proposed new compact fully convolutional network with attention module and data processing methods oriented to the features of the ISIC dataset.

2.1 On the Elements of the Proposed Network

Atrous Convolution. In the pixel-wise semantic segmentation task, as mentioned above, most of these network architectures have encoder-decoder architecture. It lowers spatial resolution and cannot completely restore it. Instead, Li et al. [20] proposed a novel 3D architecture that incorporated high spatial resolution feature maps throughout the layers. They designed a compact network architecture without down-sampling for the segmentation of volumetric images. This architecture used atrous convolution to expand the receptive field instead of the pooling layer.

Part of our network architecture draws inspiration from it. We build a compact convolutional neural network with atrous convolution. Atrous convolution maintains image resolution and computes with a high spatial resolution by inserting "holes" between pixels in convolutional kernels. The apparent advantage of atrous convolution is that it enlarges the size of the receptive field without losing spatial resolution. Chen et al. [15] used atrous convolution with up-sampled kernels for semantic image segmentation. Atrous convolution can be used to produce accurate dense predictions and detailed segmentation along object boundaries. For example, the atrous convolution rate is set to 2, the receptive field of each convolution is 3×3, and the receptive field of the entire convolution kernel is 7×7. Furthermore, it has been applied to a broader range of tasks, such as optical flow [21].

Gridding. Stacking convolution layers with the same atrous rate would have an effect on the receptive field due to the gridding. The receptive field from the same atrous convolution covers an area with non-zero values. The atrous convolution can be regarded as the standard convolution on different feature maps. If the pixels of each feature map has no further interaction, it will cause discontinuity of pixel connection. Besides, repeated stacking would further aggravate the gridding. In the convolution kernel with a large atrous rate, the receptive field is too sparse to cover any information.

Wang et al. [22] alleviated this issue by using a range of relatively prime atrous rates instead of the same atrous rate (see Fig. 1). They noted that the gridding issue would still exist if a series of atrous rates have a common factor relationship (such as 2, 4, 8, etc.). We would find that there are many pixels in the receptive field that are not used and a lot of holes appear. Proper atrous rates can increase the receptive field effectively.

Attention - ScSE Module. Hu et al. [17] proposed an architectural component, SE block, which could be integrated within any convolutional neural network model. Inspired by SE, Roy et al. [2] proposed three block for image segmentation:

- Spatial squeeze and channel excitation block - cSE as shown in Eq. 1.

$$\hat{\mathbf{I}}_{cSE} = F_{cSE}(\mathbf{I}) = [\sigma(\hat{z_1})\,\mathbf{i}_1, \sigma(\hat{z_2})\,\mathbf{i}_2, \cdots, \sigma(\hat{z_C})\,\mathbf{i}_C] \quad (1)$$

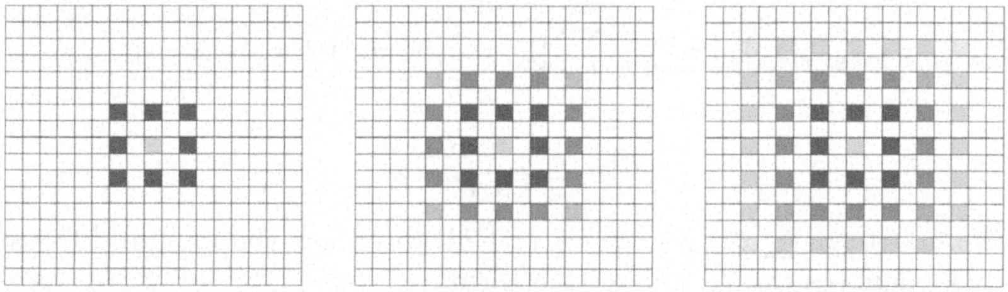

(a)

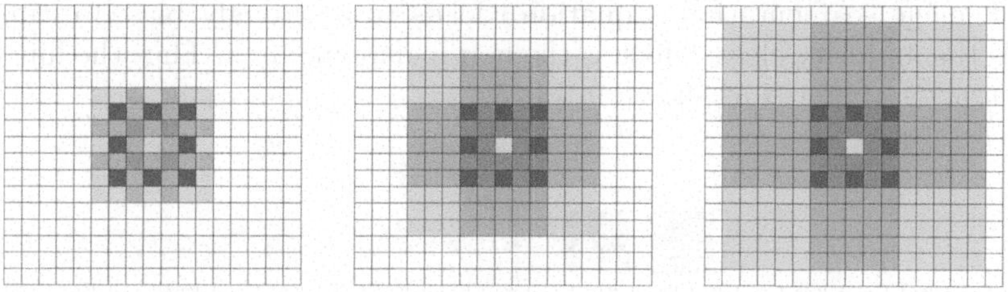

(b)

Fig. 1. Illustration of the gridding issue: (a) all convolutional layers have a atrous rate of 2; (b) avoid the gridding issue by setting relatively prime atrous rates.

where I is the input feature map $I = [i_1, i_2, ..., i_c]$, $\sigma()$ is a sigmoid layer, $\hat{z_k}$ is performed by a global average pooling layer and weights.

- Channel squeeze and spatial excitation block - sSE as shown in Eq. 2.

$$\hat{\mathbf{T}}_{sSE} = F_{sSE}(\mathbf{T}) = \left[\sigma(q_{1,1})\,\mathbf{t}^{1,1}, \cdots, \sigma(q_{i,j})\,\mathbf{t}^{i,j}, \cdots, \sigma(q_{H,W})\,\mathbf{t}^{H,W}\right] \quad (2)$$

where T is the input tensor $\mathbf{T} = \left[\mathbf{t}^{1,1}, \mathbf{t}^{1,2}, \cdots, \mathbf{t}^{i,j}, \cdots, \mathbf{t}^{H,W}\right]$, $\sigma()$ is a sigmoid layer, $q_{i,j}$ represents all channels linear combination of a spatial location (i, j).

- Patial and channel squeeze & excitation -scSE is element-wise addition of cSE and sSE as shown in Eq. 3:

$$\hat{\mathbf{U}}_{scSE} = \hat{\mathbf{U}}_{cSE} + \hat{\mathbf{U}}_{sSE} \quad (3)$$

We incorporate scSE module within the CANet.

Loss Function. We design the loss function due to unbalanced data. Inspired by Support Vector Machine (SVM) soft margin classification and large margin classification [23], the hinge loss function is uesd for the last layer of the network without any activation function.

We record positive and negative samples as ± 1. In the training data, a n-voxel volume $\{x_i\}_{i=1}^n$ and its segmentation map $\{y_i\}_{i=1}^n (y_i \in \{-1, 1\})$ are calculated in the hinge loss function as shown in Eq. 4:

$$L_{hinge}(\{x_i\},\{y_i\}) = \sum_{i=1}^{n} [1 - y_i(w \cdot x_i + b)]_+ + \lambda\|w\|^2 \tag{4}$$

$$[R]_+ = \begin{cases} R, R > 0 \\ 0, R \le 0 \end{cases}$$

where the first term $\sum_{i=1}^{n} [1 - y_i(w \cdot x_i + b)]_+$ denotes the loss, and the second term $\lambda\|w\|^2$ denotes the regularization term.

However, the training data is apparently unbalanced, which is typical of medical image segmentation. Equation 4 leads to a strongly biased estimation towards the majority class, which is the non-melanoma area. Thus the hinge loss function adds weight α as shown in Eq. 5:

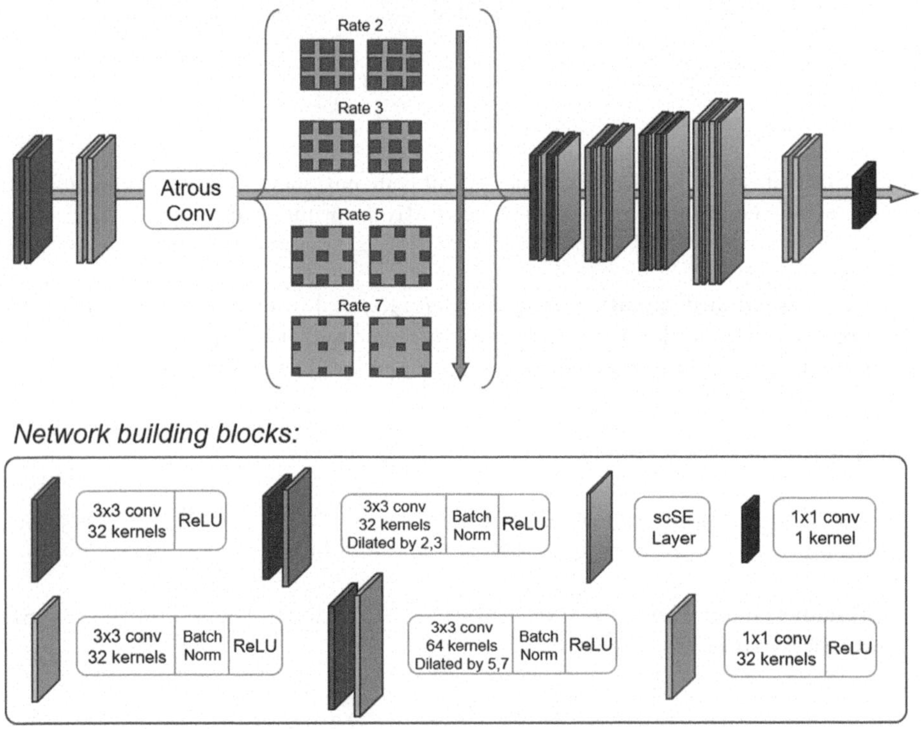

Fig. 2. Our network architecture for image segmentation.

$$L^*_{hinge}(\{x_i\},\{y_i\}) = \begin{cases} \sum_{i=1}^{n} \alpha \cdot [1 - y_i(w \cdot x_i + b)]_+ + \lambda\|w\|^2, y_i = 1 \\ \sum_{i=1}^{n} [1 - y_i(w \cdot x_i + b)]_+ + \lambda\|w\|^2, y_i = -1 \end{cases} \tag{5}$$

By choosing $\alpha > 1$, the network could pay more attention to the segmentation target and make parameters more actively optimized, so that the training network can get a reasonable segmentation model faster. To a certain extent, loss function weight could improve performance. We conduct experiments to discuss the choice of α in Sect. 3.

2.2 Network Architecture

The proposed network consists of 13 layers of convolutions (see Fig. 2). The first four convolution layers use 3×3 pixel convolutions without atrous convolution. Stacking two layers of 3×3 pixel convolution gives the same receptive field as a convolutional kernel with 5×5 pixel convolution, but parameters of them are only about half of 5×5 pixel convolution parameters. The third and fourth layer are associated with the Batch Normalization (BN) [24]. The first four layers are designed to capture low-level features of the input image.

In the subsequent 8 convolutional layers, each convolutional layer is associated with an element-wise Rectified Linear Unit (ReLU) layer, a BN layer and a scSE layer. A scSE layer could get a more accurate calibrated feature map. The kernels are dilated by the designed rates of 2, 3, 5, 7, which not have a common factor relationship. Choosing proper rates can effectively expand the receptive field and avoid the gridding issue [22]. We use atrous convolution instead of the pooling layer to efficiently enlarge the receptive field without reducing resolution. Due to the different sizes of the melanoma, the rates of atrous convolutions are gradually increased to incorporate features at multiple scales when the layer goes deeper. Except for the last layer of our network, every convolutional layer is associated with a ReLU layer. The final layer gives binary classification labels for every pixel.

2.3 Data Preprocessing

In the experiment, each network uses the processed training data set for training.

Erosion and Dilation of Image Noise. The ISIC dataset has hair noise in some dermoscopy images. Segmenting the melanoma, which is black and has many forms, requires minimizing the effects of hair noise.

We perform closing by erosion and dilation to remove the noise on the ISIC dataset. Erosion and dilation are mathematical morphology transformations [25].

Erosion uses vector subtraction as shown in Eq. 6.

$$M \ominus N = \{x, y \mid (N)_{xy} \subseteq M\} \tag{6}$$

where N denotes a structural element. M is the region to erode whose pixel values are all 1 in the binary image. It should be noted that N needs to define an origin, whose coordinate is (x, y). During the movement process of N, when the pixels of N are completely contained by M, the pixel of M covered by the origin of N is set to 1 otherwise 0.

Dilation uses vector addition as shown in Eq. 7.

$$M \oplus N = \{x, y \mid (N)_{xy} \cap M \neq \emptyset\} \tag{7}$$

where N is as the same definition as Eq. 6, and M denotes the region to dilate. During the movement process of N, when pixels of N have intersections with those of M, the pixel of M covered by the origin of N is set to 1 otherwise 0.

Data Augmentation. Training a well-performing network commonly requires a large amount of data, but datasets in the medical field are generally small. On a small dataset, the model would easily overfit. Data augmentation is a conventional method for training models with a small dataset. For each image in the training dataset, we use three augmentation functions from the following list:

- Herizontal Flip.
- Vertical Flip.
- Rotation with angle 180°.

3 Experiments

This section introduces the dataset, evaluation metrics, and experiment configurations. We conduct experiments to explore our proposed network, CANet. The experiments are presented in two parts. The first part is ablation experiments to prove the effectiveness of each element of the network. In the second part, we compare our method with the SOTA networks.

In this paper, the experiments are performed and tested with the following configurations: Intel Core i9 processor at 3.5 GHz, NVIDIA GeForce RTX 2080 GPU with Ubuntu 18.04. The learning rate is set to 0.0001 in all experiments.

3.1 Dataset

The ISIC is a well-known skin medical organization, which collects a large number of skin images and provides annotation for these images. The organization holds a skin lesion challenge every year to attract researchers in the field of computer vision to participate in, so as to improve the recognition algorithm of skin lesions and make more people realize the harm of skin cancer. In this paper, we used ISIC 2017 challenge dataset. There are 2000 skin images and the corresponding skin lesion area images marked by experts in the training set. The ratio of the training set, validation set, and testing set is 40:3:12, and the resolution of each image varies from 540 × 722 to 4499 × 6748 pixels. The dataset is a collection of real images, some of which have serious noise (see Fig. 3).

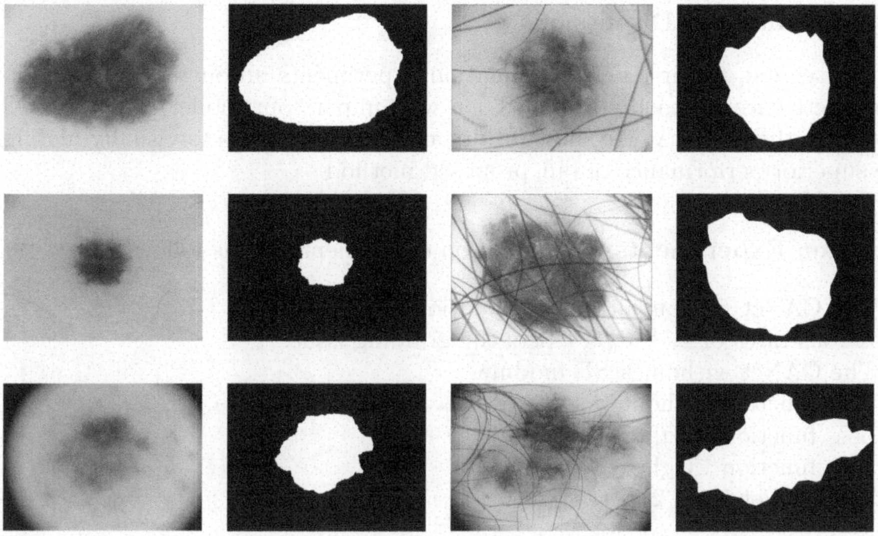

Fig. 3. Various skin lesion images in ISIC. (a) noise-free images. (b) the annotation of noise-free images. (c) noisy images. (d) the annotation of noisy images.

3.2 Performance Evaluation Metrics

A quantitative analysis of experiments is carried out based on True Positive (TP), True Negative (TN), False Positive (FP), False Negative (FN) [26]. In this work, image segmentation methods are evaluated according to the following evaluation metrics:

- **Sensitivity**.

$$Sensitivity = \frac{TP}{TP + FN}$$

- **Specificity**.

$$Specificity = \frac{TN}{FP + TN}$$

- **Accuracy**.

$$Accuracy = \frac{TP + TN}{FP + TN + TP + FN}$$

- **Jaccard Similarity Index (JSI)**.

$$JSI = \frac{TP}{FP + TP + FN}$$

- **Dice Similarity Coefficient (Dice)**.

$$Dice = \frac{2 \times TP}{2 \times TP + FP + FN}$$

3.3 Results and Discussions

In this section, we first perform ablation experiments on our network to prove the effectiveness of each element. Then we compare our model with the SOTA models in the industry. We show results and draw box-plots to visually highlight the superior performance of our proposed method.

Ablation Experiments. The ablation experiments are as follows:

- The CANet without atrous convolution.
- Atrous rates of 2, 4, 6, 8, exists the gridding issue.
- The CANet without scSE module.
- Loss function without weight α.
- Loss function weight $\alpha = 4$.
- Loss function weight $\alpha = 6$.
- The CANet ($\alpha = 2$).

Table 1 lists the mean Sensitivity, Specificity, Accuracy, Jaccard Similarity Index, and Dice scores on the test set of the ablation experiments. Comparing along the rows with the final row, it is proved that the designed atrous convolution rates 2, 3, 5, 7 is effective, which expands the receptive field and reduces the gridding effect. Attention module scSE provides a statistically significant increase in comparison to the CANet. In addition, it is necessary to set the weight of the loss function, and the weight $\alpha = 2$ is the optimal solution for the melanoma data set. Fig 4 visualizes the results of ablation experiments under the Dice scores. The CANet outperforms "No Atrous Convolution", "Rates: 2, 4, 6, 8", "No scSE Module", "No Weight α", "Weight $\alpha = 4$" and "Weight $\alpha = 6$" in Dice by 4.8%, 1.5%, 4.0%, 2.3%, 2.7% and 3.4% respectively, showing the effectiveness of each element and great segmentation performance with the melanoma in CANet.

Table 1. Ablation experiments.

Strategy	Evaluation metrics				
	Sensitivity	Specificity	Accuracy	Jaccard	Dice scores
No Atrous convolution	0.877	0.940	0.923	0.754	0.859
Atrous rates: 2, 4, 6, 8 (gridding)	0.904	0.953	0.939	0.806	0.892
No scSE module	0.879	0.938	0.920	0.765	0.867
Loss function no weight α	0.896	0.950	0.935	0.793	0.884
Loss Weight $\alpha = 4$	0.892	0.949	0.933	0.786	0.880
Loss Weight $\alpha = 6$	0.886	0.949	0.932	0.776	0.873
CANet ($\alpha = 2$)	**0.917**	**0.955**	**0.944**	**0.830**	**0.907**

The best performance is highlighted in boldface.

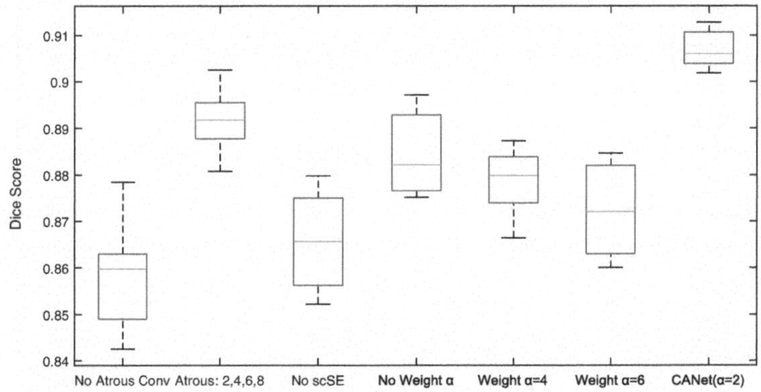

Fig. 4. Boxplot of Dice scores for ablation experiments.

Comparative Experiments. The CANet compares with the U-net [8], the SegNet [14], the FrCN [16], the Mask R-CNN [10] and the nnU-Net [19]. The required network parameters of these algorithms are provided in their papers.

Table 2. Results among CANet, Mask R-CNN, U-net, FrCN, SegNet, nnU-Net.

Network	Evaluation metrics				
	Sensitivity	Specificity	Accuracy	Jaccard	Dice scores
Mask R-CNN [10]	0.848	0.960	0.935	0.743	0.853
U-net [8]	0.672	**0.972**	0.901	0.616	0.762
FrCN [16]	0.854	0.967	0.940	0.771	0.871
SegNet [14]	0.801	0.954	0.918	0.696	0.821
nnU-net [19]	0.899	0.958	0.943	0.802	0.890
CANet	**0.917**	0.955	**0.944**	**0.830**	**0.907**

The best performance is highlighted in boldface.

Table 2 and Fig 5 compare the performance on the test set. Table 2 directly shows that our method achieves the best performance under the four metrics of Sensitivity, Accuracy, Jaccard Similarity Index, and Dice scores, and there is a small gap between our method and the best performance under the metric of Specificity. Results show that the melanoma segmentation of the CANet is 91.7% in Sensitivity and 90.7% in Dice scores for the ISIC test dataset. The CANet outperforms FrCN, U-Net, SegNet, Mask R-CNN and nnU-net in Dice by 3.6%, 14.5%, 8.6%, 5.4% and 1.7% respectively, exhibiting better performance than these classic networks. Figure 5 visualizes the results of five networks under the Dice scores. The CANet is much better than other networks in terms of mean value and stability. There is little difference between the boundary line segmented by CAnet and the boundary line marked by experts, which would be

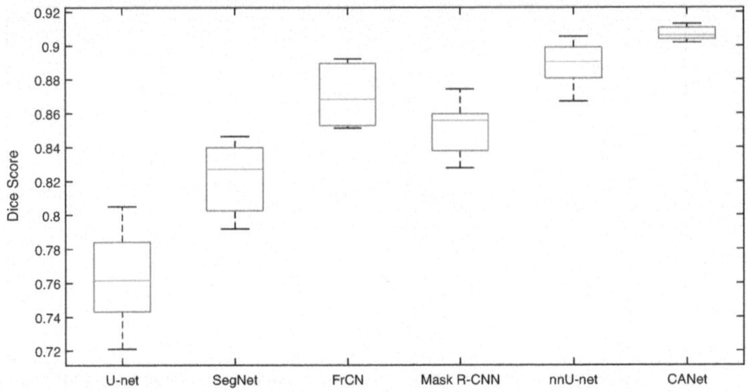

Fig. 5. Boxplot of Dice scores for six networks.

of great help to the subsequent doctors' judgment and diagnosis of the lesion area (see Fig. 6).

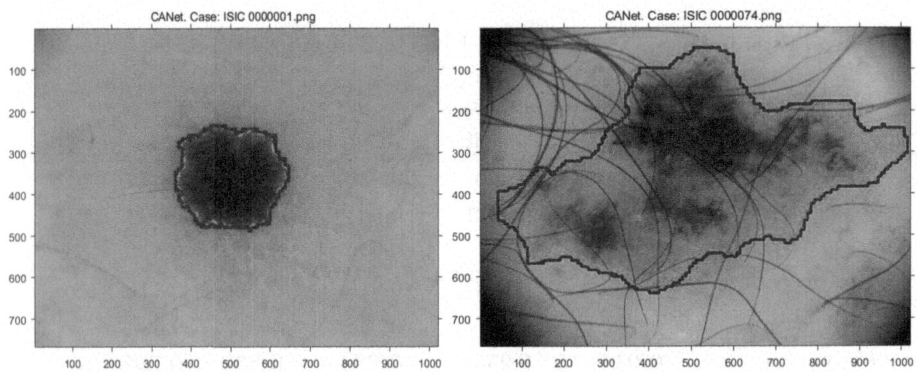

Fig. 6. Visual lesion segmentation of CANet. The segmentation results of the ground truth (green) and CANet (red). (Color figure online)

4 Conclusions

In this paper, we propose a compact attention network architecture that incorporates attention module scSE and designed atrous convolution for expanding the receptive field. On the segmentation of the melanoma, the CANet architecture performs better than the U-net, SegNet, FrCN, and nnU-net. In particular, the CANet is simpler and more compact than the SOTA segmentation network nnU-net. It is also worth noting that even in the noisy images, melanoma segmentation results are in good agreement with the ground truth. The CANet potentially provides a good point for other segmentation tasks.

In the future, we would extensively test the CANet segmentation ability in more datasets. Furthermore, we note that experts spent too much time annotating in medical images. In the subsequent research, we would try adopting a semi-automatic annotating method. The above issues would be regarded in our future research.

References

1. World Cancer Report [DB/OL]. https://www.iarc.who.int/cards_page/world-cancer-report/. Accessed 29 Feb 2021
2. Roy, A.G., Navab, N., Wachinger, C.: Concurrent spatial and channel 'Squeeze & excitation' in fully convolutional networks. In: Frangi, A.F., Schnabel, J.A., Davatzikos, C., Alberola-López, C., Fichtinger, G. (eds.) MICCAI 2018. LNCS, vol. 11070, pp. 421–429. Springer, Cham (2018). https://doi.org/10.1007/978-3-030-00928-1_48
3. Yuan, X., Ning, S., Zouridakis, G.: A narrow band graph partitioning method for skin lesion segmentation. Pattern Recogn. **42**(6), 1017–1028 (2009)
4. Schaefer, G., Rajab, M.I., Celebi, M.E., et al.: Colour and contrast enhancement for improved skin lesion segmentation. Comput. Med. Imaging Graph. Off. J. Comput. Med. Imaging Soc. **35**(2), 99–104 (2011)
5. Zhou, H., Schaefer, G., Celebi, M.E., et al.: Gradient vector flow with mean shift for skin lesion segmentation. Comput. Med. Imaging Graph. **35**(2), 121–127 (2011)
6. Wong, A., Scharcanski, J., Fieguth, P.: Automatic skin lesion segmentation via iterative stochastic region merging. IEEE Trans. Inf. Technol. Biomed. Publ. IEEE Eng. Med. Biol. Soc. **15**(6), 929–36 (2011)
7. Long, J., Shelhamer, E., Darrell, T.: Fully convolutional networks for semantic segmentation. IEEE Trans. Pattern Anal. Mach. Intell. **39**(4), 640–651 (2015)
8. Ronneberger, O., Fischer, P., Brox, T.: U-net: convolutional networks for biomedical image segmentation. In: Navab, N., Hornegger, J., Wells, W.M., Frangi, A.F. (eds.) MICCAI 2015. LNCS, vol. 9351, pp. 234–241. Springer, Cham (2015). https://doi.org/10.1007/978-3-319-24574-4_28
9. Zhao, H., Shi, J., Qi, X., et al.: Pyramid scene parsing network. In: 2017 IEEE Conference on Computer Vision and Pattern Recognition (CVPR), pp. 6230–6239. IEEE Computer Society (2017). https://doi.org/10.1109/CVPR.2017.660
10. He, K., Gkioxari, G., Dollar, P., Girshick, R.: Mask R-CNN. IEEE Trans. Pattern Anal. Mach. Intell. **42**, 386–397 (2020). https://doi.org/10.1109/TPAMI.2018.2844175
11. Peng, C., Zhang, X., Yu, G., Luo, G., Sun, J.: Large kernel matters - improve semantic segmentation by global convolutional network. In: 2017 IEEE Conference on Computer Vision and Pattern Recognition (CVPR), pp. 1743–1751. IEEE (2017). https://doi.org/10.1109/CVPR.2017.189
12. He, K., Zhang, X., Ren, S., et al. : Deep residual learning for image recognition. In: 2016 IEEE Conference on Computer Vision and Pattern Recognition (CVPR), pp. 770–778. IEEE Computer Society (2016). https://doi.org/10.1109/CVPR.2016.90
13. Kip, F.T.N., Welling, M.: Semi-supervised classification with graph convolutional networks. arXiv e-prints arXiv:1609.02907 (2016)
14. Badrinarayanan, V., Kendall, A., Cipolla, R.: SegNet: a deep convolutional encoder-decoder architecture for image segmentation. IEEE Trans. Pattern Anal. Mach. Intell. **39**(12), 2481–2495 (2017)

15. Chen, L.C., Papandreou, G., Kokkinos, I., et al.: DeepLab: Semantic image segmentation with deep convolutional nets, Atrous convolution, and fully connected CRFs. IEEE Trans. Pattern Anal. Mach. Intell. **40**(4), 834–848 (2017)
16. Al-Masni, M.A., Al-Antari, M.A., Choi, M.T., et al.: Skin lesion segmentation in dermoscopy images via deep full resolution convolutional networks. Comput. Methods Program. Biomed. **162**, 221–231 (2018)
17. Hu, J., Shen, L., Sun, G.: Squeeze-and-excitation networks. In: 2018 Proceedings of the IEEE Conference on Computer Vision and Pattern Recognition, pp. 7132–7141. IEEE (2018). https://doi.org/10.1007/978-3-030-00928-1_48
18. Stringer, C., Wang, T., Michaelos, M., et al.: Cellpose: a generalist algorithm for cellular segmentation. Nat. Methods **18**, 100–106 (2021). https://doi.org/10.1038/s41592-020-01018-x
19. Isensee, F., et al.: nnU-Net: a self-configuring method for deep learning-based biomedical image segmentation. Nat. methods **18**(2), 203–211 (2021)
20. Li, W., Wang, G., Fidon, L., Ourselin, S., Cardoso, M.J., Vercauteren, T.: On the compactness, efficiency, and representation of 3D convolutional networks: brain parcellation as a pretext task. In: Niethammer, M., et al. (eds.) IPMI 2017. LNCS, vol. 10265, pp. 348–360. Springer, Cham (2017). https://doi.org/10.1007/978-3-319-59050-9_28
21. Sevilla-Lara, L., Sun, D., Jampani, V., et al.: Optical flow with semantic segmentation and localized layers. In: 2016 Proceedings of the IEEE Conference on Computer Vision and Pattern Recognition, pp. 3889–3898. IEEE (2016). https://doi.org/10.1109/cvpr.2016.422
22. Wang, P., Chen, P., Yuan, Y., et al. : Understanding convolution for semantic segmentation. In: 2018 IEEE Winter Conference on Applications of Computer Vision, pp. 1451–1460. IEEE (2018). https://doi.org/10.1109/wacv.2018.00163
23. Tang, Y.: Deep learning using linear support vector machines. arXiv preprint arXiv:1306.0239 (2013)
24. Ioffe, S., Szegedy, C.: Batch normalization: accelerating deep network training by reducing internal covariate shift. Proc. Mach. Learn. Res. **37**, 448–456 (2015)
25. Haralick, R.M., Sternberg, S.R., Zhuang, X.: Image analysis using mathematical morphology. IEEE Trans. Pattern Anal. Mach. Intell. **9**(04), 532–50 (2009)
26. Fawcett, T.: An introduction to ROC analysis. Pattern Recogn. Lett. **27**(8), 861–874 (2006)

Tell It Your Way: Technology-Mediated Human-Human Multimodal Communication

Helena Cardoso(✉), Nuno Almeida, and Samuel Silva

IEETA – Institute of Electronics and Informatics Engineering of Aveiro, DETI – Department of Electronics, Telecomunications and Informatics, University of Aveiro, Aveiro, Portugal
{helenamncardoso,nunoalmeida,sss}@ua.pt

Abstract. Communication plays a pivotal role in our daily lives. With the advances of technology we are now able to use it to communicate with others at a distance. However, while in direct human-human communication we are able to adjust how we pass a message based on our context and the perceived context of the receiver. When we do it at a distance, using a messaging tool, one of the most popular choices, nowadays, this becomes harder. In fact, most messaging tools, such as Whatsapp or Messenger, provide some degree of flexibility regarding the way a message is sent (e.g., text, audio, image), but the receiver is limited to receiving it in the format of sender choice. In this regard, providing more flexibility in such technology-mediated communication scenarios might foster increased adaptability of these tools to multiple user abilities and contexts, and provide important alternatives for those with some disability (e.g., aphasia, blindness). The work presented here adopts a user-centered approach to design and develop a first proof-of-concept for a multimodal messaging system than enables message modality conversion regardless of the format used by the sender.

Keywords: Multimodal communicator · Technology-mediated communication · Multimodal messaging

1 Introduction

Communication plays a crucial role in the individual's social, personal and professional development, but as it is so common, sometimes we do not give it due importance. Communication is a dynamic interactive process that involves sharing information, ideas, thoughts, feelings, and values and, in our daily lives, we use a wide variety of ways to communicate with others. We say communication is successful when the person transmits the information clearly and accurately and when the receiver interprets and understands the information correctly. However,

X. Gao et al. (Eds.): MobiHealth 2021, LNICST 440, pp. 343–357, 2022.
https://doi.org/10.1007/978-3-031-06368-8_23

communication can face several obstacles to the efficient and reliable transmission of information, in many everyday contexts (e.g., a noisy environment) and, particularly, for those with speech disabilities.

The communication between humans is often multimodal since we interact with someone taking advantage of different ways that we can use to transmit our information to the recipient (e.g., speech, gestures) and, sometimes, we even use several of them at the same time. The way we communicate is often adapted to the nature of the message we want to transmit, but also to our current context, e.g., where we are and what we are doing. Additionally, we also adapt our way of communicating to what we know about the context and abilities of the receiver, e.g., if we know the receiver cannot hear us, we try, e.g., to resort to some visual form of communication (e.g., gesture, written).

Technology is increasingly present in our daily life. Through this, significant achievements were made that revolutionized the way of living in community, and thanks to its evolution, we can spend almost all day connected to everything and everyone. While video is an ever increasing possibility, most communication resorts to messaging due to its flexibility, low bandwidth requirements, and possibility of asynchronous message exchange, i.e., the interlocutors do not need to be present simultaneously. The best and most used messaging apps[1], for Android and iOS, are WhatsApp, Facebook Messenger, WeChat, and Telegram, among others. These apps provide sophisticated services, offering all kinds of interactions between users, from texting to voice and video calling to sharing images and audio. However, when technologies mediate communication, sometimes sending the message in a particular modality (e.g., audio, text, or pictograms) may not be appropriate (or understandable) for the receiver. Often, due to contextual conditions (being in a noisy place and not being able to hear the audio or driving and not being able to view the text message) or even health problems (e.g., hearing or visual impairment), this can lead to some communication difficulties. Therefore, having a messaging system that could adapt both to the sender and receiver context, preferences and abilities, enabling asymmetric use of message modalities, i.e., not limiting the message to the modality it was sent on, would improve the range of suitability of these tools.

And while technology-mediated communication supporting a versatile articulation of different forms of sending a message can be useful for all, it can provide an important support to those who have their abilities to communicate hindered due to a persistent or temporary condition. Most of the systems found on literature are limited in the number of supported modalities, typically supporting two or three conversions between modalities. Representative examples of messaging system capable of converting from speech-to-text and text-to-speech are the Stimme [2], BridgeApp [13] and ASRAR [9]. The first can also convert text to tactile feedback, the second, text to sign language and the third from text to gestures. AbleChat [5] enable the conversion from text to pictograms. These applications already provide valuable support. Nevertheless, these tools often

[1] https://www.statista.com/statistics/258749/most-popular-global-mobile-messenger-apps/.

target a small number of conversion possibilities (e.g., from pictograms to text), are tailored for a specific group of users, and can sometimes work as barriers for integration, since they are tools that are different from what everyone else around uses (or is willing to use).

One notable example of a condition hindering communication is aphasia, which often occurs after a stroke or head injury, and can affect the person's ability to speak, read, write or remember the names of objects. For these users, having multiple alternatives to send and receive messages can foster a greater adaptivity of the communication tool to their specific (often idiosyncratic) needs, which depend on the type of aphasia they have.

In this context, our research goal it to explore the interchangeable use of multiple messaging modalities in communication mediated by technology towards increased adaptability to different contexts, preferences and user abilities, adopting a vision of a communication tool designed for all. In this regard, relying on a user-centered approach, and aiming at a potential future application scenario assisting aphasics, in the scope of project APH-ALARM[2], the work presented here, establishing a ground zero for this research, is a first proof-of-concept for a communication tool supporting the exchange of messages using different modalities (e.g., text, images, audio) and introducing the ability of converting among them based on user choice or according to the user's declared abilities.

The remainder of this document is organized as follows: Sect. 2 describes the methods adopted to perform a first characterization of potential users and identify their expectations and receptivity to a multimodal communicator; Sect. 3 presents the overall steps and outcomes regarding the design and evaluation of a high-fidelity mockup of the system's interface to validate the paradigm and overall features; Sect. 4 presents the overall architecture and features for the first iteration of the multimodal communicator system; finally, Sect. 5 presents conclusions and a set of ideas for future developments.

2 Users, Scenarios and Requirements

The first stage of the work was to get further understanding of the potential target audience and of the characteristics the platform should have to be perceived as useful. Some personas and scenarios of use of the system were created, this allowed to define a list of requirements that the system must meet in the long-term. Following this way a user centered design methodology [4].

Before starting the new platform's development, a survey was performed to obtain some information about messaging use, and preferences in that context. The survey was answered by 69 persons, the main goals were to know their preferences regarding the communication systems, namely: (1) what system they usually use; (2) what modalities they know; (3) whether they are in favor of certain features; (4) if they would eventually join the new multimodal communication platform; and (5) if it solves many problems in a technology-mediated

[2] https://aph-alarm-project.com/.

communication. The analyses of the questionnaire allowed to conclude that many users frequently use communication platforms. The most used modality is the text modality, mostly because it is the one users feel most comfortable, the only one that they know how to use, or, in some cases, the only modality available in the used platform. Some people answered they would alternate the modality depending on what they want to communicate and the context around them. After explaining what was the goal of conversions between modalities, it was asked which ones they would find interesting to exist in this type of system. The most voted were the text-to-audio and audio-to-text, the least voted was pictograms-to-audio.

2.1 Personas

Personas are fictional representations of a person, since they are based on the behaviors of real people. They are created based on research to represent the different user types that might use the product. Personas provide helpful information to determine what a product should do and how it should behave [4]. With the results from the survey, 5 Personas were created trying to cover most of the questions addressed, such as context, disabilities and user preferences. Given their extent, only one Persona is presented here as an illustrative example:

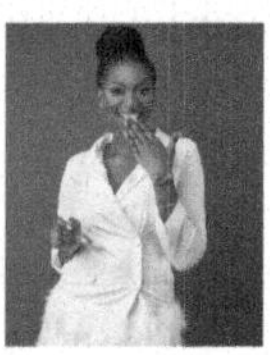

Image adapted from Wikimedia

Madalena Vagos is 30 years old, lives in Aveiro alone and was born into a large and very communicative family. Sometimes she wants to share some message with her family, but given the limitation of certain family members it would consume some time. Her uncle John lost his sight in an accident, her mother suffer from headaches, her father is always on the road, and some younger members of the family, who have access to electronics, still cannot read. Personalize a message to each member takes much time, as she works several hours as a nutritionist, Madalena wanted this function to be more optimized and not only for communication with her family members but also to communicate with all clients.

Motivation: Madalena would like to be able to send the same message to everyone, but is such a way that they could receive it in the most suited formats.

2.2 Scenarios

After defining the Personas, several scenarios were designed. These consist of small scenes illustrating how the users' motivations can be served by a new system depicting the contexts and ways of use that users will face [4]. Although several scenarios have been proposed to guide the development of the application, given their extent, only one is presented, here. As can be observed, the scenario that follows depicts Madalena (the Persona presented above) using a system addressing her motivation for a particular context.

Madalena sends Christmas wishes to the family group—Another Christmas has arrived and Madalena wants to send a Merry Christmas message to her family. She created a group with all family members in the app, wrote: "Merry Christmas to all and good entries" and send it to the family. Her uncle, who has visual problems, listens to an audio message. The message is automatically converted from the text because he has set the disability in his profile. Her younger cousin, who has autism spectrum disorder and prefers to view messages in image format rather than text, has the option image as the default modality to view the messages, so he always sees messages in image format. Her mother, due to headaches sometimes cannot read text messages or listen the messages, when is the case, she chooses to convert the message to image. Finally, while his father is driving the message is converted to audio and read aloud.

Madalena no longer needs to send a message individually in the most appropriate format for each family member since the system allows this to happen transparently.

2.3 Requirements

Requirements describe the necessary capabilities of the product. Based on the scenarios devised for the different Personas, we extracted requirements from the actions and features depicted in them [4]. The requirements were divided into two sets: functional and interaction and a summary of those deemed most relevant is presented in Table 1. These served as grounds for the design of the first prototypes.

Table 1. Overall requirements for the multimodal communication system as extracted from the scenarios identified for the different Personas.

Functional Requirements
• Allow the user to select the modality which they want to send/receive the message. • Support sending message in text, audio, image and gesture format. • Convert from one modality to another according to the users' preferences. • Convert from text to audio, text to image, audio to text, image to text, gesture to text format. • Showing the message to the user in text, audio and image format. • Adapt the modality depending on the context. • Adapt the modality depending on the users' disabilities. • Store users' preferences.

Interaction Requirements		
Modality	**Technology**	**Interaction**
Text	Touch Screen Keyboard Mouse	The application must allow users to navigate using touch inputs or mouse, depends on the device The application should allow users to write his message;
Speech	Microphone Speakers	The application should allow users to record his voice; The application should allow user to hear the message;
Image	Camera Gallery	The application should allow to take a picture; The application should allow to choose a picture from gallery;
Gesture	Camera	The application should allow to record video, to recognize the gestures;

3 High Fidelity Mockup Design and Evaluation

Following the adopted iterative user-centered design methodology, our aim was to perform short prototyping sprints followed by evaluation to inform further developments and refinements [3]. After setting the requirements for the system, those considered with a higher priority were selected for the initial prototype. At this early stage, we opted for building high-fidelity mockups to perform first validations of the design, flow, and features of the system. There are many design tools for making prototypes (e.g. Adobe XD, Proto.io). For our work, we chose the graphic editor Figma. One of the significant advantages of this editor is that it has no limitation on sharing the prototype, and someone else may be working on the same prototype. The developed mockups are high-fidelity, meaning that they are already more advanced than common paper prototypes (low-fidelity), are more aesthetically pleasing, and already support interactions (systems' flow). Thus, users have a better perception of the application, both aesthetically and functionally. This section presents the developed high-fidelity mockups, their evaluation (e.g., Heuristic Evaluation, Usability Tests) and the result of the evaluation.

3.1 First Mockup

One of the results from the initial survey taken by 69 people was that 61 persons used Messenger as a means of communication. Since many people are already acquainted with Messenger, it would be easy to handle in an application with a similar flow and interface. Therefore, the developed mockups were roughly based on the flow and element disposition adopted by Messenger.

On first use, the user has to login into the application (Fig. 1(A)). The next page shown is the Chats Page, which has a list of all the user chats (Fig. 1(B)). At the bottom of each page has a menu (Bottom Navigation), with three options: chats, friends and user profile. This menu will be present on all pages for quick access to the main pages. The friends' page (illustrated in Fig. 1(C)), displays a list of all the user's friends. The friends' profile (Fig. 1(D)) contains the usual user name, gender, avatar, birthday, but also includes information regarding the disabilities (hearing, speech or vision problems). In this page it is possible to add/remove the person to/from your friends' list and if it is already a friend, we can start a conversation. To add a new friend, the user needs to press the new button on the Friends Page and it is possible to see a list of all users registered on the application. Furthermore, on the user's profile page it is possible to see data similar to what was in the friends' profile. Adding information on disabilities to the user profile is beneficial because the system will convert the received messages to the most suitable format for their situation. For example, if the user has hearing problems, all the audio messages received will be converted to either image or text, without the user having to change each message to the desired modality.

In a private chat it is possible to send image, audio, and text messages, just like for any other chat applications that exist, these days. If the user wants to convert a message to other modality, he can click on the desired modality to convert. In this prototype, the considered conversions include text to audio or image, audio to text or image, and image to text or audio. Figure 2 illustrates examples of conversions.

Heuristic Evaluation The first step to evaluate the prototype was to conduct a heuristic evaluation. At this point, the goal was to identify major usability problems in the interface. To this end, four evaluators performed a heuristic evaluation adopting Nielsen's heuristics [10]. The evaluators were two females and two males, students of Computer and Telematics Engineering, aged 22–25 years old and with experience in performing heuristic evaluations. Each evaluator marked usability issues based on the adopted heuristics and according to a severity scale ranging from 0 to 4, in which zero consisted of a low-impact usability problem and four consisted of a high-impact usability problem. Taking into account the identity usability problems that resulted from this evaluation, the most concerning ones, with severity 4, were related to the lack of error messages and provided feedback in cases of adding or removing friends and signing out. In terms of what is related to conversions, they stated that the button to go back to the original modality was not very intuitive, and the result of the image to text conversion was not very coherent either. They also identified the lack of a landing page explaining what the application is about and introducing the user to its features, but this issue was scored as having low impact.

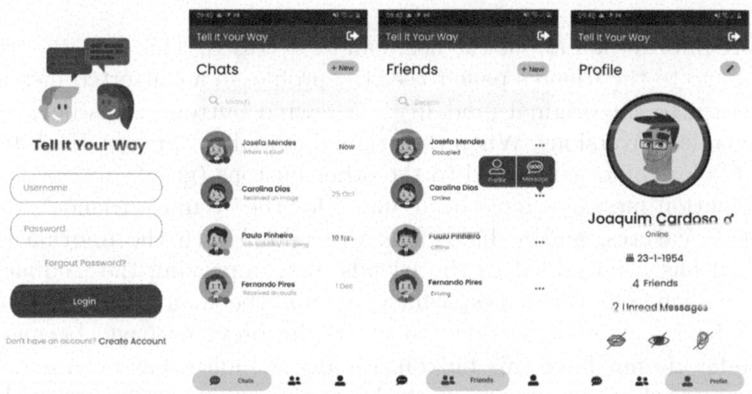

Fig. 1. Screen from the first prototype of the main pages. (A) Login page; (B) Chats page; (C) Friends page; (D) Profile page;

3.2 Refined High-Fidelity Mockup

In the second mockup several improvements were made based on the heuristic evaluation. The problem of not understanding the result of the conversion from image to text resulted from the fact that in the conversion many objects are identified, leading to the text sometimes becoming incomprehensible. To make the message a little bit more understandable, at this stage, without going into more sophisticated methods to generate a sentence, the message starts with "The image contains:".

The user's avatar in the conversation was downsized, leaving more space for the messages. It was added the "..." button in front of the user's data, through

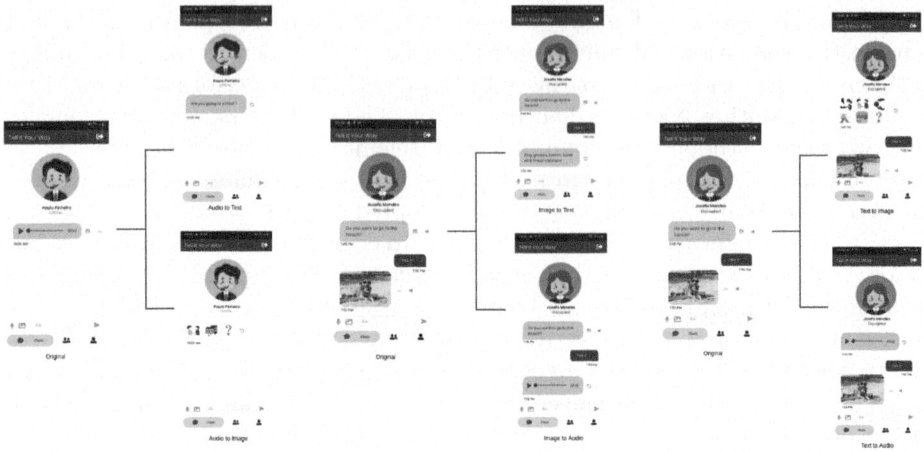

Fig. 2. Screen from the first prototype doing conversions from different modalities. (A) (1) Audio-to-Text and (2) Audio-to-Image; (B) (1) Image-to-text and (2) Image-to-audio; (C) (1) Text-to-image and (2) Text-to-audio (Color figure online)

which more information about the user can be accessed. This way, the user does not need to go to the friend's page to see the profile. In a converted message, the icon to return to the original modality – a rewind button –, has been replaced by all available conversions. When the original modality appears, the button has a different color (blue) compared to the other buttons (grey).

Confirmation messages have been added for the "remove friends" and "exit the system" features, and a dialog box was added with the information that a individual has been added to the friends' list, improving the feedback when adding a person. On the pages, which are not the main (chats, friends and profile), a back button was added to go to the previous page, because many devices today do not have this button. Finally, a tooltip has been added upon the status tag, when the user wants to know the meaning of a badge they just tap it, and the information will be displayed.

On the user profile page it was added the possibility to choose the default modality. When the user selects a default modality, all future messages will be converted to it. In the case of selecting some disability, predefined modalities will be blocked because it makes no sense for some difficulties to have specific predefined modalities (e.g., a person with a hearing impairment precludes audio as a predefined received message modality).

Usability Tests. The focus of the evaluation of the second (refined) high fidelity mockup was to understand how well users learned to use the system and how easily they were able to finish a set of tasks identified as important from the devised scenarios and requirements (see Sect. 2). The evaluation was conducted in a Concurrent Think Aloud (CTA) manner where the users were asked to narrate their thoughts as they went through the tasks. In Table 2, it is possible to see the tasks that users had to complete:

Table 2. Tasks performed by users during the usability evaluations of the second version of the high-fidelity mockup.

Tasks
1. Launch the application with personal settings;
2. Add to your profile an indication that you have hearing problems;
3. Add Liticia Dias to your friends' list and start a conversation with her
4. Remove Fernando Pires from your friends' list
5. Send an audio message to Carolina Dias
6. Send an image to Carolina Dias
7. Josefa Mendes sent you a text message, listen to it
8. Looking at the current screen, how do you know which original format the converted message was sent and go back to that original format
9. Josefa Mendes sent an image, convert it to text
10. Paulo Pinheiro sent you an audio message, see it in image format
11. See Paulo Pinheiro's profile
12. Modify the default modality to always receive messages in text format
13. Change your status to driving and check what the new default mode is
14. Logout

The participants consisted of 10 users (4 male and 6 female) of different ages, from 14 years old to 58 years old. An observation table was filled during the evaluation regarding: (1) if accomplish the task; (2) time take to accomplish the task; (3) critical and non-critical errors; (4) if felt lost; (5) if the user asked for help; and (6) perceived task difficulty. The last one was asked to the participants at the end of each task.

Participants successfully completed all the tasks, some of them with help. Results show that users encountered some obstacles/difficulties in the initial tasks and then learned how to use the application. The third task had a high perceived difficulty (3), which may be because of the complexity of the task. Some participants forgot the second part of the task, to facilitate it could be divided into two distinct tasks. Some participants gave the idea to provide an option to start a conversation from the friends' profile, right after adding a friend. In the current mockup users need to go to the friends/chats page to start a conversation. Some users had difficulties changing the profile, in task 2: even though they were able to add the hearing problem to the profile, they failed to save the change, at the end. Further analysis revealed that this was caused by the need to scroll down the page to see the save button. Task 4 was more complicated for older people, they did not know they had to go to the user's profile to remove the friend, since they were not used to social networks. Some participants had difficulty converting the first message, but after converting it, they understood how it worked. Other difficulties that were encountered by some participants, especially among the older ones, included the fact that the prototype was in

English – the users were native Portuguese – and they found the icons not very intuitive to understand. Overall, all feedback considered, we conclude that the inclusion of a tutorial or introduction may be beneficial, providing some support for the application's first use.

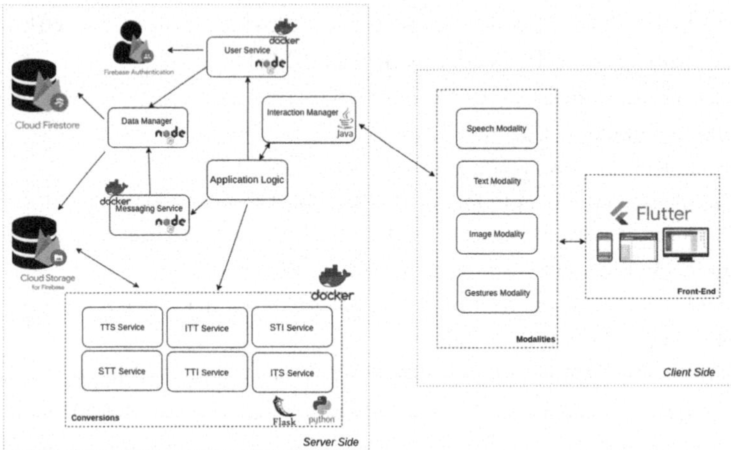

Fig. 3. Overall architecture for the developed multimodal communicator depicting the main modules and considered technologies.

System Usability Scale Questionnaire. After all tasks were completed, participants were asked to fill a System Usability Scale (SUS) questionnaire. The questionnaire consists of 10 questions with a scale ranging from 1 to 5 where 1 is strongly agree and 5 is strongly disagree. One of the benefits from using a SUS questionnaire is because this can effectively differentiate between usable and unusable systems [7]. The resulting mean SUS score, considering the 10 users, was 82.5 points, which means the system has excellent usability.

The results shows that potential users, needs a briefing explanation of the flow of the application to learn some features.

4 First Functional Prototype

After the evaluation of the second high-fidelity mockup, the following iteration initiated the development of a first functional prototype. To this effect, an overall architecture was defined and a first stage of the core element of the system – message conversions – was addressed.

4.1 Architecture

The architecture described below generically adopts the AM4I framework [1]. Designed to support the design and development of multidevice multimodal interactive systems, the adoption of this framework takes advantage of its decoupled nature where the interaction modalities and interaction management are decoupled from the application logic, supporting a variable and a dynamic number of input and output modalities. Furthermore, it is a scalable architecture so that, in the future, it will be possible to expand the context of use of the communicator into more complex interactive ecosystems, e.g., the smarthome, as a more integral part of the user's environment, overall, and important for its integration as an assistive technology.

Figure 3 presents the architecture of the proposed system. The architecture is decoupled, divided in a set of modules. They are divided by the ones running in the client-side and in the server-side.

The **client-side** provides the cross-platform front-end, able to support several different platforms to reach the most significant number of users. To this end, we choose to work with Flutter[3] since it allows creating native compiled applications for mobile devices, web, and desktops, which can potentiate the use of the system in a wider range of devices and contexts. Nevertheless, at this early stage of the work, the main focus will be on mobile due to the fact that it is an easy-to-carry device and people already use it as the primary communication choice with other users. As a simplification, in this iteration the systems' modalities are all on the client-side, but these and other modalities can run in other devices or the cloud, if required.

The **server-side**, encompasses all the logic and services for the TELL IT YOUR WAY system. Overall, it has six modules (see Fig. 3): the message conversion services, interaction manager, application logic, user service, messaging service, and data manager.

The *message conversion* module aims to translate from the modality received from one user to the modality selected by the other user. The *interaction manager* is a logical component and is responsible for receiving the events generated by the input modalities and producing new messages to be delivered to the output modalities [1]. This system proposes a single interaction manager located in the cloud, to which multiple devices can connect. It is directly connected to the *application logic*, which is the system's "brain", responsible for calling the service depending on what it receives from the interaction manager. For example, the user wants to convert a received text message to audio: this information is sent to the interaction manager, who forwards it to the Application Logic. This module will, then, call the Conversions Service to obtain the desired message conversion that will be sent to the client.

The *user service* is responsible for all user authentication, it will be possible to access and create a user's data. The user authentication is performed via Firebase authentication[4] supporting authentication using passwords, phone numbers, and well-known federated identity providers, such as Google, Facebook, and Twitter. Regarding the *messaging service*, it provides all the logic for the chat, allowing message exchange among users, in real-time. It adopts a stream protocol, and

[3] https://flutter.dev/.
[4] https://firebase.google.com/docs/auth.

an event-driven management making use of the EventSource/Server-Sent Events protocol[5]. Finally, for both User and Messaging Services, the components interact with the *Data Manager*, which is responsible for all database management. The database is a Cloud Firestore and the multimedia files are saved on a Cloud Storage. These services were developed in Node JS and Express JS.

As the Fig. 3 show, most of the components/services are deployed on docker containers, taking advantages of the simplicity and faster configurations.

4.2 Message Conversions

To provide a first level of message conversions to the first functional prototype, the literature was explored for existing works and libraries that could be considered. While the research did not cover just the technologies described ahead, these were those deemed more suitable for this stage of the development and additional reviewed solutions are not discussed for the sake of brevity.

Currently, the *message conversion* module supports six message conversions: Text-to-Speech, Speech-to-Text, Image-to-Text, Text-to-Image, Image-to-Speech and Speech-to-Image. It was developed in Python given the versatility and the large amount of libraries available supporting the envisaged conversions. To enable communication between the conversions services and the application logic, the Flask[6] library was used, a microframework (does not require private tools or libraries) that, aside from being simple and capable of doing the communication, is easy to set up and easy to start developing.

For *Text-to-Speech* we chose the Google Text-to-Speech (gTTS) library[7] that uses Google Translate's text-to-speech API. This library was selected because it supports a big set of languages, including English and European Portuguese. Therefore, it will be a great advantage, in the future, to support several languages.

The *Speech-to-Text* uses the speech recognition library[8], and it has support for several speech engines and APIs, online and offline. The API chosen was Google Speech Recognition[9], the API is free and does not require an API key to use and supports several languages.

The solution we found for Image to Text concersion was to identify all the objects in the image. There are several object detection methods, such as: YOLO (You Only Look Once), Faster RCNN, SSD (Single Shot Detector), OverFeat, among others [6]. We choose to use YOLOv3 [12] because it has good speed, high accuracy and it is open source. It is is an algorithm that detects and recognizes various objects in a picture (in real-time). The dataset used has 80 labels, coco.names[10].

5 https://www.w3.org/TR/eventsource/.
6 https://flask.palletsprojects.com/en/2.0.x/.
7 https://gtts.readthedocs.io/en/latest/.
8 https://pypi.org/project/SpeechRecognition/.
9 https://wicg.github.io/speech-api/.
10 https://github.com/pjreddie/darknet/blob/master/data/coco.names.

The conversion of text to image can be performed at different levels of complexity. For instance, the conversion of a sentence into pictograms may need to be different than just replacing every action/entity with the corresponding pictogram, since pictograms can have a more complex meaning than just a word or need to be placed in a different order than words. Additionally, recent methods have been proposed that generate images based on a textual description, e.g., DALL-E [11]. Nevertheless, and for the sake of demonstrating the concept, at this point, we opted for a first approach that just tries to replace each word by its visual representation, if it exists. To this end, we go through each word of the sentence and use Text2Picto [14] (which uses the Princeton WordNet [8] databases) to obtain the corresponding images.

Image-to-Speech and *Speech-to-Image* result from reusing some of the different conversion services, for instance, Speech-to-Image uses the Speech-to-Text and then Text-to-Image to achieve the intended result.

4.3 First Proof-of-Concept Mobile App

The implementation of the first mobile application considered the outcomes of the previous evaluations, focusing to solve the usability problems and provide a complete implementation of the provided techniques to validate the application further and enable the first assessment of their impact on users.

The current version of the Tell It Your Way application, developed with Flutter, is being tested on Android systems.

The new implementation has already solved some usability issues mentioned by the participants during the evaluation of the refined mockup. The bottom bar already appears with the icon and label of each option, making it easier for people less acquainted with these tools (in our tests, older people) to interact with it. Adding another user as a friend is no longer mandatory to access the friends' list to start a conversation with them. By adding a user as a friend, the user can quickly start a conversation with them. The save button is always visible to the user while editing his/her profile. Thus, making it possible to save changes at any time without having to scroll down to do so. Overall, the integration of the application with the current version of the message conversion services did not raise any issue and the full conversion flow is working well.

Figure 4 shows several screens for the Tell it Your Way application on Android and depicting, on the left, both sides of an illustrative situation between John and Jennifer. For the sake of simplicity, the image just illustrates how the messages sent by John can be received in a wide range of modalities by Jennifer.

John sends several messages to Jennifer, using different formats. On Jennifer's side, she receives the first message as text because it is her preferred modality. The second message is received in image format since, e.g. Jennifer was in the bus, surrounded by people and without her reading glasses. Finally, Jennifer leaves home and, while she is driving, John's third message arrives and is automatically converted to audio and read aloud.

Additionally, users can add the disabilities they have to their profile (Fig. 4b) and the messages will be shown to the user in the most appropriate modalities.

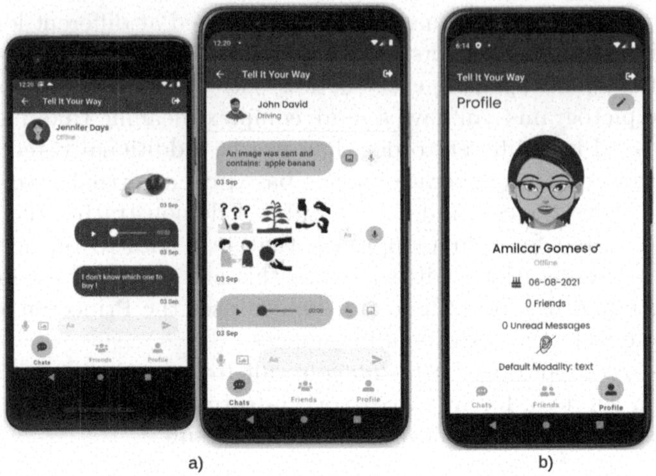

Fig. 4. Illustrative screens of the first functional prototype running on Android and depicting: (a) both sides of a conversation between John David and Jennifer Days with different messages conversions (image-to-text; audio-to-image; and text-to-audio); and (b) Amilcar's profile screen showing his preferred modality and disabilities.

5 Conclusions

In this paper we present first efforts towards a novel system to support communication between people with different needs and preferences. To this end, and adopting a user-centered design approach, we identified a set of requirements and reached a proof-of-concept that already supports sending and receiving messages in different formats and converting them to a chosen format regardless of their original modality. Our long term goal, for which this is a first stage, is to make communication mediated by technology approach the efficiency and versatility of face-to-face communication regarding an adaptation to users' preferences, abilities, and contexts.

Despite it only has been tested and evaluated with a few users, in controlled contexts, and the number and quality of the conversions can still evolve greatly, we can conclude that the presented proof-of-concept served its overall purpose, showing the potential and viability of such systems. In this context, other developments will follow that can further enrich the communication system, such as, the inclusion of an onboarding mechanism, the support for gestures, and first efforts on multilingual support.

Acknowledgement. This work was supported by EU and national funds through the Portuguese Foundation for Science and Technology (FCT), in the context of project AAL APH-ALARM (AAL/0006/2019) and funding to the research unit IEETA (UIDB/00127/2020).

References

1. Almeida, N., Teixeira, A., Silva, S., Ketsmur, M.: The AM4I architecture and framework for multimodal interaction and its application to smart environments. Sens. (Switz.) **19**(11), 1–30 (2019). https://doi.org/10.3390/s19112587
2. Amarasinghe, A., Wijesuriya, V.B.: Stimme: a chat application for communicating with hearing impaired persons. In: 2019 IEEE 14th International Conference on Industrial and Information Systems: Engineering for Innovations for Industry 4.0, ICIIS 2019 - Proceedings, pp. 458–463 (2019)
3. Bryan-Kinns, N., Hamilton, F.: One for all and all for one? Case studies of using prototypes in commercial projects. In: ACM International Conference Proceeding Series, vol. 31, pp. 91–100 (2002). https://doi.org/10.1145/572020.572032
4. Cooper, A., Reimann, R., Cronin, D.: About Face 3: The Essentials of Interaction Design, vol. 3 (2007)
5. Daems, J., Bosch, N., Solberg, S., Dekelver, J., Kultsova, M.: AbleChat: development of a chat app with pictograms for people with intellectual disabilities. In: Engineering for Society - Leuven 2016 - Proceedings, pp. 25–32 (2016)
6. Liu, L., et al.: Deep learning for generic object detection: a survey. Int. J. Comput. Vis. **128**(2), 261–318 (2019)
7. Martins, A.I., Rosa, A.F., Queirós, A., Silva, A., Rocha, N.P.: European Portuguese validation of the system usability scale (SUS). Proc. Comput. Sci. **67**, 293–300 (2015)
8. Miller, G.A.: WordNet: An Electronic Lexical Database. MIT Press, Cambridge (1998)
9. Mirzaei, M.R., Ghorshi, S., Mortazavi, M.: Helping deaf and hard-of-hearing people by combining augmented reality and speech technologies. In: Proceedings of 9th International Conference on Disability, Virtual Reality and Associated Technologies, pp. 10–12 (2012)
10. Nielsen, J.: Heuristic Evaluation. Usability Inspection Methods (1994). Edited by: Nielsen J, Mack RL
11. Ramesh, A., et al.: Zero-shot text-to-image generation. arXiv preprint arXiv:2102.12092 (2021)
12. Redmon, J., Divvala, S., Girshick, R., Farhadi, A.: You only look once: unified, real-time object detection. In: Proceedings of the IEEE Computer Society Conference on Computer Vision and Pattern Recognition, vol. 2016-December, pp. 779–788, June 2015
13. Samonte, M.J.C., Gazmin, R.A., Soriano, J.D.S., Valencia, M.N.O.: BridgeApp: an assistive mobile communication application for the deaf and mute. In: ICTC 2019–10th International Conference on ICT Convergence: ICT Convergence Leading the Autonomous Future, pp. 1310–1315, October 2019
14. Sevens, L., Vandeghinste, V., Schuurman, I., Eynde, F.V.: Less is more: a rule-based syntactic simplification module for improved text-to-pictograph translation. Data Knowl. Eng. **117**, 264–289 (2018)

Author Index

The manufacturer's authorised representative in the EU is Springer Nature Customer Service Centre GmbH, Europaplatz 3, 69115 Heidelberg, Germany. If you have any concerns regarding our products, please contact ProductSafety@springernature.com

Printed and bound by CPI Group (UK) Ltd, Croydon, CR0 4YY
30/09/2026
02225439-0018